HISTOCOMPATIBILITY TESTING

HISTOCOMPATIBILITY TESTING

Editors

Jeffrey L. Bidwell
University of Bristol

Cristina Navarrete
National Blood Service – London & The South East

ICP Imperial College Press

Published by

Imperial College Press
57 Shelton Street
Covent Garden
London WC2H 9HE

Distributed by

World Scientific Publishing Co. Pte. Ltd.

P O Box 128, Farrer Road, Singapore 912805

USA office: Suite 1B, 1060 Main Street, River Edge, NJ 07661

UK office: 57 Shelton Street, Covent Garden, London WC2H 9HE

Library of Congress Cataloging-in-Publication Data
Histocompatibility testing / edited by Jeffrey L. Bidwell & Cristina Navarrete.
p. cm.
Includes bibliographical references and index.
ISBN 1-86094-156-7
1. Histocompatibility testing. I. Bidwell, Jeffrey L. (Jeffrey Lewis) II. Navarrete, Cristina.

QR187.H57 H576 2000
616.07'9--dc21 99-087762

British Library Cataloguing-in-Publication Data
A catalogue record for this book is available from the British Library.

English version typeset using Corel Ventura™ 7.1314

☑ *This text symbol denotes individual components of a reagent mix*

First published 2000
Reprinted 2001

Printed in Singapore.

The editors wish to acknowledge their gratitude to Denny Williams, for her hard work, patience and diplomacy in helping to construct this book.

CONTENTS

PART 2: DNA-BASED HISTOCOMPATIBILITY TESTING

PART 3: CELL-BASED HISTOCOMPATIBILITY TESTING

PART 4: DONOR SELECTION

PART 5: STATISTICAL METHODS

PART 6: MINOR HISTOCOMPATIBILITY ANTIGENS

FOREWORD

HLA POLYMORPHISM: ORIGIN AND MAINTENANCE

W. F. Bodmer
ICRF Cancer and Immunogenetics Laboratory
Institute of Molecular Medicine
Oxford OX3 9DS, England

Introduction

The HLA system was discovered by virtue of the fact that it was polymorphic. The impetus for its discovery was the search for polymorphic antigens to match for transplantation, by analogy with the human red cell blood groups. The serological reagents used for the initial description of antigens, at first from multiply transfused individuals and later from multiparous women, had their activities by virtue of the existence of polymorphic differences between individuals. Furthermore, these differences were necessarily at the level of expressed proteins. Serology cannot, however, detect DNA polymorphisms that are synonymous, namely do not give rise to differences in amino acid sequences.

The extent of HLA polymorphism, apparent even from the earliest studies, made it an obvious and attractive candidate for human population studies. The first investigations using the then available relatively crude serological techniques started in the late 1960's, and included the first real field study, namely of Central African pygmies (Bodmer and Bodmer, 1970). The first of the International Workshops devoted largely to population studies, took place in 1972 and its successors, including the recent 12th Workshop, have always featured extensive analysis of HLA population data.

Origin and maintenance of polymorphisms: classical models

The ultimate origin of a polymorphic variant must be by mutation, with new combinations of mutations created by recombination or gene conversion. The mechanisms that give rise to polymorphic variants must be clearly distinguished from those which determine their propagation into a population, namely increases in frequency. Classically, it was assumed that most new mutations giving rise to functionally distinct variants of a gene would be likely to be at a selective disadvantage and so maintained in the population at a low frequency by the balance between mutation creating the variants, and selection against them and so weeding them out. The frequencies achieved by the balance between mutation and selection, even for quite high mutation rates, are generally well below 1% and so below the level that could be considered polymorphic or could explain the distribution of all but the rarest HLA alleles. Those occasional mutations which are selectively advantageous will increase in frequency relatively rapidly in the population and are the basis for evolutionary adaptation, namely evolution by natural selection. Such advantageous variants will, in general, sweep through a population relatively rapidly and only contribute to polymorphism during the relatively short period over which they increase from a low frequency to a frequency of nearly one.

Mutations that are truly selectively neutral may increase in frequency by chance, as was shown classically by R.A. Fisher and Sewall Wright. This increase will be heavily dependent on the population size and is less likely the larger the population. Sewall Wright, and following him Kimura and others emphasised particularly the contribution that these chance increases in frequency, often referred to as genetic drift, could make to the level of polymorphism. This is now accepted to be appreciable if only because of the huge number of positions along the DNA molecule where mutations can arise, and the relatively high proportions of these in introns, between genes, and in synonymous positions, all of which could be expected to be neutral. Thus, notwithstanding the low average mutation rate, which may be no more than of the order of 10^{-9} per base pair per generation, and the relatively large human population sizes, certainly of the order of at least thousands even under relatively primitive conditions, the contribution of random genetic drift to polymorphism may, in general, be appreciable. This, however, as we shall discuss, is very unlikely to be the explanation for the majority of the observed putative functionally different variants of the HLA system.

The classic mechanism for the stable maintenance of a polymorphism in a population was first analyzed by R.A. Fisher in 1922. He showed that if the heterozygote for two alleles at a single locus is fitter than either of the homozygotes, then a stable balanced polymorphism can be maintained whose gene frequencies are dependent on the relative extent to which the heterozygote is fitter than each of the two homozygotes. The classical example of such a polymorphism is with respect to the sickle cell haemoglobin variant, where homozygotes have a severe anaemia and are almost lethal under their original conditions in Africa, while the heterozygous carriers of the sickle cell gene are fitter than the homozygous normals with respect to resistance to malaria. This simple model can be generalised in a number of ways, and in particular to the situation where the heterozygotes on average over time or space are at an advantage over either homozygote, though they may at any given point in time or space, only be fitter than one of the two homozygotes. Similarly, fluctuating advantages and a tendency for a new variant always to have a selective advantage may be shown to be mechanisms by which polymorphism can be maintained, perhaps for many alleles at a single locus as in the case of the HLA system (for general background to human population genetics see Cavalli-Sforza and Bodmer, 1971).

Primary evidence for selection

The key issue is to distinguish whether the observed extensive HLA polymorphism can be explained simply by chance, namely genetic drift, or requires some form of natural selection to explain its maintenance. Genetic drift depends only on population structure, namely such features of a population as the mutation rate, population size and patterns of migration between populations. Therefore, so long as, on average, overall mutation rates for different genes are approximately the same, genetic drift should lead to comparable levels of polymorphism for all genes or DNA regions. Thus, as Luca Cavalli-Sforza first pointed out more than 30 years ago, if there is differential variability either within a gene or between genes, then this can only be explained by natural selection which can discriminate between the functional effects of different genetic variants.

As soon as the first HLA genes were cloned at the beginning of the 1980's, it became clear that some genes had many alleles while others had few or none. One of the most striking examples of this was the fact that the DRA gene for the alpha chain of the class II DR products is hardly polymorphic at all, while the DRB genes, especially DRB1, have a very large number of variants. Now that there are so many, both HLA class I and class II, genes cloned this variation in allele number per gene becomes even more striking (see for example the most recent Nomenclature Report by Bodmer *et al.* (1997)).

The determination of the HLA-A2 structure (Bjorkman *et al.*, 1987) and, through that, the identification of the peptide binding region of the HLA class I molecules and their distinctive structure, provided further striking evidence for differential variability, this time within the gene and in relation to obvious potential functional differences. Thus, it became clear, first of all that virtually all variation at the DNA level occurred in positions that gave rise to amino acid substitutions. Second came the striking observation that most of the polymorphism was in the N-terminal region where peptides were bound, and that even within this there was clear differential variability and a preference for variants to occur in exactly those positions that might most be expected to affect the differential binding of different peptides (Bjorkman *et al.*, 1987; Bodmer *et al.*, 1986). Thus, based on these various observations there can be little doubt that at least the majority of HLA variants are associated with functional differences that may in turn be associated with differential natural selection.

HLA polymorphism is old

The first evidence for the age of HLA alleles came from the fact that allo-antisera in one species, for example, the cow, recognised polymorphic differences in other species, namely humans (Iha *et al.*, 1973). This extraordinary result was at first difficult to understand, but then became easily interpreted when it was realised that there were indeed sequence homologies between polymorphic variants in quite distant species. This has been analysed most systematically in the primates. The sequences that tend to be conserved are "epitopes", namely short sequences that can be recognised, for example, by monoclonal antibodies and which presumably have functional significance in terms of their influence on peptide binding patterns. The patterns of serological reactions, especially to monoclonal antibodies, and their correlation with amino acid substitutions, indicate that an allele, defined as the sequence of a particular version of the expressed gene, can be made up of combinations of epitopes. Different alleles may be formed from different epitope combinations by recombination. This pattern of variation is especially clear for the DPA and DPB genes.

The idea that new alleles may be derived from old by recombination goes back to Fisher's interpretation of the rhesus red cell blood groups and to the earliest interpretations of the origins of the alleles of the HLA system in the mid-1960's. If different epitope combinations are present in a population at low frequencies, most probably maintained by a combination of recombination and gene conversion, then when the selective situation requires it, a new combination may quickly increase in frequency to cope with a new immune challenge. Thus, fluctuating selection can readily be responded to by extensive polymorphism and gives heterozygote advantage over time, thus maintaining high levels of polymorphism without the specific requirement that at any given time heterozygotes are always at an advantage over homozygotes. This fluctuating selection mechanism, which in general gives rise to a selective advantage for new variants, is an effective way of maintaining a high level of polymorphism without the need for increasing the number of loci in order to have an increased variety of immune responses. The long persistence of alleles across species seems most likely to reflect the existence of tried and trusted epitopes to peptide binding, and their combinations.

Haplotypes and linkage disequilibrium

Pairs of alleles at different HLA loci, such as classically A1 and B8, are often found to be associated in populations. This means that the frequency of the combination A1 and B8 is significantly higher than would be expected in the absence of any association, namely from the product of the separate frequencies of A1 and B8. This phenomenon is due to linkage disequilibrium, namely the comparatively common occurrence together on the same chromosome of the alleles A1 and B8. Ceppellini (1967) gave such combinations the now familiar name "haplotype", being the confluence of the terms haploid and genotype.

The first analysis of the population genetics of pairs of alleles at two linked loci was carried out by Jennings in 1917. He derived the classical result that the measure of the association, Δ, between alleles A and B at two loci, which is given by:

$$\Delta = \text{frequency (AB)} - \text{frequency (A) frequency (B)} \qquad (1)$$

declines to 0 at a rate 1-r, where r is the recombination fraction between the loci. Thus, after n generations of random mating and in the absence of selection:

$$\Delta_n = \Delta_0 (1-r)_n \qquad (2)$$

This result shows that Δ , and so the association between a pair of alleles in a population, decays rapidly towards 0 from its initial value unless the recombination fraction, r, is small. This, in practice for human populations, means that r must generally be less than 0.5% . For the background to this result, and other aspects of the classical results of population genetics mentioned earlier, see Cavalli-Sforza and Bodmer, 1971; and Tomlinson and Bodmer, 1995.

It is because many of the loci within the HLA region are within 1 to 0.5% recombination fraction distance of each other, that linkage disequilibrium between alleles at the HLA loci is such a characteristic feature of population data on the HLA system. Indeed, the total excess haplotype frequency for a pair of loci, which can be calculated from the sum of the linkage disequilibrium values for all pairs of alleles which show significant associations, can be used to give an overall measure of the tendency for pairs of alleles at two loci to associate (Bodmer and Bodmer, 1978). This tendency will be roughly proportional to the recombination fraction. The figure obtained at that time for HLA-B and C as compared to HLA-A and B was in the ratio of approximately 3 to 1, which is really not far from the actual situation as it is known now, either based on recombination fractions, or distance between the loci in terms of numbers of basepairs.

Haplotype frequencies are much better discriminators between populations than single allele frequencies. This point was first most clearly made in an extensive analysis of the data following the 7th International Histocompatibility Testing Workshop of 1977 (see Bodmer and Bodmer, 1978; Bodmer, 1996). Thus, for example, the haplotype A1,B8 is characteristic of Northern European populations, while the allele A1 occurs with a comparable frequency throughout caucasoid populations from Northern Europe to the Indian sub-continent. This discrimination is most probably due to the fact that the recombination fraction titrates time according to Jennings classical formula (Equation 2).

Linkage disequilibrium is also the explanation for HLA and disease associations. Thus, for example, the initially described association for insulin-dependent diabetes mellitus (IDDM) was with B15, whereas further analyses of the associations with DR and DQ alleles, clearly indicated that the primary effect probably lies with particular DQA and B allelic combinations (see, for example, Tomlinson and Bodmer, 1995). Only when an association persists across many different population groups, such as that between B27 and ankylosing spondylitis, can one assume that it is likely that the functional effect is directly connected with the allele that is associated, namely B27.

There are many factors which can lead to significant linkage disequilibrium beyond that expected due simply to the recombination fraction in the absence of selection. Selection itself can lead to transient linkage disequilibrium as first clearly analysed by Thomson *et al.* (1976). Thus, if an allele is being strongly selected for, then closely linked alleles will be pulled into the population due to linkage disequilibrium, a phenomenon that has been called "hitch-hiking". When the selection is strong, and the rate of increase of the allele therefore comparatively rapid, linkage disequilibrium can be maintained transiently over relatively large distances. The essential point is that, during a relatively rapid increase in frequency, there is not enough time for recombination to disrupt the association between the selected allele and other alleles on the haplotype initially associated with the selected allele. This is undoubtedly the major explanation for the so-called extended haplotypes or "super-types". From time to time there may well be coordinated selection for alleles at two or more different loci with immune functions on the same haplotype, leading to the types of selective interaction that might accentuate the occurrence of apparently extended haplotypes.

Other factors influencing linkage disequilibrium are:

- recent population admixture
- inbreeding
- random drift effects
- variation due to inevitably limited sizes of population samples

As shown by Cavalli-Sforza and Bodmer (1971) and Thomson *et al.,* (1976), the effects of population admixture on linkage disequilibrium, which depend on the products of the differences in allele frequencies at the two loci under consideration are generally small and dissipate rapidly, as predicted by Jennings classical formula, in the absence of linkage (when r = 1/2). Consistent observation of a particular linkage disequilibrium in different populations, such as is found for the A1,B8 combination across many populations of Northern Europe, is strong evidence against both sampling and genetic drift effects, both of which would be expected to be highly localised. Thus, the gradient in A1,B8 frequency across Europe is hard to explain other than by some form of selection (Bodmer, 1973; Thomson *et al.,* 1976). This gradient, as is the case for other haplotype combinations, is consistent with Cavalli-Sforza and colleagues stimulating proposal that such gradients reflect the gradual migration of farmers from the origins of agriculture in the Middle East spreading outwards in all directions and, in particular, to the northern most boundaries of Europe. In contrast, the frequency of the A1,B8 haplotype in Afro-Americans can readily be explained by recent admixture in the absence of any other effects, including selection.

Selective mechanisms

Since the original description by McDevitt and Benacceraf of immune response differences associated with the mouse H2 polymorphism more than 25 years ago, it has been obvious that immune response variation with respect to pathogens, whether bacteria, viruses, protozoan parasites or fungi, is likely to be the major basis for the effect of natural selection on HLA polymorphisms. This was an explanation for the maintenance of the HLA polymorphism by some form of frequency-dependent, or fluctuating selection (Bodmer, 1972). The first clear evidence for a possible role for HLA in infectious diseases was the observation by Ceppellini and co-workers (Piazza *et al.*, 1973) of an association of HLA types with malarial incidence in Sardinian villages. This association has subsequently been confirmed by Adrian Hill and his colleagues in extensive studies in Africa, though it remains weak. There are many suggestive observations on the relationship between HLA types and infections such as leprosy, tuberculosis, HPV, HIV and EBV. In no case, however, is the HLA effect unequivocally demonstrated though, of course, there are many examples of HLA restricted T-cell responses to flu and other viruses. Presumably the disadvantage due to the HLA associations now seen with auto-immune diseases, is the price we pay for earlier protection by HLA polymorphisms against infections.

There is evidence to suggest that it may be the spectrum of responses with respect to the level of expression, affinity or ability in the T-cell response repertoire which is influenced by HLA polymorphisms. Thus, whether or not auto-immune disease develops, may depend on some form of threshold effect (H. Bodmer, personal communication). These ideas can also explain why auto-immune diseases seem to be increasing in frequency so much in modern western society, whose peoples' immune systems are no longer put to work to the same extent as they were in the past for counteracting infectious pathogens. As the parasite load decreases, the risk of the T-cell activity threshold being exceeded, and leading to auto-immune disease increases. This form of antigenic competition was observed in our earliest field studies of the pygmy populations carried out with Cavalli-Sforza in the 1960's, as we then were never able to detect significant reactions in maternal antisera, in spite of clear evidence of many samples being collected from young mothers with many offspring, the most recent of which was often under one year old. The maternal allo-antisera discovered by Rose Payne and Jon van Rood, which were the basis for the original definition of the HLA polymorphism, may thus, like auto-immune disease, be products of the low parasite load of modern western society. The immune system perhaps obeys the rule that "Satan makes work for idle hands to do". This accentuates even more the contrast between the current selective load of HLA polymorphism through its effect on auto-immune disease and past protective effects with respect to, often epidemic, infections.

In spite of the fact that, for example, the overall A2 frequency seems remarkably constant throughout the world, this hides a considerable measure of variation in the frequencies of the A2 "splits". Similar stories can be told for other such variations on a theme, including for example B15 and DRB1*14. Perhaps there are dominant epitopes, such as A2 and B15 which are needed for effective resistance to key pathogen determinants. The continuing war game between host and pathogen then leads to selection of variants around a theme, both in the host and in the pathogen. This then could account for the variety of A2 and other variants. It is undoubtedly the epitopes of HLA molecules, which engender T-cell recognition, that are likely to be selected for, and not the alleles as a whole, which are, as already discussed, combinations of epitopes.

HLA and foetal maternal immunity

The survival of the foetus as a natural allograft is a classical problem of immunobiology. The lack of expression of HLA ABC molecules on the majority of trophoblasts still seems to be by far the most likely mechanism by which the foetus survives, at least initially, as an allograft. This mechanism ensures that the tissue in closest contact with the maternal circulation can neither by recognised as different by cytotoxic T-cells nor can it stimulate them to respond (Barnstable and Bodmer, 1978). HLA-G, as shown by Ellis and McMichael and others is, however, expressed on some trophoblasts, but shows very limited polymorphism. This is consistent with its role as a peptide restrictor, but without giving rise to the strong allograft responses associated with conventional HLA class I polymorphism. There is furthermore evidence that gamma-interferon can readily switch on HLA class I functional expression in the villous trophoblast, so protecting these critical cells more effectively against viral attack.

Another protection for the trophoblast may come from NK cells, whose specificity is normally inhibited by particular HLA class I products, and which can, therefore, presumably more readily attack cells that do not express classical HLA-A, B and C molecules. There must have been some intricate co-evolution of the polymorphism of NK receptors, HLA-A, B and C, polymorphic and HLA-G determinants, in order to take advantage of HLA polymorphism for withstanding pathogen onslaught, while at the same time protecting the foetus as an allograft.

Conclusions

The HLA system as originally defined by relatively crude serology but sophisticated statistics more than 30 years ago, has turned out to be the enormously complex collection of genes and variants that we can now identify at the DNA level. With this advance has come an enormous advance in our understanding of the nature of immune mechanisms, which has been paralleled by the development of plausible hypotheses for the way that natural selection acts on HLA variants. The infrastructure for our understanding of the origin and maintenance of HLA polymorphism is clearly established, but there is still much to be done in describing the explicit mechanisms by which, for example, particular HLA variants influence immune response to pathogens. It is this level of understanding that will eventually lead to more specific explanations of the way in which natural selection moulds the HLA polymorphism.

References

Barnstable, CJ and Bodmer, WF (1978) Immunology and the fetus. *Lancet* **1:** 326-326

Bodmer, WF (1972) Evolutionary significance of the HL-A system. *Nature* **237:** 139-145

Bodmer, WF (1973) Population genetics of the HL-A system: retrospect and prospect. In: *Histocompatibility Testing 1972.* (Ed. Dausset, J) pp.611-617. Munksgaard, Copenhagen

Bodmer, JG (1996) World distribution of HLA alleles and implications for disease. Variation in the human genome. CIBA Foundation Symposium **197:** 233-258

Bodmer, JG and Bodmer, WF (1970) Studies on African Pygmies IV: a comparative study of the HL-A polymorphism in the Babinga Pygmies and other African and Caucasian populations. *American Journal of Human Genetics* **22:** 396-411

Bodmer, WF and Bodmer, JG (1978) Evolution and function of the HLA system. *British Medical Bulletin* **34:** 309-316

Bodmer, WF, Trowsdale, J, Young, J and Bodmer, J. (1986) Gene clusters and the evolution of the major histocompatibility system. *Philosophical Transactions of the Royal Society of London. Series B: Biological Sciences* **312:** 303-315.

Bodmer, JG, Marsh, SGE, Albert, ED, Bodmer, WF, Bontrop, RE *et al.* (1997) Nomenclature for factors of the HLA system, 1996. *Tissue Antigens* **49**: 297-321

Bjorkman, PJ, Saper, MA, Samraoui, B, Bennett, WS, Strominger, JL *et al.* (1987) Structure of the human class I histocompatibility antigen HLA-A2. *Nature* **329**: 506-512

Cavalli-Sforza, LL and Bodmer, WF (1971) The Genetics of Human Populations. W.H. Freeman, London

Ceppellini, R, Curtoni, ES, Mattiuz, PL, Miggiano, V, Scudeller, G *et al.* (1967) Genetics of leukocyte antigens: A family study of segregation and linkage. In: *Histocompatibility Testing, 1967* (Ed. Curtoni, ES) pp.149-187. Munksgaard, Copenhagen

Iha, TH, Gerbrandt, G, Bodmer, WF, McGary, D and Stone, WH. (1973) Cross-reactions of cattle lymphocytotoxic sera with HL-A and other human antigens. *Tissue Antigens* **3**: 291-302

Piazza, A, Belvedere, MC, Bernoco, C, Conighi, C, Conte, L *et al.* (1973) In: *Histocompatibility Testing 1972* (Ed. Colombani, JD and Columbani, J) pp.73-84. Munksgaard, Copenhagen

Thomson, G, Bodmer, WF and Bodmer, J (1976) The HL-A system as a model for studying the interaction between selection, migration and linkage. In: *Proceedings of the International Conference on Population Genetics and Ecology 1975,* pp.465-498. Academic Press, New York

Tomlinson, IPM and Bodmer, WF (1995) The HLA System and the analysis of multifactorial genetic disease. *Trends in Genetics* **11:** 493-498

INTRODUCTION

IMMUNE RECOGNITION AND THE MHC

P. Travers
Anthony Nolan Research Institute
The Royal Free Hospital
Pond Street
London NW3 2QG

Introduction

How do we know who we are? This is not meant as an abstract philosophical question but as a scientific one. The function of the immune system is to protect us from assault by pathogens, and therefore it must be able to distinguish the pathogens, which it must eliminate, from self cells, which it must not.

The recognition task faced by the immune system is complicated by the diversity of micro-organisms (and some macro-organisms, such as parasitic worms) against which we must be protected. Pathogens live in different sites with respect to the body and it's cellular constituents. Some bacteria, fungi and parasites live either on the external surfaces of cells or free in the extracellular fluids. Other pathogens live within vesicles, having been phagocytosed but able to withstand the enzymatic machinery of the phagosome. Yet others can invade from these vesicles into the cytosol of the cell, and of course all viruses are obligate intracellular parasites, relying on the synthetic apparatus of the host cell for their replication. Different effector mechanisms must be applied in each of these cases to eliminate the infection; the production of neutralising and opsonising antibody for extracellular pathogens, the activation of macrophages to eliminate phagocytosed pathogens, and cytotoxic effectors to eliminate virally infected cells or those harboring intracytoplasmic pathogens. The immune system must therefore perform another recognition task in addition to identifying the presence of pathogens within the body; it must identify the compartment in which the pathogen is found to ensure that the appropriate effector mechanisms are engaged.

It is this dual requirement for the recognition both of the presence of a pathogen and its location that differentiates recognition by T cells from that by B cells and by antibody. The solution to these twin problems is to be found in the Major Histocompatibility Complex, whose products are specialised to carry information about both the presence and the location of pathogens.

The Major Histocompatibility Complex (hereafter referred to as MHC) was defined originally on the basis of mapping loci which were the most significant determinants of graft rejection, hence the terms 'major' and 'histocompatibility'. A second set of genes, the immune response (Ir) genes controlling antibody and delayed type hypersensitivity responses to protein antigens, was also mapped to the same region of the genome. With this observation came the first major division of the MHC, into what subsequently became known as class I and class II genes, initially those genes controlling graft rejection and immune response respectively. As we shall see, the MHC class I and class II genes, while evolutionarily related, and generally very similar to each other, yet have subtle differences in both structure and function.

Many genes have been identified within the genetic boundaries of the MHC, encoding complement components, cytokines and other molecules with a role in immune responses. These other genes are sometimes referred to as MHC class III genes though they are unrelated to the class I and class II genes. Yet others have no immunological function (although the function of many is as yet undetermined) and their presence in this particular part of the genome appears to be an accident of fate.

What we are concerned with here, however, is recognition by the immune system, and further discussion will be focused on the MHC class I and class II genes, and a subset of other MHC genes whose products act in concert with those of the MHC class I and class II genes to facilitate antigen recognition.

Function of MHC class I and class II molecules

The role of the MHC molecules in the immune system is , as has been alluded to above, in the presentation of antigens to T cells. The antigen receptors of T cells are unable to recognise antigen directly; they can only recognise foreign antigens in the form of short segments of peptide bound to MHC molecules. This role of MHC molecules in the presentation of antigen was first suggested by the phenomenon of MHC restricted recognition of antigens (Zinkernagel and Doherty 1974; Zinkernagel and Doherty 1997) but can now be demonstrated directly by using purified MHC molecules and purified T cell receptors (Corr *et al.,* 1994; Matsui *et al.,* 1994; Alam *et al.,* 1996; Margulies *et al.,* 1996) and has even been visualised by X-ray crystallography (Garboczi *et al.,* 1996). Neither peptide antigens alone nor MHC molecules alone can stimulate T cell responses, which require the formation of a peptide:MHC complex. However, in some specialised cases T cell receptors are able to recognise non-peptide antigens. For example, some T cells responding to mycobacterial infections have been found to recognise a lipid, mycolic acid, bound to the non-classical MHC molecule, CD1 (Beckman *et al.,* 1994).

Structure of MHC class I and class II molecules

The two distinct classes of MHC molecules that can be detected on the surface of cells differ biochemically on the basis of subunit structure (Figure 1). MHC class I molecules consist of two chains, an α or heavy chain associated non-covalently on the cell surface with β_2-microglobulin. Only the class I α chain spans the

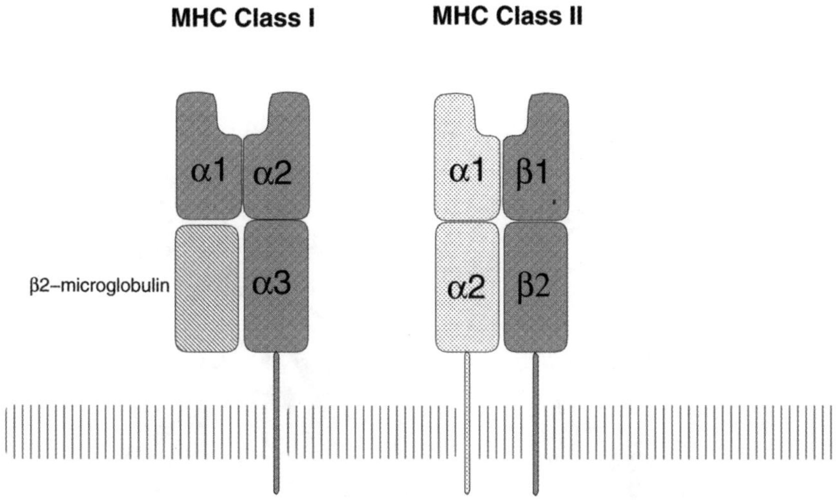

Figure 1. Schematic representation of the structure of MHC class I and class II proteins

membrane. MHC class II molecules consist of a non-covalent complex of two chains, α and β, both of which span the membrane and which are associated non-covalently on the cell surface.

The detailed structures of MHC class I and II molecules have been determined by X-ray crystallography (Bjorkman *et al.*, 1987; Bjorkman *et al.*, 1987; Madden *et al.*, 1991; Saper *et al.*, 1991; Garboczi *et al.*, 1992; Guo *et al.*, 1992; Madden *et al.*, 1992; Garboczi *et al.*, 1994; Stern *et al.*, 1994; Ghosh *et al.*, 1995; Dessen *et al.*, 1997; Smith *et al.*, 1998) and are remarkably similar (Figure 2). Each molecule contains an extracellular portion composed of four domains. In the case of MHC class I molecules, three domains (α1, α2 and α3) are contained within the α (or heavy) chain transmembrane glycoprotein while the fourth domain is contributed by a soluble protein, β_2-microglobulin. The MHC class II molecule is a heterodimer of two transmembrane glycoprotein chains, α and β; in the case of the class II molecules, each chain contributes two domains. In their general features, the structures of the class I and class II molecules are very similar. In both, the membrane distal domains, the α1 domains of MHC class I and class II molecules and the class I α2 and class II β1 domains, fold to form a long groove; the remaining extracellular domains adopt immunologlobulin folds. Comparing the two classes of MHC molecule, the class I α3 domain corresponds to the class II β2 domain and β_2-microglobulin corresponds in position with the class II α2 domain.

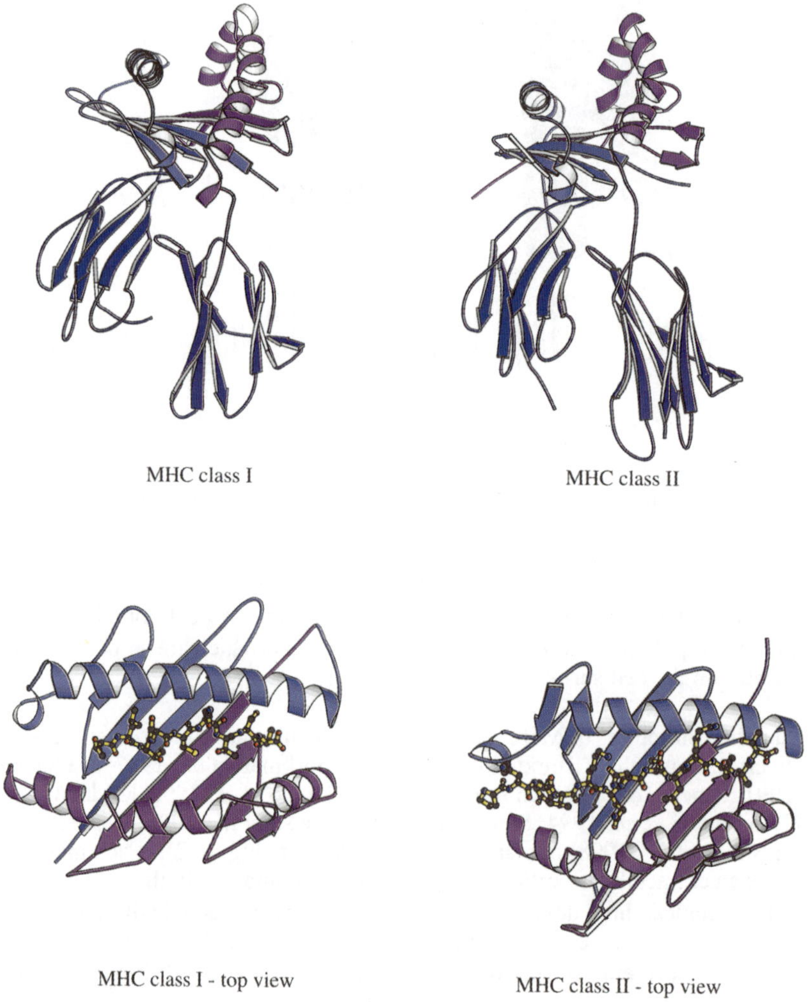

Figure 2. Detailed structures of MHC class I and II molecules

	HLA Class I	HLA Class II
Length	short (8-10)	long (13-25)
Conserved interactions	N and C termini	distributed along peptide
Side chain anchor positions	Usually P2 and PC	Often P1, P4, P6 and P9
Source	predominantly cytoplasmic protein degradation	predominantly endosomal/lysosomal protein degradation
Interaction takes place in	Endoplasmic reticulum	Endocytic compartment (MIIC)
Chaperoned by	Calreticulin, tapasin, TAP	Invariant chain, HLA-DM (HLA-DO?)

Table 1. Comparison of peptide binding to MHC class I and class II molecules

While the overall structures of class I and class II molecules are similar, there are a number of small differences that have an important effect on the way that these molecules interact with peptide antigens.

Antigen binding by MHC class I and class II molecules

The form of antigen that is bound by both class I and class II MHC molecules is as relatively short peptide fragments. Both MHC class I and class II molecules bind antigenic peptides in a cleft formed by the two membrane distal domains ($\alpha1+\alpha2$ or $\alpha1+\beta1$). In both cases, the same general principle is used, although the fine details of how the peptides are bound differ between the two classes of molecule (Madden, 1995). MHC molecules bind peptides in the first instance through conserved interactions between invariant residues on the MHC molecule and the peptide backbone. Superimposed upon these interactions, which are independent of the sequence of the bound peptide, sidechains of the peptide bind into specific pockets distributed along the peptide binding cleft and it is these interactions that allows the MHC molecules to discriminate between peptides, binding some and not others (Table 1).

MHC class I

In the case of MHC class I molecules, the peptides that are bound are predominantly short, usually octamers and nonamers, although longer peptides can be bound. The peptide is bound by both ends, with interactions between the MHC molecule and the N and C termini of the peptide (Figure 3) (Matsumura *et al.,* 1992). These interactions are critical for the ability of the class I molecule to bind peptide; peptide analogues with modified amino and carboxyl groups fail to form stable complexes with MHC class I molecules (Bouvier and Wiley 1994; Collins *et al.,* 1994; Bouvier *et al.,* 1998). In addition to these terminal interactions, which will be the same no matter what peptide is bound, MHC molecules also interact with side chains of the peptide and it is these interactions that give the different MHC molecules their differing specificities (Garrett *et al.,* 1989; Matsumura *et al.,* 1992; Young *et al.,* 1994; Strominger and Wiley 1995). For most class I molecules, the most important interactions are those between the second amino acid of the peptide (referred to as P2) and the last amino acid (depending on the length of the peptide this could be P8, P9 etc; we will designate

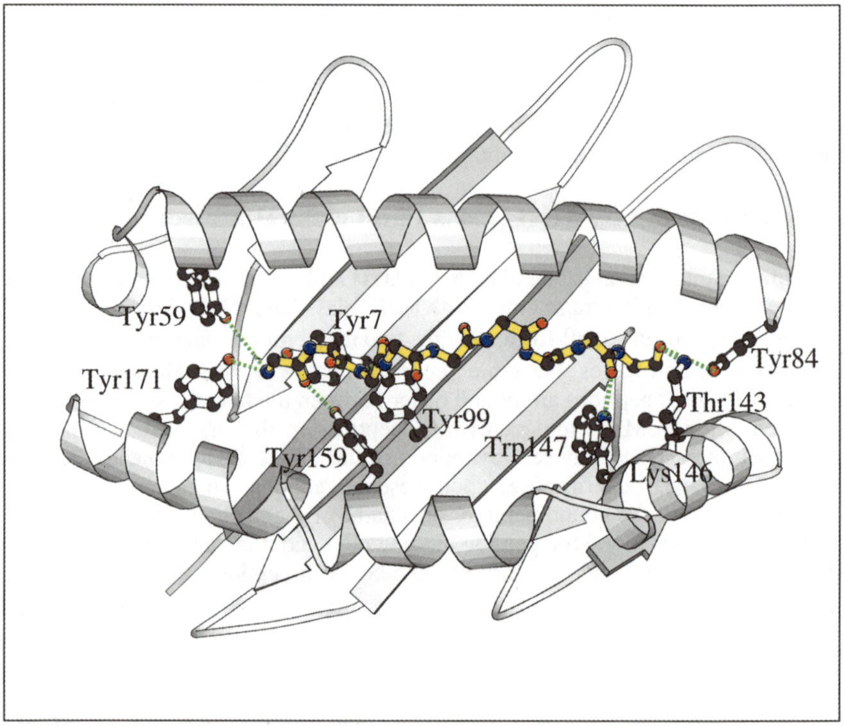

Figure 3. Peptide binding to HLA class I

this residue as PC). For some class I molecules, notably the mouse H2-K^b and H2-D^b molecules, the residue at PC-3 (ie P5 for an octamer peptide and P6 for a nonamer) is a dominant contact residue and the contribution of the P2 residue is diminished (Fremont *et al.,* 1992; Zhang *et al.,* 1992; Young *et al.,* 1994; Fremont *et al.,* 1995).

MHC Class II

Peptide binding to class II molecules differs in a number of important respects from binding to class I. The most obvious difference is in the length of the peptides that are bound (Chicz *et al.,* 1992). The majority of the peptides bound to class II molecules are greater than 13 amino acids in length and there is in principle no upper limit to the length of peptide that can be bound, with the constraint that the segment of the peptide that interacts with the class II molecule is both unfolded and accessible. This feature results from two important differences in the structure of the class II peptide binding groove compared to that of class I molecules (Stern *et al.,* 1994; Strominger and Wiley 1995). Instead of the amino terminal portion of the peptide being buried within the groove, in class II molecules an extended region of the polypeptide chain forms a short piece of parallel β sheet with the peptide backbone. This interaction has the effect of pulling up the peptide and allows the amino terminal end of the peptide to extend beyond the end of the peptide binding groove. At the carboxy-terminal end of the peptide, rather than the peptide being pulled up, the end of the α1 domain is pulled down by the α2 domain (remember that in class I molecules the end of the α1 domain continues to become the equivalent of the β2 domain). This again allows the end of the peptide to protrude beyond the end of the peptide binding groove.

Given, that the ends of the peptide no longer bind to the MHC class II molecule, how then are peptides bound? Instead of interactions focused at each end, peptides interact with MHC class II molecules along their length (Figure 4) (Brown *et al.,* 1993; Stern *et al.,* 1994). As was mentioned above, a short section of parallel β sheet is formed between the class II α chain and the peptide. In addition, the α chain contributes a number of hydrogen bonds between conserved side chains, principally asparagine residues at 64 and 71, and the peptide backbone. The β chain contributes a hydrogen bond from the conserved residues Trp61 (this interaction is identical to that between Trp147 and the PC-1 backbone carbonyl in class I:peptide complexes) and Asn 82. In some MHC molecules, the residues at positions 71, 78 and 81 are also able to interact with the peptide backbone.

As with the class I molecules, sidechains of the peptide interact with specific pockets in the class II molecules. Since the the peptides which bind to class II molecules can extend by variable lengths at both ends of the groove, it is less easy to provide a uniform nomenclature for the peptide sidechains that interact with the class II molecule. The first side chain that interacts with the class II molecule is designated P1, although this is in fact the third amino acid which interacts with the MHC molecule; it is the backbone of the preceding two amino acids which interacts. The other side chains that are bound by the class II molecule are the P4, P6, P7 and P9 residues.

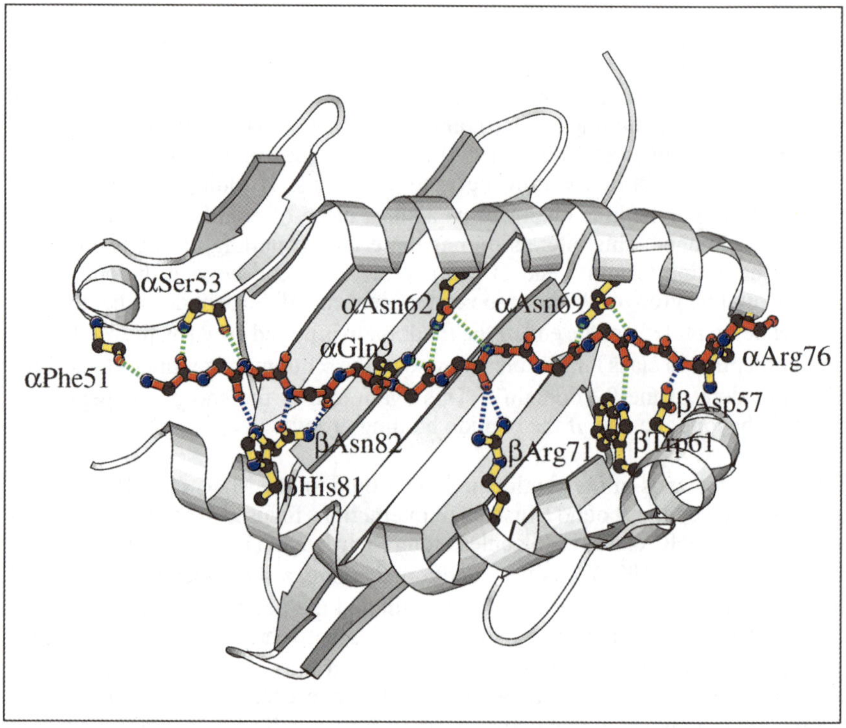

Figure 4. Peptide binding to HLA class II

One curious feature of the class II molecules is the way in which bidentate hydrogen bonds, which fix the peptide backbone in place, straddle the upward-pointing residues, the potential TCR contacts. In contrast with the peptides bound by class I molecules, where the central portion of the peptide is relatively unconstrained by the MHC molecule and can adopt a number of conformations (Madden *et al.,* 1993), it would appear that the TCRs that discriminate class II:peptide complexes do so mainly on the basis of the sequence of the peptide and less on the conformation of the bound peptide.

Synthesis and export

The biosynthesis and export of MHC molecules present a number of challenges. The MHC molecules form heterodimers that are unstable in the absence of bound peptide, and so the newly synthesised molecules must be stabilised in some way until they encounter suitable peptides. MHC class I molecules bind peptides that are derived from cytosolic proteins, and so some mechanism must exist to transport these peptides from the cytosol to the lumen of the endoplasmic reticulum, where the binding takes place. MHC class II molecules, on the other hand, bind peptides derived primarily from extracellular, secreted or membrane associated proteins that have been degraded subsequent to their endocytosis and transport, if not to a lysosome, then at least to an acidified, proteolytic compartment within the cell. This raises three issues; how is the class II molecule protected from interaction with peptides and unfolded or partially folded polypeptides in the ER, where and how does it encounter antigenic peptides and how does it get from this location to the cell surface? Not all of these problems have yet been solved, but what has been discovered reveals an exquisite system of transporters and chaperones which interact to allow the MHC molecules to bind only those peptides derived from the appropriate cellular compartment.

MHC class I molecules are synthesised in the rough endoplasmic reticulum as the separated a chain and β_2-microglobulin. As with many oligomeric proteins, MHC molecules have an immediate problem; the a chain by itself cannot fold correctly. However, as the a chain starts to fold, it interacts with a molecular chaperone, calnexin, which stabilises the partially folded a chain until it can pair with β_2-microglobulin. On pairing with β_2-microglobulin, the calnexin chaperone is replaced by a related molecule, calreticulin which encodes an ER retention signal, trapping the as-yet empty class I molecule within the ER, ready to bind peptides of the appropriate length and sequence.

The process of interaction with peptide starts with the generation of peptides from cytosolic proteins. It is not yet known what initiates the process of degradation of proteins to generate peptide fragments capable of binding to MHC class I molecules. Ubiquitination of proteins has been shown to increase the presentation of their peptides (Townsend *et al.,* 1988; Grant *et al.,* 1995) yet inactivation of the ubiquitination pathway does not decrease presentation (Cox *et al.,* 1995). Whatever the initiating signal, the actual degradation is carried out by a large proteolytic complex, the proteasome, that resides in the cytoplasm. The proteasome is a multisubunit complex, consisting of four stacked 7-membered rings encoded, in mammals, by up to 14 different genes. These subunits form a hollow barrel within which the protein is cleaved. There are at least 5 separate peptidase activities ascribed to the proteasome, although which subunits are responsible for each activity is not known. In cells treated with IFNγ, which upregulates MHC class I expression, at least three subunits of the proteasome are replaced. Two of the interferon-induced subunits, called LMP2 and LMP7, are encoded within the MHC itself while a third protein, MECL-1, is encoded on chromosome 16. Each of these three interferon-induced proteins and the constitutive subunits they replace share features with the active protease subunits of yeast and bacterial proteasomes and it is possible that they may be the only proteolytically active subunits in the proteasome. It has been suggested that the interferon-induced subunits alter the cleavage specificity of the proteasome, increasing cleavage after hydrophobic and basic amino acids and descreasing cleavage after acidic amino acids (Gaczynska *et al.*, 1994). This suggestion is attractive, as MHC class I molecules have a preference for hydrophobic and basic amino acids at the C terminal residues of peptides; however, these differences in cleavage specificity have only been seen with short peptide substrates and may not reflect the pattern of cleavage of longer polypeptides (Kuckelkorn *et al.,* 1995).

Subsequent to their production, potential antigenic peptides must be translocated from the cytosol, where the proteasome resides, to the lumen of the endoplasmic reticulum, where the class I molecule and its peptide binding site await. This process is mediated by the products of the TAP genes lying within the class II region of the MHC, which encode a transmembrane transporter protein belonging to a family of proteins known as *ATP binding cassette*, or ABC, proteins. These transporter proteins were first implicated in the delivery of peptides to class I molecules when a mutant cell line defective in the presentation of antigens in association with MHC class I proteins was found not to express one of the MHC-linked transporter genes. Moreover, restoration of the functional transporter gene restores the ability of the cell to present antigens with class I molecules. More detailed analysis of the function of the TAP molecule has shown that it is capable of transporting peptides of greater than 7 amino acids in length and with a preference for peptides of 8-12 amino acids. For longer peptides, some are transported while others are not, although what features determine whether any individual peptide will or will not be transported are not known.

The TAP molecule plays a second role, in that "empty" class I molecules, in the form of α:β_2-microglobulin:calreticulin complexes, are found associated with TAP through another MHC encoded molecule called tapasin (Ortmann *et al.,* 1997; Herberg *et al.,* 1998). These class I molecules are presumably optimally sited to interact with peptides being transported by TAP. Certainly, binding of peptides to the class I molecules causes their release from TAP complex, and allows the now fully assembled MHC class I:peptide complex to be transported from the ER, through the Golgi apparatus to the cell surface, where it is available for scrutiny by T cells.

The assembly of MHC class I molecules is thus a complex and exquisitely coordinated process whose end result is that class I molecules are retained in the ER until the can bind peptides derived from proteins degraded in the cytosol. The assembly of class II molecules is an equally coordinated process, but one whose aim is to prevent the binding of peptides from cytosolic proteins and instead facilitate the binding of peptides derived from membrane bound or extracellular proteins.

MHC class I and class II molecules resemble each other in their overall structure and function yet each presents peptides derived from very different sources, one intracellular and the other extracellular. The function of MHC class II molecules is to bind peptides generated in the intracellular vesicles of B cells and macrophages. MHC class II molecules must therefore be prevented from binding to peptides transported into the lumen of the endoplasmic reticulum by the TAP transporter. MHC class II molecules must also be prevented from binding nascent polypeptides in the ER, since the class II molecule is able to bind long unfolded peptides due to the open ends of the peptide binding groove and the endoplasmic reticulum is an environment richly endowed with such unfolded and partially folded proteins.

This is achieved by the assembly of newly synthesized MHC class II molecules together with a specialized protein known as the MHC class II-associated invariant chain (Ii). The invariant chain forms trimers, with each subunit binding non-covalently to a class II a:b heterodimer. While this complex is being assembled in the endoplasmic reticulum, its component parts are associated with calnexin. Only when assembly is completed to produce a nine-chain complex is it released from calnexin for transport from the endoplasmic reticulum. In this nine-chain complex, the MHC class II molecule cannot bind peptides or unfolded proteins, so that the peptides present in the endoplasmic reticulum are not usually presented by MHC class II molecules. Moreover, there is evidence that many MHC class II molecules are retained in the ER in the form of complexes with misfolded proteins in the absence of Ii.

The invariant chain has a second function, and that is to target delivery of the MHC class II molecules to an appropriate low pH endosomal compartment. The complex of MHC class II α:β heterodimers with invariant chain is retained for two to four hours in this compartment. During this time, the invariant chain is cleaved at several sites. The cleavage is ordered, so that the initial cleavage events generate a truncated form of the invariant chain that remains bound to the MHC class II molecule and retains it within the proteolytic compartment. A subsequent cleavage releases the MHC class II molecule, bound to a short fragment of Ii, called CLIP (for CLass II-associated Invariant chain Peptide). MHC class II molecules that have CLIP associated with them are still prevented from binding other peptides and CLIP must either dissociate or be displaced in order for the MHC class II molecule to bind processed peptide and deliver it to the cell surface.

The intracellular location at which invariant chain is cleaved and MHC class II molecules encounter peptides is not clearly defined. Newly synthesized MHC class II molecules travel to the cell surface in vesicles that, at some point after leaving the trans-Golgi network, fuse with the incoming endosomes. MHC class II:Ii complexes enter the endocytic pathway and are there exposed to an acidic, proteolytic environment in which both the the invariant chain is cleaved and pathogens and their proteins can be broken down into peptides available for binding to the class II molecule. It is likely that the cathepsins S and L are involved in these cleavage events, as mice defective in either cathepsin SA or L are defective in antigen presentation by MHC class II molecules. Ultrastructural studies suggest that there are specialised intracellular vesicles, collectively called the MHC class II Compartment (MIIC), where the final cleavage of the invariant chain and the subsequent interaction of the class II molecule with peptide occur.

Delivery of the class II molecule to the same compartments in which peptides are generated is, however, insufficient to ensure that the class II molecule actually binds the peptides. This has been become obvious by experimental observations of mutated human B cell lines in which the correct interaction of MHC class II molecules with peptide antigens does not occur. As the binding of peptide antigens to the class II molecule is required to create a stable dimer, in these mutant cells, the class II molecule dissociates readily into its component α and β chains. For this reason the mutation in these cells was called the "falling-apart" mutation. Further analysis of MHC class II molecules in the "falling-apart" mutant cell lines has shown that the CLIP peptide remains associated and peptides derived from proteins that have been internalised and degraded within the endosomal pathway do not bind.

The defect in these "falling-apart" cells lies in a class II-like molecule, called HLA-DM that lie near the TAP and LMP genes in the class II region of the MHC. The HLA-DM locus encodes an α chain and a β chain that closely resemble those of other MHC class II molecules, although, unlike other class II molecules, it does not appear to require peptide in order to generate a stable dimeric molecule. The DM molecule also differs from other MHC class II molecules in that it is not expressed at the cell surface, but rather is found predominantly in the MIIC compartment within the cell. The function of the HLA-DM molecule appears to be as an exchange protein, that binds to class II:CLIP complexes and catalyses both the release of the CLIP fragment from MHC class II:CLIP complexes and the binding of other peptides to the resulting empty MHC class II molecule. HLA-DM is also able to catalyse the release of peptides other than CLIP from MHC class II molecules, depending on the stability of the MHC:peptide complex. Peptides that make poor interactions are removed and replaced with others, allowing a continuous editing of the peptide:MHC class II complex until a peptide of sufficient affinity is bound. It is likely that this process ensures that the peptide:MHC class II complexes displayed on the surface of the antigen presenting cell will survive long enough to be able to stimulate the appropriate CD4 T cells.

One more molecule plays a role in the peptide loading of MHC class II molecules, and it is another class II-like molecule, HLA-DO. The exact function of HLA-DO is controversial as yet, but it has been observed to act as an inhibitor of HLA-DM mediated peptide exchange (Denzin *et al.*, 1997; van Ham *et al.,* 1997; Jensen 1998; Liljedahl *et al.,* 1998). However, some have found HLA-DO to have a positive role in antigen loading (Kropshofer *et al.,* 1998), enhancing the activity of HLA-DM. HLA-DO is expressed in only a subset of MHC class II positive cells, in B cells and in the thymic epithelium and why it should function in these tissues to alter peptide loading is unknown.

Thus both MHC class I and class II molecules bind antigens in a highly orchestrated process in which each class of MHC molecule is delivered to the appropriate site at which it can interact with peptides. In each case, the delivery of antigen to the MHC molecule involves other MHC encoded proteins so that it appears as though a specialised mechanism to deliver peptides efficiently has co-evolved with the MHC molecules themselves.

Genomic organisation of the MHC

Much of the major histocompatibility complex of man has been cloned and the additional use of gene mapping techniques has allowed the organisation of the gene complex to be determined directly, confirming the results of classical genetic studies (Figure 5) (Campbell and Trowsdale 1993; Trowsdale, 1993; Newell *et al.*, 1994; Trowsdale, 1995). The genes encoding the class I α chain and the class II α and β chains are linked within a gene complex covering two to three centimorgans of DNA, or about $4x10^6$ base pairs. The gene for β_2-microglobulin lies on a separate chromosome.

Within the MHC gene complex are separate regions that encode class I and class II molecules and within these regions there are many copies of class I and class II genes. In man, there are three main class I a chain genes, called HLA-A, -B and -C. There are also three main sets of class II α and β chain genes in man, called HLA-DR, -DP and -DQ This picture is complicated a little since the DR locus contains two β chain genes, both of which make functional β chain proteins that pair with the DRα chain.

MHC class I and class II genes have been identified and characterised from many vertebrate species and, with the exception of chickens, all have essentially the same organisation (Klein and OhUigin 1993; Klein *et al.,* 1993; Kaufman *et al.,* 1995; Trowsdale 1995).

A large number of class I-like genes of unknown function occur in the major histocompatibility complex (Heinrichs and Orr 1990; Bahram *et al.,* 1994; Klein and OhUigin 1994; Obata *et al.,* 1994; Watkins, 1995); the exact number differs greatly between different species and even between members of the same species. These have been termed class IB genes, and encode cell surface molecules that are expressed only in certain cells, such as T lymphocytes, Langerhans cells, or certain leukaemias. The function of class IB genes and their products is not known for certain, but some class IB products may function as the ligands for γδ T cells (Bahram and Spies 1996; Groh *et al.,* 1996; Groh *et al.,* 1998) or for the presentation of restricted subsets of peptides (Hedrick 1992; Kurlander *et al.,* 1992; Stroynowski and Lindahl 1994; Wang *et al.,* 1995; Braud *et al.,* 1998; Allan *et al.,* 1999; Braud *et al.,* 1999). The large number of genes encoding such molecules means that many different products of class IB genes can exist in a single animal. In addition, there are at least two additional class II-like molecules

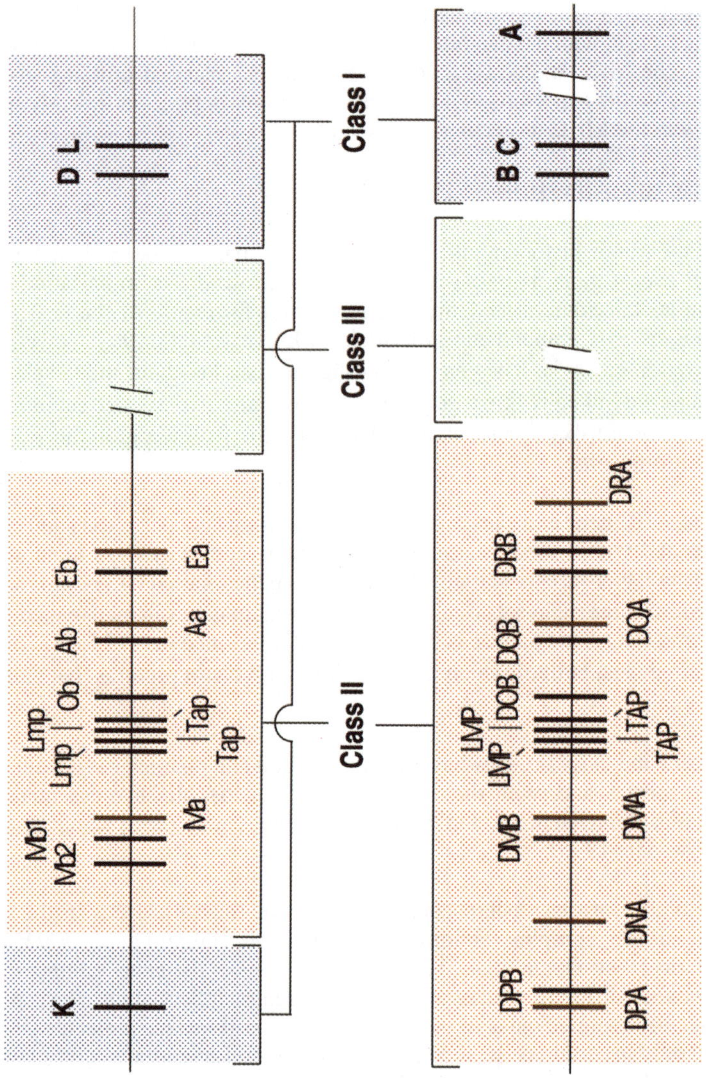

Figure 5. Map of the human MHC

encoded within the class II region, called DO (Karlsson *et al.,* 1991; Karlsson *et al.,* 1992) and DM (Kelly *et al.,* 1991). The role of the DM gene products appears to be restricted to the antigen processing pathway of MHC class II molecules, where it functions to catalyse the binding of antigenic peptides to "classical" class II molecules (Mellins *et al.,* 1991; Mellins *et al.,* 1994; Morris *et al.,* 1994; Sloan *et al.,* 1995); the fine details of how this function is carried out are not yet known, but what is known will be described later. The DO molecule appear only to be expressed in the thymus and in B cells. Its function is not yet clear, and there is a controversy over whether it functions as an inhibitor of DM or to augment DM (Denzin *et al.,* 1997; van Ham *et al.,* 1997; Jensen 1998; Kropshofer *et al.,* 1998; Liljedahl *et al.,* 1998).

MHC class I genes are expressed in most somatic cells, although the level of expression differs from one cell type to the next. Cells of the immune system express abundant MHC class I on their surface, while liver cells, for example, express relatively low levels; red blood cells express little or none. As might be expected, the level of MHC molecule expression plays an important role in T cell activation, so differences in levels of expression are known to be immunologically significant. MHC class I molecules are specialised for the presentation of viral antigens to CD8+ T cells to elicit a cytotoxic response. As viruses can infect any nucleated cell, all such cells express class I molecules.

The tissue distribution of MHC class II molecules is quite distinct from that of class I molecules (Bodmer, 1981; Ploegh *et al.,* 1981; Shackelford *et al.,* 1982; Strominger 1986), in that MHC class II molecules are found normally only on B lymphocytes, some macrophages, specialized antigen presenting cells in lymphoid tissues (dendritic cells) or the skin (Langerhans cells), and on the epithelial component of the thymus. However, expression of MHC class II molecules can be induced on many cell types by lymphokines, especially interferon (IFN) γ. This may be very important both in normal immune functioning and in autoimmunity. Under normal circumstances, the restricted tissue distribution of MHC class II molecules implies that only certain cells can present antigens in association with these molecules.

In addition to the genes encoding cell surface molecules recognized by T lymphocytes (class I, class II and perhaps class IB MHC molecules), several other genes map within the MHC. Some of these have important functions within the immune system, like the complement components C2, Factor B and C4 or the cytokines tumour necrosis factor (TNF) and lymphotoxin (LT); these have been termed class III MHC genes and are shown on the map the human MHC (Figure 5). In addition, two genes that encode a transmembrane transport protein have been mapped to the MHC class II region (Kelly *et al.,* 1992). These genes encode a dimeric transmembrane protein that is a member of a family of transport proteins known as ABC (for ATP binding cassette) transporters; members of this family are known to transport sugars, nucleotides, amino acids and large polypeptides across cell membranes. The two genes lying within the MHC encode a transport system that delivers peptides from the cytoplasm to the endoplasmic reticulum, and the genes have been designated Transporters Associated with antigen Presentation (TAP). Closely associated with the TAP genes are two proteins that form part of a large cytoplasmic complex called the proteasome, or multicatalytic proteinase complex (Monaco and McDevitt 1986; Brown *et al.*, 1991; Glynne *et al.*, 1991; Kelly *et al.*, 1991; Kelly *et al.*, 1992). This is a large assembly of some 14 distinct polypeptides that contains a number of different proteinase activities and is involved in protein degradation in the cytoplasm of the cell. MHC class I molecules bind peptides derived from cytoplasmic and nuclear proteins and the TAP and proteasome molecules encoded within the MHC exist to transport peptide fragments of cytoplasmic proteins into the endoplasmic reticulum where they can bind to MHC class I molecules.

Polymorphism

Because there are three genes encoding MHC class I molecules and four possible sets of MHC class II genes, every individual will express at least three different MHC class I proteins and four MHC class II proteins on his or her cells. In fact, however, the number of different MHC proteins expressed on the cells of most individuals is much greater, because of the extreme polymorphism of the MHC. The MHC class I and class II genes have over 100 alleles at some loci (Figure 6), with each allele being present at a relatively high frequency in the population. For these reasons, the chance that the MHC genes on both chromosomes of an individual will encode the same allele is small; that is, most individuals are heterozygous at these loci. The extensive polymorphism at each locus has the potential to double the number of distinct MHC molecules expressed by each cell in an individual and thereby increases the diversity already available through polygeny, the existence of multiple functionally equivalent genes. Thus, with three MHC class I genes and four potential MHC class II genes, a typical human will express six different MHC class I molecules and eight different MHC class II molecules on his or her cells. For the MHC class II genes the number of different products may be increased still further by the combination of α and β chains from different chromosomes (so that two α chains and two β chains can give rise to four different products). In mice, it has been shown that not all combinations of α and β chains can pair to form stable dimers and so, in practice, the exact number of different MHC class II molecules expressed will depend on which alleles are present on each chromosome.

Pairing between a class II α chain of one isotype and a β chain from another can occur (for example, DRβ pairing with DQα), but it is only seen when the correct partner fails to be expressed and it is unlikely that such combinations play any significant role *in vivo*.

All MHC products are polymorphic to a greater or lesser extent, with the exception of the DRα chain. This chain does not vary in sequence between different individuals and is said to be monomorphic. All other MHC class I and class II genes are polymorphic. This might indicate a functional constraint that prevents variation in the DRα protein, but no such special function has yet been found.

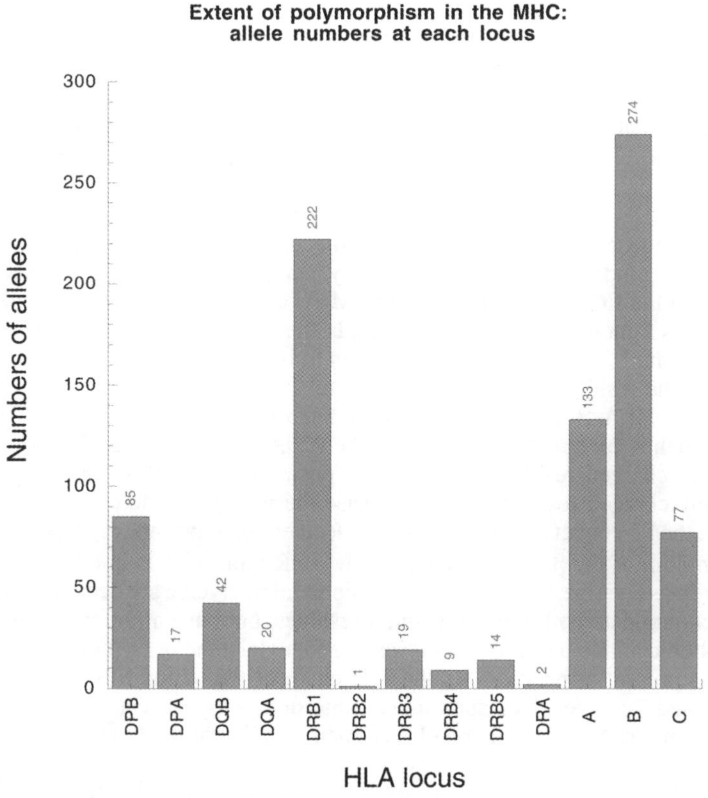

Figure 6. Extent of polymorphism in HLA

Influence of polymorphism on peptide binding

Individual MHC alleles can differ from one another by up to 20 amino acids, making each allele quite distinct. Most of these differences are localized to exposed surfaces of the outer domain of the molecule, and to the peptide-binding groove in particular. The polymorphic residues that line the peptide-binding groove determine the peptide-binding properties of the different MHC molecules.

Peptides bind to MHC class I molecules through specific anchor residues, amino-acid side chains held in pockets that line the peptide-binding groove. Polymorphism in MHC class I molecules affects the amino acids lining these pockets and thus their binding specificity. In consequence, the anchor residues differ for peptides that bind to each allelic variant. The set of anchor residues that allow binding to a given MHC class I molecule is called a sequence motif. Different allelic variants of MHC class II molecules also bind different peptides, but the more open structure of the MHC class II peptide-binding groove, and the greater length of the peptides bound in it, allow greater flexibility in peptide binding, so that it is more difficult to predict which peptides will bind to MHC class II molecules and more difficult to define motifs in the peptides which do bind.

How the sequence variation in the MHC molecules is able to change the specificity for peptide binding can be illustrated by comparing the effects of sequence changes in the first side chain pocket of MHC class I and class II molecules. In MHC class I molecules, this pocket binds the second, or P2, side chain. The residue in the MHC molecule that appears to have the greatest influence on the nature of the residue bound is residue 45 of the class I heavy chain, which, for example in HLA-B27 is glutamic acid, a negatively charged residue. The side chain which is preferentially bound by the P2 pocket of HLA-B27 is arginine, a positively charged residue. Conversely, position 45 of HLA-B44 is lysine, a positively charged residue and in this case the preferred side chain is glutamic acid. In the P1 pocket of MHC class II molecules, an important variable residue is position 86m of the β chain, which in HLA-DR molecules is present either as a glycine or as a valine. Those P1 pockets containing glycine are deep, pockets that can accommodate both large and small residues, but have a preference for large hydrophobic amino acids such as tyrosine, phenylalanine or tryptophan. When a valine is present at position 86, the side chain of the valine fills up part of the pocket, and large residues such as tyrosine or tryptophan can no longer bind; instead, smaller hydrophobic residues (leucine, valine or methionine).

The sites in MHC molecules that interact with peptide side chains all have some contribution from polymorphic residues; for example, in HLA-DR molecules, the P1, P4, P6, P7 and P9 pockets are all formed in part by variable amino acids. Moreover, all (bar one) of the most polymorphic residues in class II molecules are to be found amongst the residues forming these pockets, suggesting that the role of the polymorphism is indeed to vary the nature of the side chain-binding pockets and thus alter the specificity of the class II molecule for peptide.

Since the role of the immune system is to protect against infection, it is here we must look for the nature of the selective advantage conferred by the extensive polymorphism of the MHC proteins. Pathogens have a number of possible strategies for avoiding an immune response either by evading detection or by suppressing the ensuing response. The requirement for presentation by an MHC molecule provides at least one possible means of evasion. Although MHC molecules have a broad specificity of peptide binding, only certain peptides will bind to a given MHC molecule, and those that do not bind are not immunogenic. A pathogen could therefore escape detection by mutations that eliminated from its proteins all peptides able to bind MHC molecules. Failures in responsiveness to protein antigens by such a mechanism were reported in inbred animals, where they were called immune response (Ir) gene defects, long before the function of MHC molecules was understood. These defects could be shown genetically to map to genes within the MHC, and were the first clue to the antigen-presenting function of MHC molecules. Ir gene defects are common in inbred strains of mice because the mice are homozygous for all their MHC genes and thus express only one allelic variant from each gene locus. This process of evasion of the immune response is plainly much more difficult if there are many different MHC molecules, and the presence of different loci encoding functionally related proteins may have been an evolutionary adaptation to this strategy. Polymorphism at each locus can potentially double the number of different MHC molecules expressed by an individual, since most individuals will be heterozygotes. Polymorphism has the additional advantage that different individuals in a population will differ in the combinations of MHC molecules they express and will thus present different sets of peptides from each pathogen. This makes it unlikely that all individuals in a population will be equally susceptible to any given pathogen, thereby limiting its spread.

These arguments raise the question, if having three MHC class I molecules is advantageous, and six even more so, why are there not far more MHC class I loci? A possible explanation is that each time a new MHC molecule is added, all T cells that can recognize self peptides bound to that molecule must be removed to maintain self tolerance. It appears that the numbers of loci present in most species is roughly optimal to balance between the advantages of presenting an increased range of foreign peptides and the disadvantages of increased presentation of self peptides and the consequent loss of T cells that accompanies it.

MHC polymorphism appears to have been strongly selected by evolutionary pressures. However, for selection to work efficiently in slowly reproducing organisms like humans, there must also be powerful mechanisms to generate the variability in MHC alleles on which the selective processes act. While the generation of polymorphism in MHC molecules is not yet fully understood since it is an evolutionary problem not readily analyzed in the laboratory, it is clear that several genetic mechanisms contribute to the generation of new alleles. Some new alleles arise by point mutations, but many arise from combining the sequences of other alleles either through genetic recombination or by gene conversion, in which one sequence is replaced in part by another from a homologous gene.

Evidence for gene conversion comes from studies of the sequences of different alleles of MHC proteins, which have revealed that some changes involve clusters of several amino acids and require multiple nucleotide changes in a contiguous stretch of the gene. More significantly, the same sequences are found within other MHC genes on the same chromosome, a prerequisite for gene conversion.

Recombination between allelic variants at a single locus may, however, have been more important than gene conversion for generating MHC polymorphism. By comparing sequences of MHC allelic variants, it can be seen that different alleles represent recombination events between ancestral alleles. If one postulates a small number of ancestral alleles, most contemporary alleles can be generated by one or more recombination events occurring within polymorphic exons of MHC genes.

The effects of selective pressure in favor of polymorphism can be seen clearly in the pattern of point mutations in the MHC genes. Point mutations can be classified as replacement substitutions, which change an amino acid, or silent substitutions, which simply change the codon, but leave the amino acid the same. Replacement substitutions are seen within the MHC at a higher frequency relative to silent substitutions than would be expected, providing evidence that polymorphism is actively selected in the evolution of the MHC.

Interactions with other molecules

The specialisation of MHC molecules to present antigens from cytoplasmic versus extracellular sources is reflected in the specialisation of effector functions in the T cells that recognise class I and class II molecules respectively. Class I molecules present antigen to cytolytic T cells. Naive CTL (CTLp) become activated upon recognition of their class I+ peptide ligand and begin synthesis of a set of effector molecules, perforin and granzymes, that become localised in secretory granules. The T cell is now armed and any subsequent recognition by the T cell results in the release of the granule contents onto the surface of the target cell. Perforin,which shows homology to the late complement component C9, forms pores in the target cell membrane, allowing entry of the granzymes into the cytoplasm of the target cell which, in an as yet undefined mechanism, activate the process of apoptosis in the target cell.

Recognition of antigen in association with class I molecules results in the death of the presenting cell; recognition of complexes of antigenic peptides with MHC class II molecules however, results in the activation of the presenting cell. Class II molecules are recognised by T helper cells which, when activated, can be subdivided into two discrete subclasses defined by their patterns of cytokine secretion and consequently their effector phenotype. Naive helper T cells become activated by their first contact with antigen/class II complexes and initially secrete a broad range of cytokines including IL-2, 3, 4, 5, 10 and IFN-γ. Later, these cells differentiate either into Th1, or inflammatory T cells, which upon a second encounter with antigen secrete principally IL-2, INF-γ and TNF, and Th2, or helper T cells, which on a second encounter secrete principally IL-4, 5, 6 and 10. The cytokines secreted by Th1 cells are potent activators of macrophages, increasing their ability to kill phagocytosed microorganisms and, through the release of inflammatory mediators, to recruit macrophages, lymphocytes and neutrophils to the site of activation. The cytokines secreted by Th2 cells both activate B cells and drive their differentiation into antibody secreting cells, while cytokines from both Th cell subsets regulate the isotype switching of B cells. Moreover, activated macrophages upregulate the level of Fc receptors, particularly FcgRI, and can more efficiently phagocytose immune complexes and antibody coated pathogens. Thus the cells presenting antigen in the context of class II MHC molecules are activated by Th cells to express effector functions that are important in the elimination of extracellular microorganisms and toxins, and in the elimination of intravesicular parasites, like *Leishmania*.

The effector functions of the T cells that recognise antigen in the context of class I and class II MHC molecules are therefore quite distinct, and are tailored to eliminate pathogens from the two major compartments (intracytoplasmic *versus* extracellular and vesicular) in which they occur. It is important for the T cell, therefore, that it be able to recognise not just the antigen but also which class of MHC molecule is presenting the antigen in order for the correct effector mechanisms to be activated. However, it is not obviously the case that the T cell receptor *per se* can discriminate class I from class II molecules. Instead, this task is carried out by the coreceptor molecules, CD4 and CD8. CD4 binds to a site in the β2 domain of the class II molecule, while CD8 binds to a site in the α3 domain of class I molecules; these two sites are located in structurally homologous positions in the two MHC molecules. Thus there are *de facto* two receptors on T cells which together confer antigen/MHC specificity, the variable αβTCR and an invariant molecule, CD4 or CD8. Although T cells can be stimulated by MHC:peptide complexes binding to their T cell receptors alone, the simultaneous binding of the coreceptor molecules to the MHC molecule increases the sensitivity of the T cell some 100 fold.

References

Alam, SM, Travers, PJ *et al.* (1996) T-cell-receptor affinity and thymocyte positive selection. *Nature* **381:** 616-620

Allan, DS, Colonna, M, Lanier, LL, Churakova, TD, Abrams, JS *et al.* (1999) Tetrameric complexes of human histocompatibility leukocyte antigen (HLA)-G bind to peripheral blood myelomonocytic cells. *J Exp Med* **189**: 1149-1156

Bahram, S, Bresnahan, M, Geraghty, DE and Spies, T (1994) A second lineage of mammalian major histocompatibility complex class I genes. *Proc Natl Acad Sci USA* **91**: 6259-6263

Bahram, S and Spies, T (1996) The MIC gene family. *Res Immunol* **147**: 328-333

Beckman, EM, Porcelli, SA, Morita, CT, Behar, SM, Furlong, ST *et al.* (1994) Recognition of lipid antigen by CD1-restricted ab+ T cells. *Nature* **372**: 691-694

Bjorkman, PJ, Saper, MA, Samraoui, B, Bennett, WS, Strominger, JL, *et al.* (1987) The foreign antigen binding site and T cell recognition regions of class I histocompatibility antigens. Nature **329**: 512-518

Bjorkman, PJ, Saper, MA, Samraoui, B, Bennett, WS, Strominger, JL, *et al.* (1987) Structure of the human class I histocompatibility antigen, HLA-A2. *Nature* **329**: 506-512

Bodmer, WF (1981) HLA structure and function: A contemporary view. *Tissue Antigens* **17**: 9-20

Bouvier, M, Guo, HC, Smith, KJ and Wiley, DC (1998) Crystal structures of HLA-A*0201 complexed with antigenic peptides with either the amino- or carboxyl-terminal group substituted by a methyl group. *Proteins* **33**: 97-106

Bouvier, M and Wiley, DC (1994) Importance of peptide amino and carboxyl termini to the stability of MHC class I molecules. *Science* **265**: 398-402

Braud, VM, Allan, DS and McMichael, AJ (1999) Functions of nonclassical MHC and non-MHC-encoded class I molecules. *Curr Opin Immunol* **11**: 100-108

Braud, VM, Allan, DS, O'Callaghan, CA, Soderstrom, K, D'Andrea, A, *et al.* (1998) HLA-E binds to natural killer cell receptors CD94/NKG2A, B and C. *Nature* **391**: 795-799

Brown, JH, Jardetzky, TS, Gorga, JC, Stern, LJ, Urban, RG, *et al.* (1993) Three-dimensional structure of the human class II histocompatibility antigen HLA-DR1. *Nature* **364**: 33-39

Brown, MG, Driscoll, J and Monaco, JJ (1991) Structural and serological similarity of MHC-linked LMP and proteasome (multicatalytic proteinase) complexes. *Nature* **353**: 355-357

Campbell, RD and Trowsdale, J (1993) Map of the human MHC. *Immunol Today* **14**: 349-352

Chicz, RM, Urban, RG, Lane, WS, Gorga, JC, Stern, LJ, *et al.* (1992) Predominant naturally processed peptides bound to HLA-DR1 are derived from MHC-related molecules and are heterogeneous in size. *Nature* **358**: 764-768

Collins, EJ, Garboczi, DN and Wiley, DC (1994) Three-dimensional structure of a peptide extending from one end of a class I MHC binding site. *Nature* **371**: 626-629

Corr, M, Slanetz, AE, *et al.* (1994) T cell receptor-MHC class I peptide interactions: affinity, kinetics, and specificity. *Science* **265**: 946-949

Cox, JH, Galardy, P, Bennink, JR and Yewdell, JW (1995) Presentation of endogenous and exogenous antigens is not affected by inactivation of E1 ubiquitin-activating enzyme in temperature- sensitive cell lines. *J Immunol* **154**: 511-519

Denzin, LK, Sant'Angelo, DB, Hammond, C, Surman, MJ and Cresswell, P (1997) Negative regulation by HLA-DO of MHC class II-restricted antigen processing. *Science* **278**: 106-109

Dessen, A, Lawrence, CM, Cupo, S, Zaller, DM and Wiley, DC (1997) X-ray crystal structure of HLA-DR4 (DRA*0101, DRB1*0401) complexed with a peptide from human collagen II. *Immunity* **7**: 473-481

Fremont, DH, Matsumura, M, Stura, EA, Peterson, PA and Wilson, IA (1992) Crystal structures of two viral peptides in complex with murine MHC class I H-2Kb. *Science* **257**: 919-927

Fremont, DH, Stura, EA, Matsumura, M, Peterson, PA and Wilson, IA (1995) Crystal structure of an H-2Kb-ovalbumin peptide complex reveals the interplay of primary and secondary anchor positions in the major histocompatibility complex binding groove. *Proc Natl Acad Sci USA* **92**: 2479-2483

Gaczynska, M, Rock, KL, Spies, T and Goldberg, AL (1994) Peptidase activities of proteasomes are differentially regulated by the major histocompatibility complex-encoded genes for LMP2 and LMP7. *Proc Natl Acad Sci USA* **91**: 9213-9217

Garboczi, DN, Hung, DT and Wiley, DC (1992) HLA-A2-peptide complexes: refolding and crystallization of molecules expressed in Escherichia coli and complexed with single antigenic peptides. *Proc Natl Acad Sci USA* **89**: 3429-3433

Garboczi, DN, Madden, DR and Wiley, DC (1994) Five viral peptide-HLA-A2 co-crystals. Simultaneous space group determination and X-ray data collection. *J Mol Biol* **239**: 581-587

Garboczi, DN, Ghosh, P *et al.* (1996) Structure of the complex between human T-cell receptor, viral peptide and HLA-A2. *Nature* **384**: 134-141

Garrett, TPJ, Saper, MA, Bjorkman, PJ, Strominger, JL and Wiley, DC (1989) Specificity pockets for the side chains of peptide antigens in HLA-Aw68. *Nature* **342**: 692-696

Ghosh, P, Amaya, M, Mellins, E and Wiley, DC (1995) The structure of an intermediate in class II MHC maturation: CLIP bound to HLA-DR3. *Nature* **378**: 457-462

Glynne, R, Powis, SH, Beck, S, Kelly, A, Kerr, L-A, *et al.* (1991) A proteasome-related gene between the two ABC transporter loci in the class II region of the human MHC. *Nature* **353**: 357-360

Grant, EP, Michalek, MT, Goldberg, AL and Rock, KL (1995) Rate of antigen degradation by the ubiquitin-proteasome pathway influences MHC class I presentation. *J Immunol* **155**: 3750-3758

Groh, V, Bahram, S, Bauer, S, Herman, A, Beauchamp, M, *et al.* (1996) Cell stress-regulated human major histocompatibility complex class I gene expressed in gastrointestinal epithelium. *Proc Natl Acad Sci USA* **93**: 12445-12450

Groh, V, Steinle, A, Bauer, S and Spies, T (1998) Recognition of stress-induced MHC molecules by intestinal epithelial gamma-delta T cells. *Science* **279**: 1737-1740.

Guo, HC, Jardetzky, TS, Garrett, TP, Lane, WS, Strominger, JL, *et al.* (1992) Different length peptides bind to HLA-Aw68 similarly at their ends but bulge out in the middle. *Nature* **360**: 364-366

Hedrick, SM (1992) Dawn of the hunt for nonclassical MHC function. *Cell* **70**: 177-180

Heinrichs, H and Orr, HT (1990) HLA Non-A,B,C class I genes: Their structure and expression. *Immunol Res* **9**: 265-274

Herberg, JA, Beck, S *et al.* (1998) TAPASIN, DAXX, RGL2, HKE2 and four new genes (BING 1, 3 to 5) form a dense cluster at the centromeric end of the MHC. *J Mol Biol* **277**: 839-857

Jensen, PE (1998) Antigen processing: HLA-DO—a hitchhiking inhibitor of HLA-DM. *Curr Biol* **8**: 128-131

Karlsson, L, Surh, CD, Sprent, J and Peterson, PA (1991) A novel class II MHC molecule with unusual tissue distribution. *Nature* **351**: 485-488

Karlsson, L, Surh, CD, Sprent, J and Peterson, PA (1992). An unusual class II molecule. *Immunol Today* **13**: 469-470

Kaufman, J, Volk, H and Wallny, HJ (1995) A 'minimal essential MHC' and an 'unrecognized MHC': Two extremes in selection for polymorphism. *Immunol Rev* **143**: 63-88

Kelly, A, Powis, SH, Glynne, R, Radley, E, Beck, S, *et al.* (1991) Second proteasome-related gene in the human MHC class II region. *Nature* **353**: 667-668

Kelly, A, Powis, SH, Kerr, LA, Mockridge, I, Elliott, T, *et al.* (1992) Assembly and function of the two ABC transporter proteins encoded in the human major histocompatibility complex. *Nature* **355**: 641-644

Kelly, A, Monaco, JJ, Cho, S and Trowsdale, J (1991) A new human HLA class II-related locus, DM. *Nature* **353**: 571-573

Klein, J and OhUigin, C (1993) Composite origin of major histocompatibility complex genes. *Curr Opin Genet Devel* **3**: 923-930

Klein, J and OhUigin, C (1994) The conundrum of nonclassical major histocompatibility complex genes. *Proc Natl Acad Sci USA* **91**: 6251-6252

Klein, J, Satta, Y, OhUigin, C and Takahata, N (1993) The molecular descent of the major histocompatibility complex. *Ann Rev Immunol* **11**: 269-295

Kropshofer, H, Vogt, AB, Thery, C, Armandola, EA, Li, BC, *et al.* (1998) A role for HLA-DO as a co-chaperone of HLA-DM in peptide loading of MHC class II molecules. *EMBO J* **17**: 2971-2981

Kuckelkorn, U, Frentzel, S, Kraft, R, Kostka, S, Groettrup, M, *et al.* (1995) Incorporation of major histocompatibility complex-encoded subunits LMP2 and LMP7 changes the quality of the 20S proteasome polypeptide processing products independent of interferon-gamma. *Eur J Immunol* **25**: 2605-2611

Kurlander, RJ, Shawar, SM, Brown, ML and Rich, RR (1992) Specialized role for a murine class I-b MHC molecule in prokaryotic host defences. *Science* **257**: 678-679

Liljedahl, M, Winqvist, O, Surh, CD, Wong, P, Ngo, K, *et al.* (1998) Altered antigen presentation in mice lacking H2-O. *Immunity* **8**: 233-243

Madden, DR (1995) The three dimensional structure of peptide-MHC complexes. *Ann Rev Immunol* **13**: 587-622

Madden, DR, Garboczi, DN and Wiley, DC (1993) The antigenic identity of peptide-MHC complexes: a comparison of the conformations of five viral peptides presented by HLA-A2. *Cell* **75**: 693-708

Madden, DR, Gorga, JC, Strominger, JL and Wiley, DC (1991) The structure of HLA-B27 reveals nonamer self-peptides bound in an extended conformation. *Nature* **353**: 321-325

Madden, DR, Gorga, JC, Strominger, JL and Wiley, DC (1992) The three-dimensional structure of HLA-B27 at 2.1 A resolution suggests a general mechanism for tight peptide binding to MHC. *Cell* **70**: 1035-1048

Margulies, DH, Plaksin, D *et al.* (1996) Studying interactions involving the T-cell antigen receptor by surface plasmon resonance. *Curr Opin Immunol* **8**: 262-270

Matsui, K, Boniface, JJ, *et al.* (1994) Kinetics of T-cell receptor binding to peptide/I-E(k) complexes: Correlation of the dissociation rate with T-cell responsiveness. *Proc Natl Acad Sci USA* **91**: 12862-12866

Matsumura, M, Fremont, DH, Peterson, PA and Wilson, IA (1992) Emerging principles for the recognition of peptide antigens by MHC class I molecules. *Science* **257**: 927-934

McConnell, HM, Watts, TH, Weis, RM and Brain, AA (1986) Supported planar membranes in studies of cell-cell recognition in the immune system. *Biochim Biophys Acta Reviews on Biomembranes* **864**: 95-106

Mellins, E, Cameron, P, Amaya, M, Goodman, S, Pious, D, *et al.* (1994) A mutant human histocompatibility leukocyte antigen DR molecule associated with invariant chain peptides. *J Exp Med* **179**: 541-549

Mellins, E, Kempin, S, Smith, L, Monji, T and Pious, D (1991) A gene required for class II-restricted antigen presentation maps to the major histocompatibility complex. *J Exp Med* **174**: 1607-1615

Monaco, JJ and McDevitt, HO (1986) The LMP antigens: a stable MHC-controlled multisubunit protein complex. *Hum Immunol* **15**: 416-426

Morris, P, Shaman, J, Attaya, M, Amaya, M, Goodman, S *et al.* (1994) An essential role for HLA-DM in antigen presentation by class II major histocompatibility molecules. *Nature* **368**: 551-554

Newell, WR, Trowsdale, J and Beck, S (1994) MHCDB - Database of the human MHC. *Immunogenetics* **40**: 109-115

Obata, Y, Satta, Y, Moriwaki, K, Shiroishi, T, Hasegawa, H, *et al.* (1994) Structure, function, and evolution of mouse TL genes, nonclassical class I genes of the major histocompatibility complex. *Proc Natl Acad Sci USA* **91**: 6589-6593

Ortmann, B, Copeman, J *et al.* (1997) A critical role for tapasin in the assembly and function of multimeric MHC class I-TAP complexes. *Science* **277**: 1306-1309

Ploegh, HL, Orr, HT and Strominger, JL (1981) Major histocompatibility antigens: The human (HLA-A, -B, -C) and murine (H-2K, H-2D) class I molecules. *Cell* **24**: 287-299

Saper, MA, Bjorkman, PJ and Wiley, DC (1991) Refined structure of the human histocompatibility antigen HLA-A2 at 2.6 A resolution. *J Mol Biol* **219**: 277-319

Shackelford, DA, Kaufman, JF, Korman, AJ and Strominger, JL (1982) HLA-DR antigens: Structure, separation of subpopulation, gene cloning and function." *Immunol Rev* **66**: 133-187

Sloan, VS, Cameron, P, Porter, G, Gammon, M, Amaya, M, *et al.* (1995) Mediation by HLA-DM of dissociation of peptides from HLA-DR. *Nature* **375**: 802-806

Smith, KJ, Pyrdol, J, Gauthier, L, Wiley, DC and Wucherpfennig, KW (1998) Crystal structure of HLA-DR2 (DRA*0101, DRB1*1501) complexed with a peptide from human myelin basic protein. *J Exp Med* **188**: 1511-1520

Stern, LJ, Brown, JH, Jardetzky, TS, Gorga, JC, Urban, RG, *et al.* (1994) Crystal structure of the human class II MHC protein HLA-DR1 complexed with an influenza virus peptide. *Nature* **368**: 215-221

Strominger, JL (1986) Biology of the human histocompatibility leukocyte antigen (HLA) system and a hypothesis regarding the generation of autoimmune diseases. *J Clin Invest* **77**: 1411-1415

Strominger, JL and Wiley, DC (1995) The class I and class II proteins of the human major histocompatibility complex. *J Amer Med Assoc* **274**: 1074-1076

Stroynowski, I and Lindahl, KF (1994) Antigen presentation by non-classical class 1 molecules. *Curr Opin Immunol* **6**: 38-44

Townsend, A, Bastin, J, Gould, K, Brownlee, G, Andrew, M, *et al.* (1988) Defective presentation to class I-restricted cytotoxic T lymphocytes in vaccinia-infected cells is overcome by enhanced degradation of antigen. *J Exp Med* **168**: 1211-1224

Trowsdale, J (1993) Genomic structure and function in the MHC. *Trends Genet* **9**: 117-122

Trowsdale, J (1995) 'Both man and bird and beast': comparative organization of MHC genes. *Immunogenetics* **41**: 1-17

van Ham, SM, Tjin, EPM, Lillemeier, BF, Gruneberg, U, van Meijgaarden, KE, *et al.* (1997) HLA-DO is a negative modulator of HLA-DM-mediated MHC class II peptide loading. *Curr Biol* **7**: 950-957

Wang, CR, Castano, AR, Peterson, PA, Slaughter, C, Lindahl, KF, *et al.* (1995) Nonclassical binding of formylated peptide in crystal structure of the MHC class Ib molecule H2-M3. *Cell* **82**: 655-664

Watkins, DI (1995) The evolution of major histocompatibility class I genes in primates. *Crit Rev Immunol* **15**: 1-29

Watts, TH, Brian, AA, J. W. Kappler, JW, *et al.* (1984) Antigen presentation by supported planar membranes containing affinity-purified I-A(d). *Proc Natl Acad Sci USA* **81**: 7564-7568

Young, A, Zhang, W, Sacchettini, JC and Nathenson, SG (1994) MHC class I-peptide interactions and TCR recognition. *Cancer Surv* **22**: 17-36

Young, A, Zhang, W, Sacchettini, JC and Nathenson, SG (1994) The three-dimensional structure of H-2Db at 2.4 A resolution: Implications for antigen-determinant selection. *Cell* **76**: 39-50

Zhang, W, Young, A, Imarai, M, Nathenson, SG and Sacchettini, JC (1992) Crystal structure of the major histocompatibility complex class I H- 2Kb molecule containing a single viral peptide: implications for peptide binding and T-cell receptor recognition. *Proc Natl Acad Sci USA* **89**: 8403-8407

Zinkernagel, RM and Doherty, PC (1974) Immunological surveillance against altered self components by sensitised T lymphocytes in lymphatic choriomeningitis. *Nature* **251**: 547-548

Zinkernagel, RM and Doherty, PC (1997). The discovery of MHC Restriction. *Immunol Today* **18**: 14-17

PART 1

ANTIBODY-BASED HISTOCOMPATIBILITY TESTING

PART 1 OVERVIEWS

1. HLA NOMENCLATURE

J. Bodmer
ICRF Cancer and Immunogenetics Laboratory
Institute of Molecular Medicine
Oxford OX3 9DS, England

These days we accept HLA nomenclature as 'given', something that happens automatically. We do not try to find a local name but we send our new sequence to the Nomenclature Committee to get an official name, by which our sequence is thenceforth always known. It was not always so.

The beginning of nomenclature: serology

Even as early as the first International Workshop run by Bernard Amos in 1964, it was recognised that some standardisation of names was needed. After the third Workshop, in 1968 agreement was reached to name the system the HL-A system, a compromise between Dausset's Hu (Human) system and Bodmer's LA (Leucocyte locus A) system (WHO Nomenclature Committee 1968). Thus the letters HL-A, later changed to HLA, are not the initials of any official name, much to the puzzlement of new people entering the field. At this meeting the first eight specificities were named, leaving space for van Rood's 4a and 4b (Van Rood *et al.*, 1967). 4a and 4b had a sticky history at this time since many people thought that they were just 'broad' specificities of little use now that 'narrow' specificities had been identified. In fact, as was shown much later by sequencing, these two are epitopes in B locus and some A locus sequences and thus are the only epitopes to have a separate name.

In the second report in 1970 only four new specificities, HL-A10, 11, 12 and 13 were named (WHO Nomenclature Committee 1970). To see the size of the problem, already with only 13 serological specificities named, each one had up 10 different local names. For example, HL-A12, now HLA-B12, was known in different laboratories as 9, T12, To11, Da4, 4a, Bt-6, LC-26, styl, GE and Ao15. In the 1972 report (WHO Nomenclature Committee 1972), 10 more specificities were named and a table of equivalent nomenclature was compiled which listed the 225 local names by which the 35 officially named specificities were known in 16 laboratories (Bodmer *et al.*, 1973). The 'w' for 'Workshop' as in Bw10 was introduced to indicate a specificity which still needed a degree of confirmation.

In the 4th report in 1975 the HL-A name was modified to HLA with the letter of the locus following, as HLA-A, HLA-B and the newly named C locus HLA-C (WHO Nomenclature Committee 1975). The C locus specificities still carry the 'w' to distinguish them from the complement determinants which were being identified. In this report too the Dw or cell determined specificities Dw1 to Dw6 were named, giving us the first glimpse of what later became the D-related or HLA Class II specificities.

In the 7th Workshop in 1977 the first DR or D-related serological specificities were named DRw1 to DRw7, following the use for the first time in a Workshop of sera against Class II products (WHO Nomenclature Committee 1978). In the 1984 report two other loci DQ and DP were also named. The two chain structure of the D alleles was also identified (WHO Nomenclature Committee 1985).

The molecular revolution

By 1987 several new genes in the Class II region had been identified and the fruits of molecular typing for alleles of a gene rather than serological specificities were named (Bodmer *et al.,* 1989). Naming was kept as close as possible to the serological specificity, hence HLA-A*0201, *0202 etc. for HLA-A2 alleles. This policy of trying to match allele names to serological specificities has continued although as more new alleles and mutations which are almost equally similar to two different specificities arise, the matching with serological specificities is no longer always possible. A fifth digit, as in B*27011, was added in cases where a sequence had been shown to have a silent substitution which did not change the protein sequence.

By 1989 it was realised that with the rapid increase in new alleles it was not possible to wait until after a Workshop to name them so an interim report was produced naming the many new alleles (Bodmer *et al.,* 1990) In 1992, after the 11th Workshop, new genes and pseudo genes in both the Class I and Class II regions had been identified and the complicated genomic organisation of Class II genes, varying with different DRB1 alleles was worked out. By this time most of the report was dealing with issues at the DNA level (Bodmer *et al.,* 1992) . In 1995 two further digits were added to the allele name allowing for alleles to be named whose variation lies outside the expressed region of the sequence, such as polymorphism within the introns, 5' or 3' flanking sequences (Bodmer *et al.,* 1995). In addition an optional character 'N' was introduced indicating that the allele is not expressed. An 'L' introduced in the 1996 report indicates that the allele has low expression (Bodmer *et al.,* 1997).

The count of alleles named in the 1996 report had reached 752 with new variants coming in every day. Will there ever be an end to it or will there be a continuing stream of new mutations for rare alleles for ever? Since 1990 it has not been possible or advisable to wait for a nomenclature meeting to name new alleles, so they are now reported daily to the HLA sequence database at the Anthony Nolan Research Institute where they receive official names and listed in the monthly updates in *Tissue Antigens.*

Nomenclature in the future

As can be seen in Table 1, the number of loci identified in the HLA region is great and growing. The fact that there are many more loci in the region poses a dilemma

Name	Previous equivalents	Molecular characteristics
HLA-A	-	Class I α-chain
HLA-B	-	Class I α-chain
HLA-C	-	Class I α-chain
HLA-E	E, '6.2'	associated with class I 6.2-kB Hind III fragment
HLA-F	F, '5.4'	associated with class I 5.4-kB Hind III fragment
HLA-G	G, '6.0'	associated with class I 6.0-kB Hind III fragment
HLA-H	H, AR, '12.4'	Class I pseudogene associated with 5.4-kB Hind III fragment
HLA-J	cda12	Class I pseudogene associated with 5.9-kB Hind III fragment
HLA-K	HLA-70	Class I pseudogene associated with 7.0-kB Hind III fragment
HLA-L	HLA-92	Class I pseudogene associated with 9.2-kB Hind III fragment
HLA-DRA	DRα	DR α-chain
HLA-DRB1	DRβI, DR1B	DR β1-chain determining specificities DR1 to DR18
HLA-DRB2	DRβII	pseudogene with DR β-like sequences
HLA-DRB3	DRβIII, DR3B	DR β3-chain determining DR52 and Dw24, Dw25, Dw26 specificities
HLA-DRB4	DRβIV, DR4B	DR β4-chain determining DR53
HLA-DRB5	DRβIII	DR β5-chain determining DR51
HLA-DRB6	DRBX, DRBσ	DRB pseudogene found on DR1, DR2 and DR10 haplotypes
HLA-DRB7	DRBψ1	DRB pseudogene found on DR4, DR7 and DR9 haplotypes
HLA-DRB8	DRBψ2	DRB pseudogene found on DR4, DR7 and DR9 haplotypes
HLA-DRB9	M4.2 β exon	DRB pseudogene, isolated fragment
HLA-DQA1	DQα1, DQ1A	DQ α-chain as expressed
HLA-DQB1	DQβ1, DQ1B	DQ β-chain as expressed
HLA-DQA2	DXα, DQ2A	DQ α-chain-related sequence, not known to be expressed
HLA-DQB2	DXβ, DQ2B	DQ β-chain-related sequence, not known to be expressed
HLA-DQB3	DVβ, DQB3	DQ β-chain-related sequence, not known to be expressed
HLA-DOA †	DZα, DOα, DNA	DO α-chain
HLA-DOB	DOβ	DO β-chain
HLA-DMA	RING6	DM α-chain
HLA-DMB	RING7	DM β-chain
HLA-DPA1	DPα1, DP1A	DP α-chain as expressed
HLA-DPB1	DPβ1, DP1B	DP β-chain as expressed
HLA-DPA2	DPα2, DP2A	DP α-chain-related pseudogene
HLA-DPB2	DPβ2, DP2B	DP β-chain-related pseudogene
TAP1	RING4, Y3, PSF1	ABC (ATP Binding Cassette) transporter
TAP2	RING11, Y1, PSF2	ABC (ATP Binding Cassette) transporter
LMP2	RING12	Proteasome-related sequence
LMP7	RING10	Proteasome-related sequence

† The DOA gene has been recently renamed from its original designation of DNA, this is the only locus which has been renamed.

Table 1. Names for genes in the HLA region

for the HLA Nomenclature Committee. Since the remit of the Committee is only to name HLA and HLA-related genes, how far should we go with naming other genes in the region whose homology with HLA may be low and whose function may not yet be clear? LMP, TAP and MIC genes have already been named but what about CD1 and many other genes which have been identified within the region?

One thing is certain and that is that the willingness of the HLA community to agree on a common nomenclature and to use it has has made it a model for other areas of research to follow. Our research and clinical service has been greatly enhanced by the fact that across the world we know what each other is talking about in HLA terms and we feel hopeful that we will be able to continue to collaborate in the future.

References

Bodmer, J, Rocques, P, Bodmer, W, Colombani, J, Degos, L. *et al.* (1973) Joint report of the fifth international histocompatibility workshop. In: *Histocompatibility Testing 1972* (Ed. Dausset, J. and Colombani, J), pp.620-719. Munksgaard: Copenhagen

Bodmer, WF, Albert, E, Bodmer, JG, Dupont, B, Mach, B. *et al.* (1989) Nomenclature for factors of the HLA system, 1987. In: *Immunobiology of HLA* (Ed. Dupont, B), pp.72-79. Springer-Verlag: New York

Bodmer, JG, Marsh, SGE, Parham, P, Erlich, HA, Albert, E, *et al.* (1990) Nomenclature for factors of the HLA system, 1989. *Tissue Antigens* **35**:1-8

Bodmer, JG, Marsh, SGE, Albert, E, Bodmer, WF, Dupont, B. *et al.* (1992) Nomenclature for factors of the HLA system, 1991. In: *HLA 1991* (Ed. Tsuji, T, Aizawa, M and Sasazuki, T), pp.17-31. Oxford University Press: Oxford

Bodmer, JG, Marsh, SGE, Albert, E, Bodmer, WF, Bontrop, RE. *et al.* (1995) Nomenclature for factors of the HLA system, 1995. *Tissue Antigens* **46**: 1-18

Bodmer, JG, Marsh, SGE, Albert, E, Bodmer, WF. *et al* (1997) Nomenclature for factors of the HLA system, 1996. *Tissue Antigens* **49**: 297-321

Van Rood, JJ, van Leeuwen, A, Schippers, AMJ, Pearce, R, van Blankenstein, *et al.* (1967) Immunogenetics of the Group Four* and Nine Systems. In: *Histocompatibility Testing 1967* (Ed. Curtoni, E, Mattiuz, RM, Tosi, RM), pp.203-219. Munksgaard: Copenhagen

WHO Nomenclature Committee (1968). *Bull. WHO* **39**: 483-486

WHO Nomenclature Committee (1970). WHO terminology report. In: *Histocompatibility Testing, 1970* (Ed. Terasaki, PI), pp.49. Munksgaard: Copenhagen.

WHO Nomenclature Committee (1972). *Bull WHO* **47**: 659

WHO Nomenclature Committee (1975). *Bull WHO* **52**: 261

WHO Nomenclature Committee (1978). *Bull WHO* **56**: 461

WHO Nomenclature Committee (1985). Nomenclature for factors of the HLA system 1984. In: *Histocompatibility Testing, 1984* (Ed. Albert, ED, Baur, MP and Mayr, WR), pp.4-8. Springer-Verlag: Berlin.

2. HLA SEROLOGY

J. Bodmer
ICRF Cancer and Immunogenetics Laboratory
Institute of Molecular Medicine
Oxford OX3 9DS, England

Serology was the mainstay of HLA typing for over 30 years, from the early studies of Dausset (Dausset, 1958), Rose Payne (Payne, 1957) and van Rood (Van Rood, 1958), until at least the 11th International Workshop in 1991 when molecular typing was first used in a Workshop (Sasazuki, 1992).

Dausset first observed leucoagglutinins in the serum of transfused patients and Rose Payne and van Rood observed them in the serum of women who were pregnant or had recently borne children.

The methods

The tests in the beginning were, perhaps naturally, based on leucoagglutination of mixed white cells. The amounts of serum used were by today's standards enormous - three drops of serum which was about 90 μl if you were lucky and more if the pipette was broken and therefore dispensing larger amounts.

Many other methods were used and compared, including complement fixation of platelets and cytotoxicity assays. All the methods used different conditions and often were targetting different cells, mixed lymphocytes, platelets or lymphocytes. Much time and effort in the 1960's was devoted to comparing methods and results, since it was not clear whether a given serum would react in the same way giving the same result using different target cells and different methods. We were then at the stage we are at present with molecular typing, everybody used a slightly different method to achieve hopefully the same result but, worse than today, everybody gave different names to the antigens they found. As discussed in the Overview on HLA nomenclature above, this potentially crippling problem was solved by the series of International Histocompatibility Workshops and the Nomenclature reports which followed them.

However an excellent typing method was developed by Terasaki (Terasaki and McLelland, 1964), the microcytotoxicity assay. This method, using only 1 μl of serum, compared with the earlier very much larger amounts, was a blessing as it enabled a given serum to test many more people then previously. When fluorescent labelling was added to Terasaki's method by Bodmer in 1967 (Bodmer *et al.*, 1967) the method became the gold standard for a generation.

This meant that laboratories could concentrate on the results of typing, the genetics and the effects in transplantation, disease and different populations and be fairly sure that everybody using the same reagents would have comparable results.

The sources of antibodies

Antisera

As the early workers in the field had found, multiply transfused patients and pregnant women were good sources of HLA antibody. A problem was that any given serum might contain not only one but several antibodies to different HLA specificities. It might seem that pregnancy sera might tend more to be monospecific than transfusion sera as the variety of stimulation would be less. In fact although many of the very best sera were pregnancy sera, for example Gillespie, Rose Payne's famous HLA-A1 serum which was used through many Workshops, there were monospecific antisera produced in multiply transfused patents as well. A serum which Rose Payne identified was from a child of 13 who had an anaemia and had had many units of blood over many years but still produced a monospecific HLA-A2 serum.

However, many of the sera which were available were multispecific and so great care was needed in analysing them. The first analysis which identified different specificities was by van Rood who looked not at the individual serum reactions but the reactions of a set of sera which were shown to share a common antibody, using Chi-squared values to separate the sera into clusters each defining a different specificity. This method was followed to identify alleles of the LA, later HLA-A locus, and further to identify clusters of sera giving reactions at the same locus, negative association with another cluster, or a different locus (Payne *et al.,* 1964). It was based on the only computer program that Julia Bodmer ever wrote and in the first 20 sera of Rose Payne gave clusters for LA1, LA2 and 4A, now HLA-A1, HLA-A2 and Bw4.

Another method of achieving monospecificity was by absorbing out from sera the unwanted antibodies leaving the one of choice. This method was recommended in the early days to prove monospecificity but in fact was extremely difficult to do accurately since sometimes you left behind some secondary antibody and sometimes you lost all the antibodies.

It was clear that a more certain and specific source of antibodies was needed. Attempts were made by immunising HLA typed volunteers with a particular antigen (Payne *et al.,* 1970) but results again were variable and the ethics of deliberate immunisation with incompletely characterised material was perhaps doubtful, particularly by today's standards. Another method was to immunise a woman who had a particular pregnancy antibody with the corresponding antigen to boost the antibody. This worked quite well but was rather limited in scope.

Monoclonal antibodies

Many of us believed that the goose which was going to lay the golden eggs had arrived with the development of the technology to produce monoclonal antibodies (Kohler and Milstein, 1975). Many people started to try to make antibodies and to begin with there was great success (Brodsky *et al.*, 1979). However it soon became clear that it was extremely difficult to design experiments which would produce narrow polymorphic antibodies, although some did appear, particularly when made by immunising women *post partum* (Kosinski *et al.*, 1987). It seemed particularly difficult to make monoclonal antibodies against HLA Class I determinants. By contrast, whereas anti-Class II antisera were nearly always polyspecific containing antibodies to both DR and DQ determinants, and often to Class I as well, most of which had to absorbed out to produce a 'monospecific' antibody, many very good monoclonal antibodies were made against HLA-Class II determinants (De Kretser *et al.*, 1982; Bodmer *et al.*, 1985). The 8th Workshop in 1980 was the first to include monoclonal antibodies, produced by Ceppellini and Trucco and increasing numbers have been used since then. It is ironic, that after all the efforts by many laboratories to produce monospecific antibodies to polymorphic HLA determinants, that they only became widely available, mostly from commercial companies, at careful dilutions of multispecific monoclonals, after the advent of molecular typing.

The place of serology today and in the future

Now and in the foreseeable future there will always be a place for HLA antibodies. The great difference between serological and molecular typing is that molecular typing can only identify the genes which code for the different specificities, whereas serological typing shows what is actually expressed on the cell surface. There are enough cases in which an HLA allele is not expressed to make serology an important tool in transplantation typing. A more general application is in histopathology in which HLA antibodies, particularly monoclonal antibodies, are used to identify HLA expression, or lack of it on tumour cells (Bodmer, 1993). It appears that loss of HLA surface expression is one of the ways in which tumour cells can escape the immune response and thereby proliferate.

Finally, an interesting note: despite the fact that pregnancy and transfusion HLA antisera were often polyspecific, serological reaction patterns were able to establish the genetics of the HLA system, which specificities were coded at which locus, which were in linkage disequilibrium, and the pattern of inheritance of HLA alleles in families, without error.

References

Bodmer, WF, Tripp, M and Bodmer, J. (1967) Application of a fluorochromatic cytotoxicity assay to human leukocyte typing. In: *Histocompatibility Testing 1967* (Ed. Curtoni, ES, Mattiuz, PL and Tosi, RM), pp.341-350. Munksgaard: Copenhagen.

Bodmer, WF, Browning, MJ, Krausa, P, Rowan, A, Bicknell, DC *et al.*(1993) Tumor escape from immune response by variation in HLA expression and other mechanisms. *Ann New York Acad Sci* **690**: 42-49

Bodmer, J, Heyes, J and Lindsay, J. (1985) Study of monoclonal antibodies to the HLA-D region products DQw1 and DRw52. In: *Histocompatibility Testing 1984* (Ed. Albert, ED, Baur, MP, and Mayr, WR), pp.432-438. Springer-Verlag, Berlin

Brodsky, F, Parham, P, Barnstable, C, Crumpton, M and Bodmer, W. (1979). Monoclonal antibodies for analysis of the HLA system. *Immunol Rev* **47:** 3-61

Dausset, J. (1958) Iso-leuco-anticorps. *Acta Haematol* **20:** 156-166

de Kretser, TA, Crumpton, MJ, Bodmer, JG and Bodmer, WF. (1982) Two-dimensional gel analysis of the polypeptides precipitated by a polymorphic HLA-DR1, 2, w6 monoclonal antibody: evidence for a third locus. *Eur J Immunol* **12:** 600-606

Kohler, G and Milstein, C. (1975) Continuous culture of fused cells secreting antibody of predefined specificity. *Nature* **256**: 495-497

Kosinski, S, Ferrara, G, Yang, S and Hammerling, U. (1987) A human monoclonal-antibody against HLA-A25. *Tissue Antigens* **29**: 177-183

Payne, R. (1957) Leukocyte agglutinins in human sera. *Arch Intern Med* **99**: 587

Payne, R, Tripp, M, Weigle, J, Bodmer, WF and Bodmer, J. (1964) A new leukocyte isoantigen system in man. *Cold Spring Harbor Symp Quant Biol* **29**: 285-295

Payne, R, Bodmer, J, Bodmer, W and Shanbrom, E. (1970) Characterisation of HL-A antisera produced by planned immunization. In: *Histocompatibility Testing 1970* (Ed. Terasaki, PI), pp.207-220. Munksgaard: Copenhagen.

Sasazuki, T. (1992). Introduction to the DNA Component.In: *HLA 1991* (Ed. Tsuji, K), pp.395-518. Oxford University Press: Oxford

Terasaki, P and McLelland, J. (1964) Microdroplet assay of human serum cytotoxins. *Nature* **204**: 998

Van Rood, JJ, van Leeuwen, E and van Leeuwen, A (1958) Leukocyte antibodies in sera of pregnant women. *Nature* **181**: 1735

CHAPTER 1

HLA TYPING BY ALLOANTIBODIES AND MONOCLONAL ANTIBODIES

G. M.Th. Schreuder
Dept of Immunohematology and Blood Bank
Building 1, E3-Q
Leiden University Medical Centre
PO Box 9600
2300RC Leiden, The Netherlands

Introduction

HLA antigens or HLA specificities (Table 1.1) have been defined by serological typing using the complement dependent lympho-micro-cytotoxicity test. For HLA typing, viable lymphocytes are used as targets and are tested with sets of selected alloantisera and monoclonal antibodies (mAb). Rabbit serum is used as source of complement. Lysed cells are stained, and the results are generally read with an inverted microscope. One of the major drawbacks in serological typing is the need for viable lymphocytes. Thus, there is a need for careful selection of anti-coagulants, isolation, freezing and thawing procedures, and also special requirements for long distance shipping of specimens.

The HLA system encodes class I and class II molecules. The class I molecules carrying the HLA-A, -B, and -C specificities, are expressed on virtually all nucleated cells including all peripheral blood lymphocytes (PBL). The class II specificities, HLA-DR, DQ and DP, are only expressed on cells specialised in antigen presentation, such as B cells, monocytes and activated T cells. Because B cells only constitute some 15 % of PBL, several techniques have been devised to enrich the class II-bearing cells in test suspensions.

The intricacy of the HLA system is due to the fact that each HLA molecule consists of several antigenic determinants or *epitopes* (a group of several amino acids) which are often shared among different HLA molecules. An immune response against foreign HLA, either due to pregnancy, transfusion or transplantation, can result in antibodies against any of the epitopes on the different HLA molecules, as long as these epitopes are foreign to the host.

This complicates the selection of alloantibodies as typing reagents and also the interpretation of the results. For example: the A2 specificity is identified by antibodies that recognise anti-A2+A69, anti-A2+B17 and anti-A2+A28 (Parham *et al.,* 1987). This means that although HLA-A2 is very well identified serologically, antibodies that recognise only A2 do not exist.

A	B	B	C	DR	DQ
A1	B5	B49(21)	Cw1	DR1	DQ1
A2	B7	B50(21)	Cw2	DR103	DQ2
A203	B703	B51(5)	Cw3	DR2	DQ3
A210	B8	B5102	Cw4	DR3	DQ4
A3	B12	B5103	Cw5	DR4	DQ5(1)
A9	B13	B52(5)	Cw6	DR5	DQ6(1)
A10	B14	B53	Cw7	DR6	DQ7(3)
A11	B15	B54(22)	Cw8	DR7	DQ8(3)
A19	B16	B55(22)	Cw9(w3)	DR8	DQ9(3)
A23(9)	B17	B56(22)	Cw10(w3)	DR9	
A24(9)	B18	B57(17)		DR10	
A2403	B21	B58(17)		DR11(5)	
A25(10)	B22	B59		DR12(5)	
A26(10)	B27	B60(40)		DR13(6)	
A28	B2708	B61(40)		DR14(6)	
A29(19)	B35	B62(15)		DR1403	
A30(19)	B37	B63(15)		DR1404	
A31(19)	B38(16)	B64(14)		DR15(2)	
A32(19)	B39(16)	B65(14)		DR16(2)	
A33(19)	B3901	B67		DR17(3)	
A34(10)	B3902	B70		DR18(3)	
A36	B40	B71(70)			
A43	B4005	B72(70)		DR51	
A66(10)	B41	B73			
A68(28)	B42	B75(15)		DR52	
A69(28)	B44(12)	B76(15)			
A74(19)	B45(12)	B77(15)		DR53	
A80	B46	B78			
	B47	B81			
	B48				
		Bw4			
		Bw6			

Table 1.1. Complete listing of recognised serological HLA specificities. Splits are given with their respective broad antigens in parentheses.

There are frequent and rare HLA antigens, their distribution often being race dependent. The above variables should be considered when reagents are selected for inclusion in typing trays.

The scarcity of alloantisera as typing reagents prompted several investigators to embark on the production of monoclonal antibodies (mAb) against HLA. Initially only mouse mAb became available, mostly directed against public epitopes (shared by many different HLA specificities). Eventually also human mAb were produced (Mulder *et al.,* 1993). At present a variety of mAb against many of the

HLA specificities have been identified and sets of monoclonal typing reagents are commercially available (Tongio *et al.,* 1997, Navarrete *et al,* 1997).

DNA based typing techniques are employed in addition to, or even as replacement of serology. For class II typing this has resulted in an increase of typing quality and reproducibility. Class I typing is still mostly performed by serology, although an increasing number of laboratories is using molecular techniques in addition. An intelligent combination of both techniques will enable a laboratory to identify the relative advantages and disadvantages of each of these techniques, resulting in increased quality of typing.

Clinical relevance

HLA typing serves many different purposes. Serological typing identifies polymorphism at the cell surface level. For a number of questions this method will be more relevant than molecular typing. For each purpose the optimal typing method should be selected carefully.

Organ transplantation

HLA matching is beneficial in organ transplantation as it prolongs both graft and patient survival. HLA-A,-B and -DR "broad" specificities are generally accepted for typing and matching. This level can be reached by serological typing methods or by low resolution molecular typing. In practice HLA matching is only used for kidney and high risk cornea transplantation. Heart transplantation recipients would also benefit from matching but the time necessary for HLA typing and subsequent organ allocation exceeds the acceptable cold ischaemia time of the organ.

Bone marrow transplantation

HLA matching is essential in bone marrow transplantation. Serology can be applied effectively to type the patients' family. When no HLA identical family donor is available bone marrow donor registries may be searched. These registries are based on HLA phenotypes of volunteer bone marrow donors. Their typings were mostly obtained by serological methods, especially where class I is concerned. Once HLA 'identical' donors are selected for a certain patient high resolution typing methods should be applied to select the best matched donor. It is therefore essential that patient and donor are typed in the same laboratory by the same techniques.

HLA-AB typing for platelet transfusion

Patients refractory to platelet transfusion will need platelets expressing HLA antigens, to which no alloantibodies are present. Often it is possible to define the specificity or even the epitopes to which the patients' antibodies are directed (see Chapter 2). If there is not sufficient time for extensive screening, one needs to select platelet donors that are HLA compatible to the patient, or provide crossmatch-negative platelets.

HLA-B27 typing

Due to the high prevalence of B27 among patients with ankylosing spondylitis (AS), over 90% in most populations, B27 typing is used to confirm clinical diagnosis. A number of different alleles appears to encode the serologically defined B27 specificity, the predominant being B*2705. For clinical purposes the identification of B27 by serological methods suffice. Problems with B27 typing by serology can occur due to cross reactivity with B7, B22 and B47. The use of monoclonal antibodies may help, but often such B27 specific moabs fail to react with some B*27 alleles (Lopez-Larrea *et al.,* 1997). Recently the B7Qui (now B2708) was identified as a low frequency specificity occurring also in Caucasoid populations. (Hildebrand *et al.,* 1994). Since this B27 variant carries the Bw6 epitope, and is more reactive with B7 than with B27 sera, it will be regularly mistyped as B7 by serology. Its relation to AS is not yet known.

HLA typing for disease association studies

HLA is involved in a number of autoimmune and other diseases. The majority of HLA typings requested for HLA and disease studies concern research projects and should be performed at the allelic level at least for class II. However in several instances serology can be sufficiently informative. Clinicians may ask for HLA typing to confirm clinical diagnose. Dialogue between clinicians, researchers and tissue typers is essential. Typing resolution, clinical purpose and cost aspects should be taken into account to select the optimal typing technique for each question.

In narcoleptic patients a high prevalence of DR2 has been defined. However DNA typing revealed stronger associations with the DQB1*0602 allele, which is in linkage disequilibrium wit DRB1*15 in most populations. Serological DR2 typing is feasible but should be extended to the DR15 and DR16 splits.

In rheumatoid arthritis (RA) the major positive association is with DR4, but an epitope shared between most DR4, DR1 and DR10, and some DR14 alleles has been described as a susceptibility determinant in RA (HV3 aa 67-71). This epitope is also detectable by serology. In RA it is thought that HLA influences severity of the disease. Clinicians may want to know if their patients are DR4 positive and, if homozygous, for which alleles.

In diabetes and coeliac disease sometimes HLA typing is requested. Here the DR3, DR4, DQ2 and DQ8 are the antigens of interest. Since only few laboratories will be able to perform reliable serological DQ subtyping, molecular techniques should be applied for these questions.

HLA and cancer research

In some cancers one or more HLA alleles may not be expressed at the cell surface. With the use of immunohistological techniques HLA specific mAb can be successfully applied for identification of single antigens that are expressed in tissue sections (Garrido *et al.,* 1997).

Methods

The principle of cytotoxicity is that lymphocytes of the individual to be typed are incubated with a set of HLA specific typing sera. Rabbit serum as complement source is added. This allows lysis of cells that express HLA antigens to which specific antibodies have bound. With vital dyes such as eosin, trypan blue, or with fluorescent dyes the lysed and non-lysed cells can be discriminated by inverted phase contrast or fluorescent microscopy.

An excellent summary with detailed protocols for HLA class I and II typing by cytotoxicity is given by Darke and Dyer (1993). Here, some of the most important aspects will be mentioned.

Antisera

For typing purposes antisera have to be selected very carefully. Pregnancy sera are the predominant source for alloantisera. This requires extensive screening procedures, and is only performed in few laboratories. Class II sera generally have to be absorbed with platelets to remove additional class I antibodies. Monoclonal antibodies can be used successfully as typing reagents, especially for class II because platelet absorption is of course not needed.

Carry-over is a problem when using mAb typing trays. Unless cells are added with a no-touch technique (e.g. shooting, automatic dispenser) one or two negative control sera should be placed next to each mAb. Sets of allosera and/or mAb can be obtained commercially (One Lambda, C-six, Pel Freez). Several organisations may have sets or selected sera available to laboratories participating in transplant projects (Eurotransplant, UK Transplant, France Transplant, etc.). Sera and mAb can often also be obtained from the laboratory of origin.

Positive (eg. anti-Bw4 and Bw6) and negative control sera should be included in each typing tray.

Typing trays should contain antibodies to all antigens that occur regularly in the population. Preferably an antigen should be recognised by at least two antisera. If no monospecific sera are available one can chose several sera with different cross reactivity patterns: e.g. combination of several B40+ sera allows reliable B40 subtyping and may also discriminate B48 (Table 1.2). Specificities can only be defined by negative reactions towards some split sera such as B61 in Table 1.2. In B locus typing the use of Bw4 and Bw6 sera is recommended. All B locus antigens carry either the Bw4 or the Bw6 determinant (Table 1.3). Some B antigens are split

	Antigens						
Antisera	**B60**	**B61**	**B47**	**B48**	**B13**	**B7**	**B27**
B40+B13+B47	+	+	+	–	+	–	–
B40+B7+B48	+	+	–	+	–	+	–
B60+B7	+	–	–	–	–	+	–
B60+B48	+	–	–	+	–	–	–
B13	–	–	–	–	+	–	–
B27+B47	–	–	+	–	–	–	+

Table 1.2. Selection of sera for B40 subtyping

Bw4: B5, B13, B17, B27, B37, B38(16), B44(12), B47, B49(21), B5102, B5103, B51(5), B52(5), B53, B57(17), B58(17), B59, B63(15), B77(15)

Bw6: B7, B703, B8, B14, B18, B22, B2708, B35, B39(16), B3901, B3902, B40, B4005, B41, B42, B45(12), B46, B48, B50(21), B54(22), B55(22), B56(22), B60(40), B61(40), B62(15), B64(14), B65(14), B67, B70, B71(70), B72(70), B73, B75(15), B76(15), B78, B81

Table 1.3. Distribution of Bw4 and Bw6 on HLA-B antigens

by this determinant only. Bw4 sera tend to cross react with A9, A25 and A32, due to shared epitopes.

HLA-C typing for Cw1-Cw10 is possible, but with notoriously low reproducibility. Many C locus alleles do not have a serological equivalent, resulting in a relatively high proportion of blanks. Anti-C sera are scarce.

Alloantisera often are mixtures of antibodies directed against antigens that are in linkage disequilibrium. Examples are A25+B18, B14+Cw8, B15+Cw3, DQ1+DR2, DQ2+DR7, DQ3+DR4, DQ7+DR11, DR8+DQ4. Sets of sera are dispensed in 'Terasaki' test trays at 1µl or 0.5µl volumes under oil to prevent evaporation. Trays should be labelled clearly and are frozen until use.

Lymphocytes

In general viable lymphocytes are obtained from whole blood by Ficoll gradient centrifugation. As anti-coagulants sodium free-heparin, ACD, EDTA or defibrination are in use. If lymphocytes can not be isolated the same day, samples should be stored at room temperature. During sample shipment extreme heat and cold should be avoided. In case of cadaveric donor typing lymphocytes can also be obtained from spleen or lymph nodes. Isolated PBL can be frozen at –90°C or lower with DMSO and stored until further use. Frozen and thawed cells are more sensitive in cytotoxicity than freshly isolated PBL.

For class II typing B lymphocytes are needed. Since they constitute only some 15% of regular PBL, B cell enrichment is necessary. T cells can be depleted using sheep red blood cells, nylon wool columns, or magnetic beads loaded with T or B cell specific antibodies. Some class II cytotoxicity methods do not require B cell enrichment. Since B cells tend to stick more easily to glass and plastic tubing, special care should be taken to prevent B cell loss.

Cell suspensions with relatively many monocytes will make DQ typing more difficult, because monocytes do not express DQ.

Cells are resuspended in RPMI + 10% fetal calf serum (FCS). Cell suspension from PBL for regular class I typing normally contain $2x10^6$ cells/ml. For class II the number of cells largely depends on the technique in use. Viability of cells should be above 90% for reliable typing. Media and FCS should be clean without yeast or debris.

Complement

Rabbit serum is used as complement source in cytotoxicity. Two factors in the serum are important: complement and naturally occurring antibodies that react non-specifically with human lymphocytes. Both factors can vary widely among animals and can be influenced by e.g. feeding and season. For those reasons rabbit serum should be pooled from many animals.

Before use, titration of rabbit serum using well characterised test sera should be performed to compare the strength and reactivity of the different batches of complement. Suitability of a complement batch should be tested for each type of cytotoxicity method and target cell type (e.g. class I/II, PBL frozen/fresh, B cell line, spleen cells). Some complement batches do not react very well with certain mAb. Complement can be obtained freeze dried and frozen from several companies (Pel Freez, C-six, BioScope etc.). Complement should be thawed or reconstituted shortly prior to use; once thawed it should not be re-frozen for future use.

Incubation time and temperature

In cytotoxicity two incubation steps are generally necessary. For class I typing 1 μl cell suspension is incubated with 1 μl serum for 30 min at room temperature. After adding 5μl complement to each well the mixture is incubated for 60 min at room temperature. Now the reaction is stopped by staining and fixation. Class II tests use prolonged incubations: 60 min before and 120 min after addition of complement. However many different protocols are in use depending on cell type and staining method.

Shorter incubation will result in decreased reactivity. Room temperature as the incubation temperature is not very critical, however temperatures below 18°C and above 22°C should be avoided.

Typing equipment

In cytotoxicity 1 μl of cell suspension is added to each well of the typing tray. Several companies supply dispensers for cells and serum, either manually (*e.g.* Hamilton, Robbins) or automatic (*e.g.* Greiner, One Lambda, Robbins etc.). An advantage of automatic cell dispensers is prevention of carry-over, a major problem when using high titred sera and mAb. Automatic dispensers often only fit particular test trays. Typing trays should be centrifuged to spread the serum (and cells) over the bottom of the wells. Special mineral oil may be needed when serum and cells fail to mix easily in the wells.

Dyes and microscopes

In general dye exclusion methods are used to differentiate dead and live cells. Even without a vital dye live and dead cells can be discriminated using inverted phase contrast microscopy. This is done in some laboratories to check if prolonged incubation is indicated. Special skill is needed for this method.

Normally vital dyes are used. Fluorescent dyes render the assay more sensitive as compared to the eosin or trypan blue staining. Reactions are stopped by formaldehyde fixation or EDTA.

Automatic reading systems have been developed, which have the advantage of objective reading and reducing clerical errors. Moreover reading results can be interpreted and transferred automatically to other databases. The disadvantages are that cell suspensions have to be clean, with well adjusted cell counts and have to be dispensed very carefully and evenly through the trays. An additional centrifuge step of the trays may be necessary to spread the cells evenly over the bottom of the wells. Positive and negative control sera have to be chosen very carefully, because of differences in fluorescent background between alloserum and mAb-diluent mixtures. For example in our laboratory class II typing is performed using the propidium iodide/ethidium bromide double staining method, and results are read on a PATIMED Leitz microscope (Naipal *et al.,* 1984). We use unseparated PBL at a concentration of 12 x 10^6 cells/ml, a mouse anti-human B cell serum (Cedarlane) as positive control. Allosera and mAb are tested in separate trays. As negative control for the mAb tray we use the mAb diluent, but in the allo-tray we use a negative human serum.

Interpretation

HLA typing means assignment of HLA specificities to a complex of serum reactions. In class I typing lymphocytes should express at least one but not more than two of each of the HLA-A, -B and -C antigens as listed in Table 1.1. With a normal typing set nobody will have problems to type an HLA-A1, A2, B7, B8 individual.

Cross-reactivity

Problems occur when one has to decide between one or two antigens, that show cross reactivity. An HLA antigen or specificity is defined by (a combination of different) antigenic determinants. Cross-reactivity is caused by the fact that antigenic determinants or epitopes are shared between different specificities (Table 1.4), and that one antigen can cross react with different groups of antigens. For example anti-B5 sera may cross react with B53. To discriminate between B5 and B53 one needs also B5 sera that do not react with B53, and B35+B53 sera that do not react with B5. Interpretation becomes even more complicated if the cell sample carries a combination of these antigens.

HLA-A
A1 A36
A1 A3 A11
A1 A11 A24 A80
A2 A28
A10 A19
A25 A32
A28 A33 A34

HLA-Cw
Cw4 Cw6
Cw5 Cw8

HLA-DR
DR1 DR10
DR3 DR5 DR6 DR8
DR4 DR7 DR9

HLA-B
B5 B35 B53 B78
B5 B35 B53 B18 B15 B21 B70
B7 B27 B42 B67 B2708 B81
B22 B17 B42
B40 B13 B47 B48 B81
B60 B48 B81
B41 B21
B14 B8 B18 B39
Bw6 B13

Between loci
A2 B17
B46 Cw3
Bw4 A9 A25 A32
DR4 DQ3
DR11 DR8 DPw3

Table 1.4. A few examples of crossreactivity of HLA antigens

Splits and associated antigens

Many of the HLA 'broad' specificities have 'splits'. Originally splits were defined by sera that failed to identify a proportion of individuals with a certain antigen. In Table 1.1 split antigens are shown with their respective broad antigens. Splits from some broad antigens can both (or all) be identified specifically by antisera. For example the B51 and B52 splits of B5. Monospecific B51 sera do exist. Some B5+35+53 antisera are only reactive with B51 and negative towards B52, whereas some B21 sera cross react with B52.

The A68 and A69 splits of A28 are very difficult to identify serologically. First of all A69 is very rare in Caucasoid populations. A68 or A69 specific sera do not exist. A69 was originally described using the BB7.2 mAb which recognises A2+A69 (Parham 1987). Also many anti-A2 allosera appear to react with A69. It should be clear that A28 can not be split by serology in the presence of A2.

B61 cannot be typed in the presence of B60, because no B61 specific sera have been found. In general a split (like B61) can be safely defined when broad (B40) sera are positive and the other split (B60) sera are negative. Several of the antigens and splits of the B locus can be discriminated using Bw4 and Bw6 antisera. Examples are the splits of B12, B16 and B21 (Table 1.3).

More recently the WHO Nomenclature Committee also defined associated antigens (Bodmer *et al.,* 1997). These are antigens encoded by distinctive alleles which can be distinguished from all other allelic products by specific serum reactions. Since many laboratories will not have the proper sera to distinguish these associated antigens they will most likely be typed as regular antigens. Examples are: A203 and A210, associated with A2, A2403 with A9, B5102 and B5103 with B5, B703 with B7, B3901 and B3902 with B16, B4005 with B21, B2708 with B27. As mentioned before the B2708 can be easily mis-assigned as B7.

As already stated above HLA-C locus typing by serology is incomplete. A large number of C alleles have been identified by molecular techniques. Although some alleles give specific serum patterns with some antisera (Bunce *et al.,* 1997), they have not been assigned official serological names. There is strong linkage disequilibrium between HLA-B and -C at the serologic and also at the allelic level. Detection of exceptional B and C combinations can of course occur but should be treated with caution.

HLA-Class II typing

One of the complicating factors of class II typing is the varying number of gene products that are expressed at the cell surface. A DR haplotype can express one or two DR molecules and this depends on the specificity (Table 1.5). Moreover the linkage disequilibrium between DR and DQ is much stronger than between HLA-A and B. The most common haplotypes in Caucasoid populations are shown in Table 1.5, together with examples of some haplotypes that are seen in other populations. For example DR4-DQ2 is more often seen in Mediterranean populations and DR9-DQ2 is sometimes seen in Blacks. During routine typing rare combinations of DR and DQ will be encountered, but should always be treated with caution.

Variations in the number of expressed DR antigens can also be detected by serology. DR7-DQ2 haplotypes carry the DR53 antigen, but most DR7-DQ9

DR	DR	DQ	
DR1	–	DQ5(1)	
DR15(2)	DR51	DQ6(1)	
DR16(2)	DR51	DQ5(1)	
DR17(3)	DR52	DQ2	
DR4	DR53	DQ7(3)	
DR4	DR53	DQ8(3)	
DR11(5)	DR52	DQ7(3)	
DR12(5)	DR52	DQ7(3)	
DR13(6)	DR52	DQ6(1)	
DR13(6)	DR52	DQ7(3)	
DR14(6)	DR52	DQ5(1)	
DR7	DR53	DQ2	
DR7	–	DQ9(3)	
DR8	–	DQ4	
DR9	DR53	DQ9(3)	
DR10	–	DQ5(1)	
DR103	–	DQ5(1)	
Some other haplotypes, common in other populations:			
DR1404	DR52	DQ5(1)	(Eastern Europe)
DR4	DR53	DQ2	(Mediterranian)
DR18(3)	DR52	DQ4	(Black)
DR4	DR53	DQ4	(Oriental)

Table 1.5. Common Caucasian HLA-DR/DQ types

haplotypes do not express the DR53 at the cell surface, although they have the DRB4 gene.

Expression of DRB5 alleles is also heterogeneous. Occasionally a DR1-DQ5 haplotype can express the DR51 antigen. Such phenotypes look like DR1+DR2 triplets when typed by serology. In Africa the DR2'LUM' haplotype is found that has DR15-DQ6, but lacks the DRB5 gene and is thus DR51 negative. Non expression of DRB5 has recently been described on a DR15-DQ6 haplotype (Voorter *et al.,* 1997).

As mentioned earlier alloantisera are often directed against class II haplotypes. Especially in allo anti-DQ sera extra anti-DR is almost always present, but difficult to detect, and therefore often leading to errors in DQ typing. For example if an anti-DQ2 serum contains anti-DR3, it is almost impossible to detect DR3 without DQ2 (e.g. DR3-DQ4) combinations. Likewise DQ2+DR7 sera make it difficult to type the DR7 - DQ9 combination. DQ4 sera are scarce and may also contain DR8.

Class II mAb have been successfully produced and have provided useful reagents for DR and DQ typing. Cross reactivity in class II is extensive, and often due to amino acid (aa) sequences which are shared between alleles of different loci. For example, the mAb FK7.3.19.1 is a perfect anti-DR52 but also reacts with DR3 because of sharing of aa 77:N in DR3 and DR52 molecules. For several mAb the possible aa for recognition have been sorted out (Marsh *et al.,* 1992, Navarrete *et al.,* 1997). It is now also possible to identify DR103 using mAb MP10 (12w506 - ITAFER) reacting with DR103(+1+2+9+10). Allosera show very similar patterns which are now much better understood. Intelligent use of this knowledge will also allow recognition of certain alleles by serology.

Some examples:

- DRB1*1404 shares an HV1 sequence with DR8 and DR12 by which it can be clearly distinguished from DR14
- DRB1*1402 and *1406 share an HV3 sequence with DR1 and most DR4 alleles to which good antisera are available
- DRB1*0415 is a DR4 allele with a DR11 specific sequence, to which DR11 antisera and mAb react

Homozygosity versus non/low expression

Identifying only one antigen does not guarantee homozygosity. Family typing, preferably of the parents, is needed to prove that the antigen segregates on both haplotypes. Often antigens may be "hidden" in certain combinations. Depending on the composition of the typing tray one can predict which antigens may not be typable in which combinations. To mention a few: A30 in the presence of A31, A66 in the presence of A26, B52 in the presence of B51, B42 in the presence of B7, B70 in the presence of B35 and B15, DR16 in the presence of DR15, DR103 in the presence of most other DR, but especially DR1 and DR2. Incidentally family typing can reveal blanks at a certain locus. Through these findings, an increasing number of alleles that are not detectable or which are detectable only at low levels at the cell surface by standard serological techniques, have been identified. Quite a few have been detected at the A locus, but also non-expression of B15, DR51 and DQ1 has been reported (Parham, 1997a,b). Their nomenclature shows this by adding an "N"(non-) or "L"(low-expression) to their allele number (e.g. A*0215N, A*2402102L, A*2409N, B*1526N). Until it is completely clear to what extent these alleles form products that can be seen by immune cells, donors with these alleles should only be used with great caution in bone marrow transplantation.

The mutations that are involved in the non-expression of the alleles are often located outside exon 2 and 3 sequences. This means that most DNA based typing kits will not detect these alleles as irregular. It will remain necessary to perform serological typing to confirm expression of antigens on cells of individuals that have only been typed by molecular methods.

HLA nomenclature: Serology - DNA equivalents

HLA-A, B and C antigens that were originally defined by serology formed the basis of the naming of the class I alleles. Class II nomenclature is more complicated. Nomenclature of HLA-DR (D-Related) antigens was originally based on HLA-D (as defined by homozygous typing cells (HTC) in mixed lymphocyte reactions). Sequencing of these HTC gave the names of the first DRB1 alleles. At present DNA of all regularly occurring HLA antigens has been sequenced and the respective alleles have been named.

Variants of serological specificities that are readily identifiable by many laboratories received serological nomenclature. This has often led to further splits of known specificities. Examples are the splits of B15: B62, B63, B75, B76 and B77. Further studies have shown that such serological splits can be encoded by a number of different alleles. Thus, in the nomenclature there is not a one to one relation between serological specificities and allele names.

Now that many more individuals from different populations have been studied, often only by DNA based techniques, the number of class I and II alleles is increasing rapidly. These new alleles may be extremely rare, or they may be specific to certain populations. As long as lymphocytes that express these new alleles have not been tested by serology it is not easy to decide to which specificity they match best. We know that certain sequences may be very similar as far as amino acids are concerned but may differ significantly in serological reactivity pattern: e.g. B4005, encoded by the B*4005 allele reacts in serology like B50(21) and not like B40. Historically B70 was identified as a specificity different from B15. However the allele sequences are so similar that they received B*15 nomenclature. These few examples show that it has become very complicated to link generic DNA typing results with serology.

A "Dictionary" has been produced to compare alleles and their known serological specificities (Hurley *et al.,* 1997). This listing can help to find HLA matched donors for patient in need of bone marrow transplantation, especially when the patient appears to have one or more infrequent alleles. HLA typings in databases that have been accumulated through many years need to be comparable irrespective of the technique used. We hope that in the near future software will become available that can combine molecular and serological data in an intelligent way.

References

Bodmer, JG, Marsh, SGE, Albert, ED, Bodmer, WF *et al.* (1997) Nomenclature for factors of the HLA system, 1996. *Hum Immunol* **53**: 98-128

Bunce, M, Vilches, C, Marsh, SGE, van den Berg-Loonen, EM, Pazderka, F *et al.* (1997) AHS#9: all HLA-C alleles. In: *Genetic diversity of HLA: functional and medical implication* Vol I. (Ed. Charron, D), pp.83-88. EDK, Paris

Darke, C, and Dyer, P. (1993) Clinical HLA typing by cytotoxicity. In: *Histocompatibility testing: a practical approach.* (Ed. Dyer, P and Middleton, D), pp.51-80. Oxford University Press, Oxford

Garrido, F, Cabrera, T, Accolla, RS, Bensa, JC, Bodmer, WF *et al.* (1997) HLA and cancer: 12th International Histocompatibility Workshop study. In: *Genetic diversity of HLA: functional and medical implication* Vol I. (Ed. Charron, D), pp.445-452. EDK, Paris

Hildebrand, WH, Domena, JD, Shen, SY, Marsh, SGE, Bunce, M *et al.* (1994) The HLA-B7Qui antigen is encoded by a new subtype of HLA-B27 (B*2708). *Tissue Antigens* **44**: 47-51

Hurley, CK, Schreuder, GMT, Marsh, SGE, Lau, M, Middleton, D *et al.* (1997) The search for HLA-matched donors: a summary of HLA-A*, -B*, -DRB1/3/4/5* alleles and their association with serologically defined HLA-A,-B,-DR antigens. *Tissue Antigens* **50**:401-418

Lopez-Larrea, C, Alvarez, V, du Toit, E, Fan, L, Grosse-Wilde, H *et al.* (1997) AHS#5: HLA-B7, B27, B22, B42, B47, B73, B81, B703. In: *Genetic diversity of HLA: functional and medical implication* Vol I. (Ed. Charron, D), pp.56-62. EDK, Paris

Marsh, SGE, Moses, JH and Bodmer, JG (1992) HLA class II sequence polymorphism detectable by serology. In: *HLA 1991* Vol I. (Ed. Tsuji, K, Aizawa, M, and Sasazuki, T), pp.610-620. Oxford University Press, Oxford

Mulder, A, Kardol, M, Blom, J, Jolley, WB, Melief, CJM, *et al.* (1993) Characterization of two human monoclonal antibodies reactive with HLA-B12 and HLA-B60 respectively, raised by in vitro secondary immunization of peripheral blood lymphocytes. *Human Immunology* **36**: 186-192

Naipal, A, D'Amaro, J, Bruning, JW, van Leeuwen, A and van Rood, JJ (1984) Automated reading of propidium iodide lymphocytotoxicity tests for HLA-DR, MB, MT typing. *Tissue Antigens* **24**: 302.

Navarrete, C, Brown, C, de Lange, P and Schreuder, GMT (1997) 12th IHW HLA class II monoclonal antibody study. In: *Genetic diversity of HLA: functional and medical implication* Vol I. (Ed. Charron, D), pp.11-17. EDK, Paris

Parham, P, Lawlor, DA, Salter, RD, Lomen, CE, Bjorkman, PJ *et al.* (1987) HLA-A,B,C: Patterns of polymorphism in peptide-binding proteins. In: *Immunobiology of HLA* Vol II (Ed. Dupont, B), pp.10-33. Springer-Verlag, New York

Parham, P. (1997a) Definition and importance of HLA class I null alleles: a new role for serological HLA class I typing. In: *Genetic Diversity of HLA; Functional and medical implication* Vol II. (Ed.Charron, D), pp.28-34. EDK, Paris

Parham, P. (1997b) Filling in the blanks. *Tissue Antigens* **50**: 318-321

Tongio, MM, Doxiadis, I, Laforet, M, Schreuder, GMT, Froelich, N *et al*. (1997) 12th IHW HLA class I monoclonal antibody study. In: *Genetic Diversity of HLA: Functional and medical implication* Vol I. (Ed. Charron, D), pp.7-11. EDK, Paris

Voorter, CEM, Roeffaers, HET, du Toit, ED, and van den Berg-Loonen, EM (1997) The absence of DR51 in a DRB5-positive individual DR2ES is caused by a null allele (DRB5*0108N). *Tissue Antigens* **50**: 326-333

CHAPTER 2

SCREENING FOR HLA-SPECIFIC ANTIBODIES

C. Brown and C. Navarrete
Department of Histocompatibility & Immunogenetics
NBS - London & The South East
North London Centre
Colindale Avenue
LONDON NW9 5BG

Introduction

HLA antibodies were first identified as the result of an investigation of a non-haemolytic febrile transfusion reaction (NHFTR) occurring in a patient following a blood transfusion. This reaction was later found to be due to the presence of alloantibodies found in the patient reacting with lymphoctyes present in the transfused product. From then on the clinical relevance of HLA antibodies has been clearly established.

Alloantibodies may be produced in any situation that expose the host to HLA alloantigens including pregnancy, transplantation, blood transfusion and planned immunisation. However, the affinity and avidity of the antibody responses produced will be dependent on the route of immunisation and persistence and type of immunological challenge, as well as the immune status of the host.

Development of HLA-specific antibodies

Pregnancy

In approximately 20% of human pregnancies the mother produces cytotoxic antibodies directed against the paternally derived mismatched HLA antigens and this is influenced by the number of previous pregnancies, whether brought to term or aborted. Fetal material often enters the maternal circulation at parturition or during pregnancy and with subsequent pregnancies there is often a maturation of the antibody response resulting in high titre, IgG, high affinity HLA specific antibodies. Although these IgG antibodies can cross the placenta they have been shown to be harmless to the fetus, in contrast to platelet or granulocyte specific antibodies.

Sera from multiparous women have historically been the main source of HLA specific typing reagents as in pregnancy it is possible to obtain antibody responses directed against specific paternal HLA antigens present in the fetus.

Transplantation

The antigenic stimulus provided by an allograft will depend upon the degree of HLA mismatch between donor and recipient. Allografts are normally accompanied by immunosuppressive therapy and this can affect the development and/or nature of antibodies produced. Antibodies in allograft recipients may have a narrow or broad range of specificities, depending on previous HLA mismatches and sensitisation events, and although they are predominately IgG, some IgM antibodies are also produced.

Blood transfusion

The presence of leucocytes in transfused blood or blood products may result in the formation of HLA antibodies. The antigenic load of a single transfusion may be smaller than the exposure to an allograft or multiple pregnancies and the production of HLA specific antibodies is more often in response to multiple transfusions. The recipient also receives a greater number of donor exposures as some products such as platelets are pools derived from up to 4 separate donations. Antibodies more commonly detected in multi-transfused patients are multispecific IgM and IgG and these are mostly directed at public epitopes. The immune status of the recipient is an important factor as many patients may be immunosuppressed as part of their treatment which will influence both the development and maturation of the immune response.

The use of leucodepleted (LD) blood and blood products can prevent primary alloimmunisation induced by direct allorecognition of HLA antigens. However, LD blood is not very effective in preventing alloimmunisation in an already sensitised recipient in whom the indirect pathway of HLA allorecognition can still operate.

Planned immunisation

In the past, donor and recipient pairs were selected for a particular HLA mismatch for planned immunisation and a number of potent HLA specific antibodies were produced. The deliberate immunisation of healthy individuals with donor lymphocytes or skin graft to produce HLA typing reagents would, nowadays, be difficult to justify ethically. Planned HLA immunisation is carried out as a form of treatment for women who have recurrent spontaneous abortions; these women are immunised with lymphocytes from their partners or third party to attempt to induce an immunomodulatory response that results in the maintenance of the pregnancy.

Clinical relevance of HLA-specific antibodies

Solid organ transplantation

Pre- and post-transplant monitoring of HLA-specific antibodies directed against donor antigens in renal and cardiac recipients is important, since these have been associated with hyperacute rejection of the graft (Lobo *et al.*, 1995).

Bone marrow transplantation

The influence of HLA antibodies in the success of bone marrow transplantation has not been well documented, but the presence of donor reactive HLA specific antibodies in the recipient has been identified as a significant risk factor for patients undergoing bone marrow transplantation (Anasetti *et al.,* 1989). Leukaemic patients with donor specific antibodies reacting with T or B cells in a cytotoxic crossmatch had a reported higher incidence of graft failure than those with a negative crossmatch. Pre-formed cytotoxic antibodies can increase the incidence of graft failure in patients with aplastic anaemia (Hansen *et al.,* 1981). However it is primarily in the post bone marrow transplant setting, where patients receive multiple transfusions, that recipients experience problems due to HLA specific antibodies leading to refractoriness to random platelet transfusions and thus requiring transfusions of HLA-matched platelets (see below).

Transfusion reactions

HLA specific antibodies have been shown to cause non-haemolytic febrile transfusion reactions (NHFTR) and have also been implicated in the development of transfusion related acute lung injury (TRALI), of which both conditions are potentially serious hazards of blood transfusions. Furthermore, HLA alloimmunisation is one of the most common causes of platelet destruction in patients who are immunologically refractory to random platelet transfusion.

1. *Non-haemolytic febrile transfusion reactions*

This condition occuring in approximately 5% of transfused patients is characterised by fever and chills and a rise in temperature of more than 1 or 2°C in patients during or shortly after transfusion. The presence of HLA and granulocyte specific antibodies in the blood product have been demonstrated and the majority of NHFTRs occur following platelet transfusion. More recently a number of cytokines including TNFα, IL-6 and IL-8, present in the transfused product, have also been implicated.

2. *Transfusion related acute lung injury*

This reaction, characterised by acute respiratory distress, pulmonary edema and severe hypoxia is a rare but serious complication of transfusion. The development of TRALI has been associated with the presence of HLA and other leucocyte specific antibodies including granulocytes, in the transfused plasma or blood product.

3. *Immunological refractoriness to random platelet transfusion*

Multiple transfusions of random donor platelets can cause an alloimmune response in the recipient leading to a significant reduction in platelet survival and lack of a significant rise in platelet count following platelet transfusions. HLA alloimmunisation is the major cause of immunological refractoriness and, in particular, the presence of cytotoxic HLA-specific antibodies correlate strongly with refractoriness to random donor platelet transfusion. HLA antibodies may be detected in 50% of multi-transfused patients with bone marrow failure.

The most effective treatment for refractory patients is the transfusion of HLA matched or cross matched negative platelets. The rapid determination of the HLA antibody status of the refractory patient can be an important aid to the diagnosis of alloimmune refractoriness.

Non-HLA antibodies

Autoantibodies

The presence of lymphocytotoxic autoreactive antibodies in patients' sera is not thought to be of clinical significance in solid organ transplant recipients (Ting and Morris 1983; Ettenger *et al.,* 1983) and for patients receiving HLA matched platelets but very little is known about their relevance in the destruction of platelets. The importance of autoreactive antibodies relates to the fact that they can cause a false positive crossmatch and therefore the laboratory screening strategy must identify these antibodies (Chapman *et al.,* 1986). Fortunately the majority of these lymphocytotoxic autoantibodies are IgM and can be identified by screening with and without DTT. In addition, they react with PBL from random donors but are negative, or react weakly, with B-CLL cells.

Monocyte/endothelial cell antibodies

Non-HLA antibodies reacting with a common epitope found specifically on peripheral blood monocytes, endothelial cells and macrophages have been described (Moraes and Statsny 1977). In addition, antibodies reacting specifically with endothelial cells have also been described and the clinical significance of these antibodies has now been clearly established in both renal and heart transplant recipients. Molecular characterisation of the endothelial cell specific antigens is not yet available but preliminary studies have indicated that the endothelial cell target antigen detected by antibodies present in kidney transplant recipients is approximately 97-100 kD, whereas the antibodies found in heart transplant patients react again a 56-57.5 kD endothelial cell antigen.

Monocyte/endothelial and endothelial specific cell antibodies may be detected by the LCT, ELISA or flow cytometric methods using a panel of well characterised peripheral blood monocytes or the endothelial cell lines ECV304 (Takahashi & Sawaki, 1992), EAHy.926 and HUVEC (Perry *et al.,* 1998).

Epithelial cell antibodies

The presence of antibodies reacting with donor epithelial cells in paediatric renal recipients has been shown to be associated with transplant failure (Harmer *et al.,* 1990; Martin *et al* 1991). These antibodies are IgM and can be detected in the LCT or by flow cytometry using the epithelial cell line A549 provided that the patient's serum is well characterised and the autoreactive and HLA IgM antibodies can be clearly distinguished from those reacting with the epithelial cells. The cell line A549 expresses HLA class I but not HLA class II antigens and therefore the serum with any suspected HLA class I activity (IgM or IgG) could be absorbed out with platelets in order to remove any HLA class I activity. In this way any residual reactivity will be due to the presence of epithelial cell specific antibodies.

Anti-idiotype antibodies

Antibodies directed against immunoglobulin variable domains have the potential of blocking antibody activity. The clinical significance of these anti-antibodies or anti-idiotype antibodies is unclear. The detection of anti-idiotype antibodies can be achieved using modifications of the LCT or more specialised techniques (Reed and Suciu-Foca, 1995).

Screening for HLA-specific antibodies

The aim of a screening programme is to detect and identify HLA specific antibodies but the approaches will differ when testing patients' sera and when screening for typing reagents.

Procedures for identifying antibodies in the patient's sera

These must be designed to detect all relevant antibodies using techniques as sensitive as those used for crossmatching. Screening results should provide data on antibody specificity; HLA class I or class II, public, private or auto and the strength of reactivity. This data will be used to:

- Predict the likelihood of finding an HLA compatible organ or platelet donor in a random population
- Identify donor HLA antigens likely to give a positive crossmatch, 'unacceptable antigens', thus avoiding unnecessary testing, organ transport and prolonged cold ischaemia time.

The screening approach should aim to provide a comprehensive history of the patients' antibody status which will aid the interpretation of equivocal or unexpected positive results.

Procedures for screening sera to be used as reagents

These procedures differ from the above in that the aim is to identify high affinity/avidity antibodies that consistently react with cells bearing a specific HLA antigen. These typing sera are normally used in the standard microlymphocytoxicity test and should be extensively screened with well characterised panel cells including donors from different ethnic groups.

DNA based techniques for HLA typing are rapidly replacing serological typing resulting in a dramatic reduction in this activity.

Variations of the complement dependent lymphocytotoxicity (LCT) technique are currently used routinely for antibody screening but flow cytometric and ELISA based techniques are being used more widely, often in conjunction with the LCT. The isolation and cryopreservation of lymphocytes are techniques required for the cytotoxicity and flow cytometric assays and are briefly described below. In addition careful consideration must be given to panel selection and collection of serum samples for all three techniques and this will also be discussed.

1. *Isolation of mononuclear cells from whole blood*

This is one of the basic procedures of an H&I laboratory. Lymphocytes present in the mononuclear cell (MNCs) population are required for serological typing, cytotoxic and flow cytometry based screening techniques and cellular assays. Therefore it is important that appropriate care is taken at this stage. Freshly drawn venous blood may be defibrinated directly or taken into anticoagulant leaving the option for defibrination.

1.1. *Principle of the technique*

The separation of MNCs from whole blood can be achieved by the addition of compounds that aggregate erythrocytes thereby increasing their sedimentation rate. This principle was adapted by Boyum (1968) with the development of a single step centrifugation technique using a mixture of Ficoll, a high molecular weight sucrose polymer and sodium metrozoate (Isopaque) as the aggregation and separation medium. Briefly, whole blood is layered onto Ficoll-Isopaque at a density of 1.077 and centrifuged. At this density the mononuclear cells (lymphocytes and monocytes) remain at the interface of the Ficoll-Isopaque/plasma, whilst the other blood components (red cells and granulocytes) pass through, leaving the serum or plasma above.

1.2. *Defibrination*

The technique described for the removal of fibrin from blood to avoid coagulation, will result in the removal of platelets, which can interfere with the HLA class I typing cytotoxicity test, but some lymphocytes may also be lost.

- Place 10 glass beads, 3mm diameter, into a 250ml conical flask.
- Add 30 ml of freshly drawn blood and rotate the flask immediately until a clot has formed around the beads (5-10 min).
- The blood can now be manipulated without clotting.

Citrated blood:

Add 1.8ml calcium gluconate (10%) and 25 units thrombin (1000U/ml), per 10ml blood to the flask.

Heparinised blood:

Add 1.8ml protamine sulphate and 25 units thrombin (per 10ml blood) to the flask.

1.3. *Isolation of mononulear cells from defibrinated blood*

- Dilute blood with an equal volume of Hanks BSS.
- Layer 10ml of blood onto 3.5 - 4.0ml of Ficoll-Isopaque.
- Centrifuge at 800g for 20 min with the brake off.
- Aspirate cells at the Ficoll-Isopaque /plasma interface into a clean centrifuge tube and add Hanks BSS, a ratio of 1 cells : 2 Hanks BSS should be sufficient to ensure the cells are washed.
- Centrifuge at 400g for 5 min with the brake on.
- Discard the supernatant and resuspend the cells in Hanks BSS.
- Centrifuge at 400g for 5 min with the brake on.
- Resuspend in 1.0ml of RPMI.
- Count and assess viability of lymphocyte suspension

1.4. *Isolation of lymphocytes from blood in anticoagulant*

- Dilute blood with an equal volume of Hanks BSS containing 3.3% citrate.
- Layer 10ml of blood onto 3.5-4.0ml of Ficoll-Isopaque.
- Centrifuge at 800g for 20 min with the brake off.
- Aspirate cells at the Ficoll-Isopaque /plasma interface into a clean centrifuge tube and add Hanks BSS, a ratio of 1 cells : 2 citrated Hanks BSS should be sufficient to ensure the cells are washed.
- Centrifuge at 400g for 5 min with the brake on.
- Discard the supernatant and resuspend the cells in Hanks BSS.
- Centrifuge at 400g for 5 min with the brake on.
- Resuspend in 1.0ml of RPMI.
- Count and assess viability of lymphocyte suspension.

1.5. *Isolation of mononulear cells from lymph node or spleen*

This technique has been extensively described in Chapter 4 of this volume and by McCloskey *et al.,* (1993).

2. *Cryopreservation of mononuclear cells*

Mononuclear cells from individuals selected for the screening panel should be frozen as soon as possible after isolation in suitable aliquots and maintained in liquid nitrogen (LN_2).

The rate of freezing must be controlled to prevent the formation of harmful ice crystals damaging the cells. This may be achieved using a controlled rate freezer or suitable freezing containers that allow a gradual exchange of temperature and the use of the cryoprotectant dimethyl sulphoxide (DMSO). The initial phase of cooling is most crucial; the cells are cooled at a rate of –1°C/minute from 4°C to –30°C and then at a rate of –10°C/minute from –30°C to –100°C. The cells can then be transferred to liquid nitrogen.

Lymphocytes may be stored in 2ml cryovials or microcentrifuge tubes (Beckman). The concentration of lymphocytes in each tube will be dependent upon the number required for each test but in general up to $5x10^6$ cells/Beckman and up to $10 x10^6$ cells/2ml cryovial can be stored.

Two different freezing mixtures are required for lymphocyte cryopreservation, and they should be prepared in advance and kept cold (on ice) if used on the same day, otherwise they can be stored below –20°C.

2.1. *Serum*

- Human AB or Fetal Calf Serum (FCS) may be used.
- Prepare an 80% serum mixture with RPMI e.g. 4ml AB serum + 1 ml RPMI - keep on ice

2.2. *DMSO*

Prepare a 20% DMSO mixture with RPMI e.g. 1ml DMSO + 4ml RPMI - keep on ice (care should be taken when preparing DMSO as heat is produced).

The lymphocytes are resuspended in the serum mixture and an equal volume of DMSO mixture is added dropwise whilst agitating the tube to ensure mixing the two solutions. Thus, the final concentration of the freezing reagents are DMSO 10%, serum 40% and RPMI 50%. The cell suspension is then transferred to Beckman tubes or cryovials.

If large numbers of Beckman tubes are to be filled, a multi-dispenser can be used but it is important to cool all reagents including the multi-dispenser and the Beckman tube holder.

Example

12 x10^6 lymphocytes are required to be frozen at concentration of 2x10^6/Beckman for the screening panel. The total volume in each Beckman is 250µl. Requirements are thus:

☑ 12 x10^6 lymphocytes

☑ 6 Beckman tubes

☑ 6 x250µl = 1.5ml of freezing mixture (i.e. 750µl 80% AB serum + 750µl 20% DMSO)

- Mix and dispense 250µl of the cell suspension into 6 labelled Beckmans
- Transfer Beckmans to a controlled rate freezing machine or process as in 2.3 or 2.4, below.

2.3. *Cryopots (Nalgene^{TM}) method*

- Fill cryopots with isopropanol.
- Place Beckmans (or cryovials) into pots and transfer immediately to a –70°C to –80°C freezer for a minimum of 4 hours before transferring to liquid nitrogen for long term storage.

2.4. *Expanded polystyrene box method*

The box should be at least 5cm larger than the rack it contains and should be pre-cooled to 4°C.

- Place rack containing Beckmans (or cryovials) into the box
- Transfer the box immediately to a –70°C to –80°C freezer overnight before transferring to liquid nitrogen for long term storage.

These methods are useful if small numbers of Beckmans or cryovials have to be frozen and less expensive than a controlled rate freezer.

2.5. *Thawing of Frozen Lymphocytes*

When thawing cryopreserved lymphocytes it is important that the DMSO is removed as quickly as possible again to prevent the formation of harmful ice crystals damaging the cells. The cells should be thawed rapidly in a 37°C waterbath and immediately transferred to RPMI +10% FCS or AB serum and washed. The second and subsequent washes may be performed in RPMI or HANKS BSS. The washing procedure is the same as is used when isolating lymphocytes.

3. *Screening panels*

Three types of panels can be used to screen for the presence of HLA-specific antibodies: random, selected, or a mixture of both.

3.1. *Random panel*

The percentage of panel cells with which a serum reacts is termed the %PRA (panel reactive antibodies) and can be used to predict the chance of finding a compatible platelet donor or obtaining a negative crossmatch for a solid organ transplant patient. The disadvantages of using random panels are that not all HLA antigens may be represented in the panel and the more common antigens and haplotypes may be over represented making identification of antibody specificity difficult. Furthermore, panels will vary and therefore comparable results may not be achieved for a single serum sample. However, the results should reflect reactivity with the local ethnic population. Laboratories involved in HLA typing of healthy volunteers for bone marrow registries may screen a patient's serum with cells of donors as they are typed.

3.2. *Selected panel*

This is the more commonly used panel for screening since it ensures that the majority of known HLA specificities are represented in the panel. Three important features of the HLA system; extensive polymorphism, linkage disequilibrium and cross reactivity must be taken into account when designing a selected panel.

Cell donors must be selected to cover most of the known HLA specificities avoiding common haplotypes wherever possible and cells possessing two highly crossreactive antigens (at the same locus) should be avoided as they may not be informative (see Table 2.1)

Panel Cell ID	HLA TYPE					
#001	A2	A28	B7	B55	Cw7	Cw3
#002	A25	A32	B18	B51	Cw5	Cw1
#003	A68	A30	B45	B57	Cw8	
#004	A1	A31	B27	B39	Cw4	Cw3

Table 2.1. HLA types of possible cell panel donors

In Table 2.1,

- Cell #001 & #002 : A2 & A28, B7 & B55; A25 & A32 are highly crossreactive. Furthermore A2-B7 and A25-B18 are in strong linkage thus these donors would not be ideal panel cells.
- Cell #003 & #004: The HLA A & B locus specificities of both these donors are not crossreactive and in European Caucasoids the common linkages are seen with: A1-B8, A30-B13 or B18 and A31-B51 or B60, therefore these would be more informative panel cell donors.

HLA-A,B, C & DR homozygous cells can be informative in patients with high PRA to help with the exclusion of particular antigens, although the double dose of a single antigen can also make cells more sensitive to specific killing in the LCT. Homozygosity of the cells should always be confirmed using DNA techniques and/or family studies where possible.

An example of a selected panel is shown in Table 2.2.

	ID	A	A	B	B	Cw	Cw	DR	DR	DQ	DQ
CLL	1	1	2	71	57	3	6	1	8	5	4
	2	2	32	38	67	5	-	18	4	4	8
	3	3	69	41	8	7	-	16	1	6	7
	4	11	23	44	27	4	5	15	13	6	-
	5	25	24	58	37	3	6	17	7	2	9
	6	30	74	52	56	1	-	4	15	8	6
	7	31	26	75	49	7	8	11	10	7	5
	8	32	34	62	60	3	4	12	7	7	2
	9	33	3	44	18	2	7	13	17	6	2
	10	29	68	39	55	1	7	14	9	5	9
PBL	11	1	68	51	50	6	-				
	12	36	74	52	42	-	-				
	13	80	66	53	27	4	2				
	14	2	33	7	49	7	-				
	15	3	32	8	62	7	9				
	16	23	30	7	51	3	-				
	17	24	31	44	18	7	5				
	18	25	29	13	38	6	-				
	19	26	69	64	63	8	-				
	20	34	23	65	44	8	4				
	21	11	2	63	56	7	1				
	22	68	30	45	57	8	-				
	23	1	33	62	55	9	-				
	24	2	3	37	61	6	2				
	25	3	24	35	13	4	6				
	26	23	66	78	47	1	6				
	27	24	29	46	60	1	3				
	28	25	31	39	8	7	-				
	29	26	1	60	35	3	4				
	30	11	32	72	65	2	8				

Table 2.2. Example of 30 panel cells, consisting of 10 B-CLL cells and 20 PBL. Refer also to Table 2.3.

The PBL from donors 11 to 30 in Table 2.2 are used to detect HLA class I antibodies. However, B-cells comprise 10-15% of peripheral blood lymphocytes and express HLA class II in addition to class I antigens. A panel of B-cells (donors 1-10 in Table 2.2) covering most of the HLA-DR and DQ specificities may also be required. The PBL from patients with B-cell chronic lymphocytic leukaemia (B-CLL) are a good source of B-cells for screening as they can comprise up to 50-95% of PBL depending on the stage of the disease (Navarrete *et al.*, 1986). Therefore the percentage of B-cells must be checked each time the patient is bled. The use of flow cytometry for antibody screening has simplified the use of EBV transformed B-cells as a source of HLA class II positive targets as careful selection of complement is required when using these cell in the LCT.

A		B		B		C		DR/DQ	
A1	4	B5		B53	1	Cw1	4	DR1	2
A2	5	B7	2	B54(22)		Cw2	4	DR103	
A203		B703		B55(22)	2	Cw3	2	DR2	
A210		B8	3	B56(22)	2	Cw4	6	DR3	
A3	5	B12		B57(17)	2	Cw5	3	DR4	2
A9		B13	2	B58(17)	1	Cw6	7	DR5	
A10		B14		B59		Cw7	9	DR6	
A11	3	B15		B60(40)	3	Cw8	5	DR7	2
A19		B16		B61(40)	1	Cw9(w3)	2	DR8	1
A23(9)	4	B17		B62(15)	3	Cw10(w3)	3	DR9	1
A24(9)	4	B18	2	B63(15)	2			DR10	1
A2403		B21		B64(14)	1			DR11(5)	
A25(10)	3	B22		B65(14)	2			DR12(5)	1
A26(10)	3	B27	2	B67	1			DR13(6)	2
A28		B2708		B70				DR14(6)	1
A29(19)	3	B35	2	B71(70)	1			DR1403	
A30(19)	3	B37	2	B72(70)	1			DR1404	
A31(19)	3	B38(16)	2	B73				DR15(2)	2
A32(19)	4	B39(16)	2	B75(15)	1			DR16(2)	1
A33(19)	3	B3901		B76(15)				DR17(3)	2
A34(10)	2	B3902		B77(15)				DR18(3)	1
A36	1	B40		B78	1				
A43		B4005		B81				DR51	
A66(10)	2	B41	1					DR52	
A68(28)	3	B42	1	Bw4				DR53	
A69(28)	2	B44(12)	4	Bw6					
A74(19)	2	B45(12)	1					DQ1	
A80	1	B46	1					DQ2	3
		B47	1					DQ3	
		B48						DQ4	2
		B49(21)	2					DQ5(1)	3
		B50(21)	1					DQ6(1)	4
		B51(5)	2					DQ7(3)	3
		B5102						DQ8(3)	2
		B5103						DQ9(3)	2
		B52(5)	2						

Table 2.3. Frequency of occurence of individual HLA alleles in the 30 panel cells (refer above to Table 2.2).

The use of different targets for antibody screening is discussed more fully later on in this chapter and summarised in Table 2.7.

The numbers of cells to be included in the panel will depend on the patient group being tested. The 30 cell panel shown in the example above would provide a basic screen for the detection, but not for the full characterisation of HLA specific antibody. For patients immunologically refractory to random platelet transfusions, testing HLA class II specific antibodies are not important. In these cases the cell panel may be smaller than that used for screening patients on a renal transplant waiting list where class II antibodies may be taken into account. A possible strategy would be to perform an initial screen, using a reduced cell panel to identify broad antibody reactivity and then to use a second panel and /or selected cells to refine the identification of antibody specificity.

4. *Handling serum and reagent samples*

4.1. *Patients*

Serum samples should be collected 10-14 days after each sensitisation event, such as blood transfusion, and at intervals relevant for the patient group. For example; heart transplant patients are not normally transfused whilst on the transplant waiting list and should be screened less frequently than patients who may receive blood transfusions for anaemia. Refractory patients receiving frequent platelet transfusions will require regular screening. Whatever protocol is used, the frequency of screening should allow the laboratory to build up a comprehensive history of the patients' antibody status so that appropriate organ or platelet donors can be selected. Post transplant monitoring protocols must also be designed to obtain serum samples at relevant intervals and during rejection episodes.

4.2. *Reagents*

4.2.1. *Normal donors*

Screening pregnancy sera for the procurement of HLA typing reagents is a labour intensive and costly process. Only approximately 20% of pregnant women produce cytotoxic HLA specific antibodies and of these only approximately 1% may be useful typing reagents. The effectiveness of a screening programme can be improved by limiting the screening to only multiparous women and using a paternal cell sample to perform a crossmatch, or a reduced number of panel cells for the initial screen, biased toward the specificities required. Samples taken during the antenatal period may be used to identify potentially useful reagents and the placenta can also be used as source of typing reagents. Much of the maternal immunisation occurs at parturition and HLA specific antibodies can be detected in post- natal samples, months, and in some cases years, after delivery.

Although serological typing is rapidly being replaced by DNA based typing techniques, serological reagents may still be required for antigen expression studies.

Serum samples should be stored below –20°C in appropriate volumes to reduce the number of times the serum is thawed and re-frozen. Sera should be thawed immediately before it is required and, once thawed, kept below 8°C (e.g. in a fridge) until used. Freeze-thawing and high temperatures may cause loss of antibody activity in the complement dependent LCT, in particular, affecting the formation of anti-complementary factors such as microbial products and aggregated gamma globulin.

4.2.2. *Monoclonal antibodies*

Monoclonal antibodies directed against most of the HLA class I and II specificities are available and provide a more consistent, stable source of typing reagent. Whether monoclonal reagents are obtained from ascitic fluid or supernatants of hybridoma cell cultures they normally require careful dilution to maintain consistent activity in the LCT. Additional measures to those used for handling serum must be employed to prevent cross-contamination and loss of activity (Kennedy *et al.,* 1987), thus:

- Use disposable tips where possible
- Avoid centrifugation of supernatants which may result in loss of activity
- Store supernatants undiluted but in suitable aliquots that will minimise freeze-thawing
- The ascitic fluid may need to be initially diluted and stored at a concentration to enable ease of use

4.3. *Manipulation of HLA typing reagents*

4.3.1. *Absorption*

The HLA class I reactivity from a serum selected for its specific anti-class II activity can be absorbed using pooled platelets since HLA class II antigens are not normally expressed on platelets. Platelets greater than 5 days old are not normally used for transfusion but may be stored for months at 4°C in PBS containing azide prior to use in absorption procedures.

To absorb 1ml of serum:

- Wash pooled platelets twice with PBS.
- Prepare 3 x1.5ml aliquots of pooled platelets (in tubes with at least 2.5ml capacity).
- Spin all 3 tubes at very high speed to produce a packed platelet pellet of at least 1ml.
- Remove supernatant ensuring that the pellet is as dry as possible.
- Add serum to packed platelets and mix.

- Incubate at room temperature for 30 min, mixing at regular intervals or continuously on a roller
- Spin tube at very high speed as before to pellet the platelets
- Keep the supernatant and transfer it to the second tube containing packed platelets
- Repeat the procedure as before for the second and third tube of packed pooled platelets
- After the third absorption the serum may be spun until it has been clarified, frozen in suitable aliquots and rescreened

Cells may also be used to remove any unwanted HLA reactivity but careful selection of the cell donor and characterisation of the serum reactivity is required to confirm the specificity of the absorption. A minimum of 10 million cells are required to absorb 1ml of serum.

4.3.2. *Serum dilution*

For high titre HLA antibodies or in order to identify HLA specific antibodies in some multispecific sera, it is sometimes advisable to titrate these samples using serum from human blood group AB donors to dilute out the reactivity with a low titre antibody. It is important to carefully and extensively screen the AB serum for the possible presence of HLA specific antibodies. Dilutions may also be used to increase antibody activity in those instances where the high titre antibody inhibits complement dependent cytotoxicity. This prozone effect can be abolished using diluents with such as complement fixation test diluent (CFT), PBS or RPMI 1640.

4.3.3. *Antibody concentration*

A number of techniques are available for concentrating low titre antibodies such as the use affinity columns and precipitation with ammonium sulphate, caprylic acid and even antibody bound to beads. A weak antibody directed against a rare specificity or a monospecific antiserum are both good candidates for concentrating if sufficient antiserum is available.

A detailed costing of all procedures involved in procuring serological reagents should be made before undertaking such a task as comparable commercial alternatives are available.

4.4. *Preparation of screening plates*

When an appropriate number of serum samples have been collected they can be dispensed into 60 or 72 well microtitre plates. The sera should be tested neat and in dilution (e.g. 1:1) to avoid the affects of prozone. Appropriate positive and negative control reagents should be included on the plate particularly if both class I and II antibodies are to be detected with a number of different targets.

If the cells are to dispensed manually, the design of the plate layout should take into account those samples known to have strong cytotoxic antibodies to avoid the effects of carry over. Dyes such as phenol red can be used to aid visualisation of serum on the clear plastic plates e.g. 1µl phenol red (1%)/200µl serum.

5. *Lymphocytotoxicity*

The most widely used technique for the detection of HLA antibodies is the microlymphocytotoxicity assay, developed by Terasaki & McClelland (1964) and standardised by the NIH, USA. Equal volumes of serum and cells are mixed and incubated to allow the formation of immune complexes, rabbit complement is then added and there is a further incubation step. Activation of complement via the classical pathway by complement fixing antibodies that have reacted with cell surface molecules will result in the disruption of the cell membrane. There are a number of ways to detect this cytotoxic reaction.

5.1. *Methodology*

- Thaw the screening plate containing the patients' serum immediately prior to use.
- Dispense 1µl of lymphocyte suspension (2 x10^6/ml) in to each well of the microtest plate using a 50µl syringe or automated dispenser. Ensure cells and serum are mixed which can be achieved by centrifuging the plates for 30 sec at 1000 rpm or using the 50µl syringe, but care must be taken to prevent cross contamination between wells (see procedures for screening monoclonal antibodies).
- Incubate for 60 min at room temperature.
- Add 5µl of pooled rabbit complement.
- Incubate for 120 min at room temperature.
- Stop the reaction and stain the cells by the addition of 1µl of stain, containing EDTA/acridine orange/ethidium bromide/haemoglobin.
- Read the test with an inverted fluorescence microscope using an ultra violet light source.

The plates may be kept in the fridge and read several hours later if necessary but wide variations in reading times should be avoided.

5.2. *Typing reagents*

When screening for HLA typing reagents. e.g. for HLA class I, using PBL, the incubation times should be adjusted to those used for typing as given below.

- Incubate cells and serum for 30 min at room temperature.
- Add 5µl of pooled rabbit complement.

- Incubate for 60 min at room temperature.

If typing is carried out with lymphocytes isolated using immunomagnetic beads the incubation times for screening should also be adjusted.

5.3. *Interpretation of the LCT*

Ethidium bromide (EB) and acridine orange (AO)

Live cells actively take up AO and under ultra violet (UV) light appear green. Disruption of the cell membrane allows the entry of EB which binds to DNA and these dead cells appear red under uv light.

5.3.1. *Alternatives to ethidium bromide and acridine orange*

5.3.1.1. *Carboxyfluoroscein diacetate (CFDA)/ ethidium bromide*

In this technique the lymphocytes are incubated with CFDA then used in the cytotoxicity test. CFDA leaks out of damaged cells and EB enters. As with EB/AO dead cells appear red and live cells appear green.

5.3.1.2. *No stain*

This requires a high quality phase contrast microscope to distinguish between live and dead cells and plates must be read at the end of the incubation period as the reaction is not stopped. Live cells appear small and refractile with a pale blue/green cytoplasm and an orange centre surrounded by a white halo. Dead cells appear slightly larger than live cells with a dark cytoplasm with little or no halo around the cells.

5.3.1.3. *Eosin or trypan blue*

The disrupted cell membrane allows the entry of these stains into dead cells so that dead cells appear red or blue respectively under visible light. These stains can cause cell damage so the cells must be fixed with neutral formaldehyde after staining.

5.3.2. *Scoring of reactions*

The reactions are scored by estimation of the percentage of dead cells in each well after establishing base line values in the negative and positive controls (Table 2.4).

5.4. *IgM and IgG discrimination*

The reducing agent dithiothreitol (DTT) can be used to distinguish between IgG and IgM reactivity in the lymphocytotoxicity test. The addition of DTT results in the breakdown of the intersubunit disulphide bonds in the IgM molecule leading to the loss of cytotoxicity due to IgM. Prolonged exposure or excess DTT can

Cell Death %	Score	Interpretation
0-10	1	Background cell death, Negative
11-20	2	Doubtful Negative
21-50	4	Weak Positive
51-80	6	Positive
81-100	8	Strong Positive
	0	Unreadable / invalid

Table 2.4. Interpretation of percentage cell death in the LCT reaction.

breakdown the intramolecular disulphide bonds and inactivate complement but this can be inhibited by the addition of cystine.

Screening sera with DTT:

The sera must be tested with and without DTT to allow meaningful analysis of the results.

Techniques have been described that rely on the addition of DTT to the serum or lymphocyte suspension. Both methods (see 5.4.1 and 5.4.2) yield similar results.

5.4.1. *Addition of DTT to the lymphocyte suspension*

- This method has the advantage of not diluting the serum
- Remove an aliquot of the lymphocyte suspension sufficient for the number of plates to be screened.
- Centrifuge for 5 min at 2000rpm
- Resuspend in RPMI containing 0.01M DTT
- Test duplicate plates using lymphocyte suspension with and without DTT in the lymphocytotoxicity assay adding 0.1ml of cystine to 0.9ml of complement to inhibit any further DTT activity.

5.4.2. *Addition of DTT to the serum*

This involves some dilution of the sera and two methods have been described.

5.4.2.1. *Method 1*

The dilution effect is minimised by using 0.1M DTT added directly to the serum.

- Mix 5μl of 0.1M DTT with 45μl of serum and dispense serum onto screening plate. The concentration of DTT in the serum is now 0.01M.
- The procedure for the LCT may be followed as previously described. After the addition of cells the final concentration of DTT will be 0.005M.
- Add 0.1ml of cystine (24mg/ml) to 0.9ml complement to prevent any further breakdown of disulphide bonds in the antibody molecules.

5.4.2.2. *Method 2*

- This method dilutes the serum with an equal volume of DTT but involves an additional incubation step at 37°C to ensure breakdown of the IgM pentamer.
- Mix 1μl of 0.01M DTT with 1μl of serum on a microtest plate and incubate for 30 min at 37°C.
- The procedure for the LCT may be followed as previously described. After the addition of cells the final concentration of DTT will be 0.0025M.
- Add 0.1ml of cystine (24mg/ml) to 0.9ml complement to prevent any further breakdown of disulphide bonds in the antibody molecules.

LCT without DTT	LCT with DTT	Interpretation
Positive	Positive (no change in strength of reaction)	IgG
Positive	Positive (weaker strength of reaction)	IgG + IgM
Positive	Negative	IgM
Negative	Positive	possible IgM blocking antibodies

Table 2.5. Interpretation of DTT testing results

5.5. *Analysis of serum reactivity*

The basic principles of analysis apply whatever methodology or approach is used for antibody detection and identification. The pattern of positive reactions between the test serum and the donor panel of known HLA type is recorded. The specificity of the serum may be explained as the best correlation between the positive reactions with the donor panel and the HLA antigens present on the positive donors. The correlation between serum reactivity and HLA specificity will not always be absolute as the immune response is not normally monoclonal. Patients' sera will contain an array of antibodies with different affinities directed against the different epitopes that make up the HLA specificity. Typing sera are selected for, and sometimes manipulated to give, a restricted operational specificity but patients should be screened to reveal all the HLA specificities contained in their sera.

The polyclonal nature of the immune response together with the extensive polymorphism of the HLA system, the effects of linkage disequlibrium and the marked degree of cross-reactivity between different HLA antigens can present considerable problems in the analysis of serological reaction patterns and the assignment of HLA specificity to a particular serum. Careful attention should also be paid to the cell type, panel and the limitation of the technique when documenting results of serum analysis.

Analysis of patterns of reactivity can be assisted by recording the donor HLA type and serum cytotoxicity scores in an appropriate format such as a cell/serum matrix. If an informative panel has been used it should be possible, where there is a clear cut specificity, to determine antibody specificity by a process of elimination. When performing a manual analysis it is useful to have a record of the number of times each antigen is represented on the panel (see Table 2.2).

Statistical methods may be used to provide an objective assessment of serum reactivity. A 2 x 2 contingency table can be used to calculate the Chi-squared value (χ^2). For example:

		Cells	
		+	-
Serum	+	a	b
	-	c	d

Where for serum with putative specificity "Z":

- a = +/+, number of cells positive for "Z" that react with the test serum (true positive)
- b = +/–, number of cells negative for "Z" that react with the test serum (false positive)
- c = –/+, number of cells positive for "Z" that do not react with the test serum (false negative)
- d = –/–, number of cells negative for "Z" that do not react with the test serum (true negative)

The χ^2 value can be calculated from the following formula:

$$\chi^2 = \frac{(ad - bc)^2 \times (a + b + c + d)}{(a + c) \times (a + b) \times (c + d) \times (b + d)}$$

If the presence of a specific HLA antigen does not correlate with a positive reaction, i.e. the events are independent, the χ^2 value will be low. If the two events are dependent then χ^2 will be high. In the perfect serum there would be no false positives nor false negatives and will equal the total number of comparisons, *n*, but in practice *n* is approached but not reached. This type of analysis is often performed when assessing reagents rather than patients' sera but the χ^2 value will vary with the value of *n* so the correlation coefficient or *r* value is calculated to give an objective assessment of serum performance for a particular specificity independent of *n*.

$$r = \sqrt{\frac{\chi^2}{n}}$$

The ideal tissue typing reagent would have an *r* value of 1.0 but in practice a value of 0.9 for a common specificity is achievable. Other factors have to be considered when selecting typing reagents for example, a lower *r* value may have to suffice for a serum detecting a rare specificity. Most sera contain more than one specificity and in these cases the specificity with the highest χ^2 value is assumed to be the main specificity then these donors are excluded from further analysis and the χ^2 is calculated for the remaining cell serum reactivity. This "Tail" analysis can be repeated until all reactivity is accounted for or no significant χ^2 values can be obtained.

5.6. *Cross reactive group (CREG)/public epitope analysis (PEA)*

It has been known since the 1960s when many of the HLA antigens were being defined that alloantibodies can react with additional HLA antigens other than that of the immunising cell. Determinants shared by many HLA antigens were termed 'public epitopes', e.g. Bw4, Bw6 and 'private epitopes' where specific for a particular HLA molecule. In addition epitopes shared by a discrete group of HLA antigens CREG have been defined by reactivity with alloantibodies and some have been confirmed by reactivity with HLA specific monoclonal antibodies. A number of workers have described a series of public epitopes by analysis of the serum reactivity of a large group of renal patients and now PEA or CREG analysis has become an important tool in analysing serum and in particular, those with high panel reactivity (Takemoto *et al.,* 1992).

HLA-A
A1, A36
A1, A3, A11
A1, A10, A11(A25, A26, A34, A66)
A2, A28(A68, A69)
A2, A9, A28(A68, A69, A24)
A10, A11
A25, A32
A10, A28, A33
A29, A43
A30, A31

HLA-B
B5, B35, B51, B52, B53
B7, B27
B7, B22, B27, B40, B42, B48(B54, B55, B56, B60, B61)
B8, B14, B16, B18, B51, B59(B64, B65, B38, B39)
B12, B13, B21, B44, B45, B49, B50
B15, B17, B21, B35, B70, B62, B63, B57, B58, B49, B50, B71, B72
B27, B13, B47

HLA-C
Cw4, Cw6
Cw5, Cw8

HLA-DR
DR1, DR10
DR3, DR5, DR6, DR17, DR18, DR11, DR12, DR13, DR14

INTERLOCUS HLA-A/B
A2, B17
A9, A23, A24, A25, A32, Bw4

INTERLOCUS HLA-B/C
B46, Cw3

Table 2.6. Serologically defined cross reactive groups

High PRA

The United Kingdom Transplant Support Service Authority's (UKTSSA) definition of a highly sensitised patient is a patient with a serum sample giving a PRA of 85% and this level of reactivity can present a number of problems in defining antibody specificity. The serum may contain non specific IgM antibodies so it essential that a screen with DTT is carried out.

There may be weaker antibodies whose reactivity may be removed with titration to reveal the specificity of the main stimulating antigen. There may also be antibodies directed against public epitopes. Consideration of the HLA types of cell donors who are negative with sera with high PRA will yield more useful information regarding acceptable and unacceptable mismatches.

Computer programmes that will perform statistical analysis of reaction patterns are available. They can cope well with mono or duo specific antibodies but more complex patterns of reactivity will require additional knowledge of both the HLA system and previous sensitisation events e.g. allografts or pregnancies.

Example

Data that may be recorded when performing an analysis of serum reactivity:

- HLA type of the patient or serum donor (if available).
- HLA type of the stimulator e.g. husband, partner and/or graft.

- Panel reactive antibodies (PRA)

  i.e. $\frac{\text{number of positive reactions}}{\text{total number of cells tested}} \times 100$

- Reaction frequency (RF) for a specificity X

  i.e. $\frac{\text{number of true positives for antigen X}}{\text{number of panels cells expressing antigen X}} \times 100$

- Reaction strength (i.e. the percentage of true positive reactions with cytotoxicity scores of 8). This may be calculated for the serum overall or for a particular HLA specificity.

  i.e. $\frac{\text{number of true positives (score 8) for antigen X}}{\text{number of panel cells expressing antigen X}} \times 100$

- Antibody isotype: IgG and /or IgM
- Antibody specificity: e.g. anti- HLA-A2
- Auto antibody status
- Non-HLA antibodies: e.g. anti-endothelial

6. *Antibody Screening by Flow Cytometry*

The routine use of flow cytometric techniques for antibody screening can be regarded as a relatively recent development in the HLA field. Flow cytometry was initially investigated as an alternative crossmatch technique by Garovy (1983) and was shown to be more sensitive than the cytotoxic crossmatch (see Chapter 4). The increased sensitivity may be attributed to a number of factors one of which is the additional reactivity due to the detection of non-cytotoxic antibodies which may be HLA specific. As with the LCT screening, cells and serum are mixed and incubated to allow the formation of immune complexes, the bound antibody is detected by using secondary anti-human immunoglobulin antibodies labelled with flourescent marker such as FITC or RPE. The flow cytometer is then used to identify the different cell populations based on their morphology and whether they have bound antibody present in the serum being tested.

6.1. *Methodology*

The method described is used locally with a Becton Dickinson (BD) FACSCAN or FACSORT. The reagents are from specific manufacturers and each reagent batch standardised for the test. These variables should be investigated and optimised locally.

6.1.1. *Preparation of lymphocyte pools*

Select 16 cell donors to cover all the major cross reactive groups and design a scheme to prepare 4 pools containing lymphocytes from 4 donors.

Example

- Isolate lymphocytes as detailed previously and adjust the cell concentration to 2.5×10^6/ml in PBS containing 1% FCS.
- Pool equal volumes of lymphocytes from 4 donors

The pooled cells may be cryopreserved at this stage as previously described or used directly.

If frozen pooled lymphocytes are used the cells are thawed, washed twice in RPMI with 10% FCS and resuspended in the same medium at 2.5×10^6/ml.

The incubation of cells and serum can be performed using U-bottomed microplates for large numbers, or individual tubes. 50µl of cell suspension is required for each test so the number of cells required should be calculated beforehand.

Each serum should be tested in triplicate.

- Mix 50µl of cell suspension with 50µl of serum and incubate for 45 min at 37°C.
- Wash 5 times in PBS/1% FCS (or 3 times when using tubes)
- Add 50µl of FITC anti-IgG to each cell pellet, mix and incubate in the dark for 30 min at room temperature
- Wash 3 times in PBS/1% FCS
- Resuspend in 175µl of PBS/1% FCS and transfer to glass tubes (when using microplates) suitable for use with the flow cytometer e.g. 50 x 70mm can be used with BD flow cytometers.
- The samples can now be passed through the flow cytometer acquiring a minimum of 10,000 events.

6.2. *Analysis and Interpretation of results*

Once all the samples have been processed, the data can be analysed using the following procedure:

- Using a dot plot of FSC (forward scatter) *versus* SSC (side scatter) draw an analysis region around the lymphocytes

- Produce a histogram of the FL1 fluorescence of the cells contained within the lymphocyte region
- Using the geometric histogram statistic option record the median fluorescence values of FL1
- Calculate the mean + 3SD of the median fluorescence intensity values of the 4 negative controls.

Test sera with median fluorescence values greater than the mean + 3 SD of the negative controls are considered as positive.

To detect antibodies reacting with only T or B cells, a modification of the above procedure (usually performed using tubes) can be used:

After the addition of FITC and the completion of cell washes

- Add 10µl of PE conjugated anti-CD3 for T cells or anti CD19 or 20 for B cells to the appropriate tubes and mix.
- Incubate at 4°C for 20 min in the dark
- Add 4ml of PBS/1% FCS to the tubes and centrifuge at 900g for 3 min
- Remove supernatant and resuspend the lymphocytes in 250µl of PBS/1% FCS.
- The samples can be processed using a flow cytometer (acquiring 25,000 events).

Draw an analysis region around (R1) the lymphocytes using a dot plot of FSC *versus* SSC. Lymphocytes are distinguished by their size and granularity.

From the cells in R1 produce a FL1/FL2 dot plot and draw a region (R2) on this dot plot to include T or B cells that have been stained red.

Thus, from the selected lymphocytes, T or B cells can be distinguished if they have a high FL2 value. Furthermore, T or B cells that have bound patient antibody will have also have a high FL1 value.

To obtain this information from the flow cytometer construct a logical gate of R3 = R1 and R2 and produce an FL1 histogram of cells within R3.

Using the geometric histogram statistic option record the median fluorescence values for FL1.

From the results of the 4 negative control sera calculate the mean + 3 SD. This can be used as the cut off between positive and negative but the definition of positive and the clinical significance must be assessed together with local information comparing cytotoxic crossmatching with flow cytometric techniques and retrospective analysis of transplant outcome (Harmer *et al.,* 1996).

T and B lymphocytes that have bound alloantibody can be distinguished simultaneously by the use of a third fluorochrome RPE-CY5.

6.3. *Advantages/disadvantages*

The main advantages of flow cytometric techniques are the increased sensitivity when compared to the LCT and the detection of non-complement fixing antibodies allowing the early detection of sensitisation.

Flow cytometric techniques may also detect non-HLA, lymphocyte reactive antibodies but the clinical relevance of these antibodies is unclear.

6.4. *Modifications of flow screening technique*

- Azide (0.01%) may be added to the diluent and washing reagent to prevent any capping and internalisation of antibody/antigen complexes
- The number of cell donors in each pool may be increased, but in very large pools positivity due to reactivity with a single donor within the pool may not reach the threshold level
- Single donor preparation instead of pooled lymphocytes may enable the determination of antibody specificity where the panel reactivity is not high . However, this can be a labour intensive process if the flow cytometer does not have an automatic sampler and if there is no cell washer for all the tubes
- EBV transformed B cell lines can be used instead of PBL and can ensure a constant supply of cells with uncommon phenotypes, allow standardisation of the panel and allow more control of the process maintaining the cell panel. Large numbers of donor lymphocytes may be obtained from buffy coats produced as a by-product of processing blood donations at blood transfusion centres
- FlowPRA^{TM} - microparticles coated with purified HLA class I and class II antigen are commercially available for the detection HLA specific antibody in serum. The beads and serum are mixed and any bound antibody is detected with a flourescent anti-human IgG and the flow cytometer can be used to quantify the intensity of flourescence on the beads. The recent development of microparticles coated with purified HLA antigen should overcome the problem of false positive due to non-HLA antibodies.

6.5. *Quality control*

6.5.1. *Control sera*

Negative control sera from 4 untransfused males, blood group AB who have tested negative for the presence of lymphocyte reactive antibodies and frozen in suitable volumes are used .

These are highly selected negative control sera and may not be representative of the normal population. Pooled AB serum may also be used but the individual donors should be pre-screened for lymphocyte reactivity.

Positive controls: Locally, both a strong and a weak positive control alloantiserum are used to ensure that the performance of the test is adequately monitored. These are stored frozen in suitable volumes.

6.5.2. *Conjugates*

Each batch of conjugates should be titrated and standardised to allow comparison of data.

6.5.3. *Calibration of the flow cytometer*

Beads are commercially available to enable the optical alignment of the flow cytometer and also the performance of the wavelength detectors to be checked.

7. *Antibody screening by Enzyme Linked Immunosorbent Assay (ELISA)*

ELISA based techniques have often been the technique of choice for antibody detection for a number of antigen systems, particularly where there has been a requirement for testing large numbers of samples.

The basic principle of the technique is as follows: HLA antigen is purified and immobilised on a microwell plate, directly or via an antibody directed against a non polymorphic region of the HLA antigen. Any patient's antibody bound specifically to the immobilised antigen can be detected with an enzyme linked secondary antibody which upon addition of specific substrate catalyses a colour change reaction which is detected in an ELISA reader.

Commercial kits are available for the detection of HLA class I specific antibody and two approaches have been used for immobilisation of antigen and antibody detection:

1. HLA antigen is isolated from the platelets of a large panel of donors of different ethnic origin (GTI QuikScreen). In this test the antigen is bound to the microwell under conditions that will preserve its protein activity. The aim is to ensure that in every well there is HLA antigen present covering all the main HLA class I specificities in sufficient quantity to react with specific antibodies in patient sera.

This ELISA test can only be used to determine the presence or absence of HLA specific antibody.

2. HLA antigen is isolated from a selected panel of cell or platelet donors or cell lines from these donors (SangStat.-PRA-STAT, GTI QuikId or Lambda antigen tray LAT™M). Antibodies directed against the non polymorphic region of the HLA class I molecule i.e. the α3 domain, are used to immobilise the HLA antigen to the microwell ensuring the more polymorphic α1 and α2 domains are available for antibody binding. The test is designed to cover all the major HLA specificities at least once, thus it should be possible to determine antibody specificity in those sera which show a restricted panel reactivity. PRA-STAT ELISA (Harmer *et al.*, 1997) and the LAT™M test can also detect HLA class II antibodies.

7.1. *Methodology*

Detailed methodology is provided with each kit and the basic principle will be given.

- Equilibrate reagents and plates
- Prepare negative and positive controls
- Dilute patient sera
- Add sera to be tested to ELISA plate as detailed in method
- Incubate & wash off any unbound patient antibody
- Add enzyme linked anti-IgG (IgG,A,M) reagent
- Incubate & wash
- Add enzyme substrate
- Incubate
- Stop reaction
- Read the absorbance at the specified wavelength

7.2. *Analysis and Interpretation of results*

The manufacturers may give a value or ratio where the patient serum should be considered as positive: e.g. twice the mean of the negative control values for GTI-QuikScreen, but these should be evaluated locally with retrospective analysis of crossmatch and screening data (Lucas *et al.*, 1997; Kerman *et al.*, 1996). Duplicates wells should not differ by greater than 20% of the mean of the 2 values.

The specificity of the conjugate should be taken into account when reporting results as not all the commercial kits detect IgM antibodies.

7.3. *Advantages/disadvantages*

ELISA detects both cytotoxic and non-cytotoxic HLA specific antibodies and not irrelevant autoreactive antibodies or ATG (anti-thymocyte globulin). The technique is technically simple, the read-out is objective and it lends itself to mass testing.

7.4. *Antibody targets*

There are numerous polymorphic structures on the cell surface that are potential targets for antibody and patients may produce antibodies directed against one or more of these structures. Pre-formed antibodies directed against HLA antigens and endothelial antigens have been shown to be associated with loss of allografts. Patients' sera may also contain antibodies that are thought not to be important for graft survival but react with lymphocytes so it is important that appropriate targets are selected to determine the specificity of antibodies detected.

Table 2.7 shows a number of targets that have been used for the detection of HLA specific antibodies. The use of purified HLA antigens removes any ambiguity regarding antibody specificity provided that the antigen structure is maintained in its preparation.

Antibody target	HLA specificity of the antibodies detected	Antibody isotype	Technique most commonly used for detection
Peripheral blood lymphocytes	Class I (+/- class II) non-HLA auto	IgG, IgM	Cytotoxicity Flow cytometry Immunofluorescence
T cells	Class I non-HLA auto	IgG, IgM	Cytotoxicity Flow cytometry
B cells	Class I and II non-HLA auto	IgG, IgM	Cytotoxicity Flow cytometry
Spleen cells	Class I and Class II	IgG, IgM	Cytotoxicity Flow cytometry Immunofluorescence
CLL cells	Class I and Class II	IgG, IgM	Cytotoxicity Flow cytometry
EBV cell lines	Class I and Class II	IgG, IgA	Flow cytometry
Endothelial	Class I and Class II	IgG, IgA	Flow cytometry
Epithelial	Class I and Class II	IgG, IgA	Flow cytometry
Soluble antigen*	Class I or Class II	IgG, IgA	Flow cytometry ELISA
Purified HLA antigen	Class I or Class II	IgG, IgM, IgA	ELISA

Table 2.7. Targets for detection of HLA-specific antibodies

8. *Screening strategies*

It is clear that there are a number of factors that can influence the choice of strategy employed for antibody screening. It is important that the technique used for screening should be at least as sensitive if not the same technique as that used for crossmatching.

Detection of antibody by ELISA can be relatively inexpensive but the cost of identification of specificity by ELISA may prevent its routine use by many laboratories. Antibody screening strategies will also be influenced by the patient group being tested.

8.1. *Patients immunologically refractory to random platelet transfusion*

The most significant cause of immunological refractoriness to random donor platelet transfusion is the presence of cytotoxic HLA class I specific antibodies in the patient's serum. As previously mentioned these are multi-transfused patients and IgG antibodies are most important. Thus, a possible strategy would be to:

- test all patients by ELISA for HLA class I antibody detection
- test those ELISA positive samples to identify HLA specificity by cytotoxicity

This would also detect non cytotoxic HLA specific antibodies but their role in immunological refractoriness is unclear.

8.2. *Patients awaiting solid organ transplantation*

The detection and identification of both HLA class I and class II specific antibodies will be important for this group of patients.

Lymphocytotoxicity can be used to both detect and identify HLA specific antibodies - but non-cytotoxic antibodies would not be detected and are relevant for those patients requiring second renal allografts.

Flow cytometric screening techniques are very sensitive and will detect antibodies that will react with T-cells and B-cells, most of which will be HLA class I or II specific. If automated sampling is used this is a good antibody detection technique but positive samples would require further screening for antibody identification.

ELISA techniques for detection of HLA specific antibodies are relatively inexpensive but ELISA for antibody identification is much more expensive and where a significant proportion of the waiting list is sensitised, the cost may be unacceptable. Careful consideration would need to be given to the crossmatching technique that was employed as the use and clinical relevance of ELISA will require evaluation in more transplant centres (Worthington *et al.,* 1998; Zaer *et al.,* 1997).

In practice, laboratories use a combination of techniques as at present there is no one technique that will provide all the relevant information.

9. *Troubleshooting*

9.1. *Isolation of mononuclear cells*

Problem	Possible Cause	Action
Diffuse layer of lymphocytes	Poor blood/Ficoll interface	Re-layer lymphocytes ensuring that the interface with Ficoll is not disturbed.
Granulocytes in the lymphocyte layer	Ventilated organ donors or old samples	Pre-treat sample with carbonyl iron incubate at 37°C
Red cells in the lymphocytes layer	Often seen in particular patient groups e.g. haemoglobinopathy patients, or due to nucleated red cells e.g. cord blood samples	Treat blood sample with Red Out ™ to agglutinate red cells. Dextran 110 causes red cells to rouleau and pass to the bottom of the centrifuge tube as with agglutinated red cells.

9.2. *IgM and IgG discrimination*

Problem	Possible solution
IgG-positive control negative	Check concentration of DTT. Check cystine was added to complement
IgM control positive with DTT. Patient with high titre IgM	Pre-incubation of serum and DTT at 37°C may be required. Check concentration of DTT

Summary

The detection and identification of HLA antibodies has progressed from a relatively crude, non-specific lymphocytotoxicity technique to sensitive flow cytometric methods to highly specific ELISA techniques. The clinical relevance of cytotoxic HLA antibodies has been clearly established in patients receiving solid organ transplants and immunologically refractory to random platelet transfusion. The non-cytotoxic HLA antibodies detected by flow cytometry or ELISA are more relevant in patients requiring a second allograft.

The role of HLA antibodies in the acute and chronic phases of graft rejection needs to be clarified and therefore post transplant monitoring will become crucial to establish such role (Abe *et al.,* 1997).

The screening strategies and techniques used for the detection of HLA antibodies will depend upon the group of patients involved, i.e. awaiting solid organ transplantation, immunologically refractory to random platelet transfusion, women with recurrent abortions to name but a few. The importance of accurate, reproducible and relevant data cannot be understated as decisions made from this data can influence many facets of patient care.

References

Abe, M, Kawai, T, Futatsuyama, K, Tanabe K, Fuchinoue, S *et al.* (1997). Postoperative production of anti-donor antibody and chronic rejection in renal transplantation. *Transplantation*, **63**: 1616-1619

Anasetti, C, Amos, D, Beatty, PG, Appelbaum, FR, Bensinger, W *et al.* (1989) Effect of HLA compatibility on engraftment of bone marrow transplants in patients with leukemia or lymphoma. *N Engl. J. Med*, **320**: 197-204

Boyum, A (1968) Isolation of mononuclear cells and granulocytes from human blood. *Scand. J. Clin. and Lab. Invest*, **97**: 77

Chapman, JR, Taylor, CJ, Ting, A and Morris, PJ (1986) Immunoglobulin class and specificity of antibodies causing positive T-cell crossmatches. Relationship to renal transplant outcome. *Transplantation*, **42**: 608-613

Ettenger, RB, Jordan, SC and Fine, RN (1983). Cadaver renal transplant outcome in recipients with autolymphocytotoxic antibodies. *Transplantation*, **35**: 429-431

Garovoy, MR, Rheinschmidt, MA, Bigos, M, Perkins, H and Colombe, B (1983). Flow cytometry analysis: a high technology crossmatch technique facilitating transplantation. *Transplant Proc*, **15**: 1939-1944

Hansen, JA, Clift, RA, Mickelson, EM, Nisperos, B and Thomas, ED (1981) Marrow transplantation from donors other than HLA identical siblings. *Human Immunology*, **1**: 31-40

Harmer, AW, Haskard, D, Koffman, GC and Welsh, KI (1990) Novel antibodies asociated with unexplained loss of renal allografts. *Transplant International*, **3**: 66-69

Harmer, AW, Garner, S, Bell, AE, Anyanwu, C, Cavanagh, G *et al.* (1996). Evaluation of the flow cytometric crossmatch. Preliminary results of a multicentre study. *Transplantation*, **61**: 1108-1111

Harmer, AW, Heads, AJ and Vaughan, RW (1997). Detection of HLA class I and class II specific antibodies by flow cytometry and PRA-STAT screening in renal transplant recipients. *Transplantation*, **63**: 1828-1832

Kennedy, LJ, Bourel, D, Dejour, G, Fauchet, R and Bodmer, JG (1987). A European workshop to investigate technical problems of using HLA monoclonal antibodies in microlymphocytotoxicity assays. *Tissue Antigens,* **29**: 43-54

Kerman, RH, Susskind, B, Buelow, R, Regan, J, Pouletty, P *et al.* (1996) Correlation of ELISA-detected IgG and IgA anti-HLA antibodies in pretransplant sera with renal allograft rejection. *Transplantation*, **62**: 201-205

Lobo, PI, Spencer, CE, Stevenson, WC and Pruett, TI (1995). Evidence demonstrating poor kidney graft survival when acute rejections are associated with IgG donor-specific lymphotoxin. *Transplantation*, **59**: 357-360

Lucas, DP, Paparounis, ML, Myers, L, Hart, JM and Zachany, AA (1997). Detection of HLA class-I specific antibodies by the QuikScreen enzyme linked immunosorbent assay. *Clinical and Diagnostic Laboratory Immunology*, **4**: 252-257

Martin, S, Brenchley, PE, Postlethwaite, RJ, Johnson, RWG and Dyer, PA (1991) Detection of anti-epithelial cell antibodies in association with paediatric renal transplant failure using a novel microcytotoxicity assay. *Tissue Antigens*, **37**: 152-155

Martin, S and Harmer, A (1999) Crossmatching by Lymphocytotoxicity and Flow Cytometry. In: *Histocompatibility Testing* (Ed. Bidwell, JL and Navarrete, C), pp.125-143. Imperial College Press, London

McCloskey, DJ, Brown, J and Navarrete, C (1993). Serological typing of HLA-A, -B, and -C antigens. In: *Handbook of HLA Typing Techniques*, (Ed. Hui, KM and Bidwell, JL), pp.175-247. CRC Press, Boca Raton

Moraes, JR and Statsny, P (1977). Human endothelial cell antigens: molecular independence from HLA and expression in blood monocytes. *Transpl Proc*, **9**: 605-607

Navarrete, C, Fernandez, N, Alonso, MC and Festenstein, H (1986) Ontogenic and functional implications of the differential expression of HLA-DQ antigens on leukemia cells. *Human Immunology*, **16**: 52-68

Perry, C, Brenchley, PEC, Johnson, RWG and Martin, S (1998). An association between antibodies specific for endothelial cells and renal transplant failure. *Transplant Immunology*, **6**: 101-106

Reed, E and Suciu-Foca, N (1995). Anti-idiotype assay. In: *ASHI Laboratory Manual,* Third Edition. (Ed. Phelan, DL, Mickelson, EM, Noreen, HS, Shroyer, TM, Cluff, DM *et al.*), pp.ID8.1-ID8.10. ASHI.

Sumitran-Karuppan, S and Möller, E (1996). The use of magnetic beads coated with soluble HLA class I or class II proteins in antibody screening and for specificity determination of donor reactive antibodies. *Transplantation*, **61**: 1539-1545

Takahashi, K and Sawasaki, Y (1992) Rare spontaneous transformed human endothelial cell line provides useful research tool. *In Vitro Cell Dev Biol,* **28A**: 380-382

Takemoto, S, Gjertson, DW and Terasaki, PI (1992). HLA matching: A comparison of conventional and molecular approaches. In: *Clinical Transplants 1992*, (Ed. Terasaki, PI and Cecka, JM), pp.413-434. UCLA.

Terasaki, PI and McClelland, JD (1964). Microdroplet assay of human serum cytotoxins. *Nature*, **204**: 998-1000

Ting, A and Morris, PJ (1983). Successful transplantation with a positive T and B cell crossmatch due to autoreactive antibodies. *Tissue Antigens*, **21**: 219-226

Worthington, JE, Thomas, AA, Dyer, PA and Martin, S (1998). Detection of HLA-specific antibodies by PRA-STAT and their association with transplant outcome. *Transplantation*, **65**: 121-125

Zaer, F, Metz, S and Scornik, JC (1997) Antibody screening by enzyme-linked immunosorbent assay using pooled soluble HLA in renal transplant candidates. *Transplantation*, **63**: 48-51

CHAPTER 3

DETECTION OF SOLUBLE HLA

V. Rebmann and H. Grosse-Wilde
Institute of Immunology
University Hospital of Essen
Germany

Introduction

In 1970, van Rood (van Rood *et al.*, 1970) was the first to show that HLA class I antigens exist in a soluble form (sHLA-I) in serum. This was demonstrated by the neutralisation of HLA-A2 antibodies with serum of an HLA-A2 positive individual. In the same year Charlton and Zmijewski (1970) found that soluble HLA-B7 antigens (sHLA-B7) were present in the lipoprotein fraction of human serum. Although Gussow and Ploegh (1987) denied the biological relevance of soluble HLA antigen, three international meetings on sHLA (Pouletty *et al.*, 1993; Grumet *et al.*, 1994; Puppo *et al.*, 1997), and a growing number of clinical studies since these meetings, have clearly underlined the important role of sHLA molecules in infection and autoimmune diseases, in tumours and in transplantation.

Here, we summarise the most clinically and biologically significant features of sHLA molecules, focus on the detection methods of sHLA molecules with respect to their molecular structures, and try to give practical guidelines for the detection of sHLA molecules.

Structures of sHLA molecules and their biological role

Structure of soluble HLA class I and class II antigens

Membrane-anchored HLA class I antigens are composed of cytoplasmic, transmembrane, and extracytoplasmic segments. With the exception of HLA-C antigens, HLA class I heavy chains are predominantly associated with beta-2-microglobulin (β2m) and endogenously-derived peptides at the cell surface. However, studies of sHLA-I antigens in body fluids revealed a higher heterogeneity of molecular size and molecule structures than their respective membrane-anchored ones. Purification of serum sHLA-I molecules by size exclusion chromatography revealed two sHLA-I-specific peaks with approximately molecular weights of 50 kD and of 150 kD, indicating that sHLA-I exists as a heterodimer with β2m, and as higher order multimers in serum (Reisfeld *et al.*, 1976). In the urine of renal transplant recipients, only one sHLA-I peak was found with an approximate size of 44 kD: this could further be dissociated into components of β2m and of sHLA-I heavy chain (Vincent *et al.*,

1976). Original reports of the sHLA-I molecular weight variants by SDS-PAGE analysis demonstrated that sHLA-I heavy chains exist mainly in three different molecular weight forms (Krangel 1984, 1985, 1986, 1987; Dobbe *et al.,* 1988) (Figure 3.1).

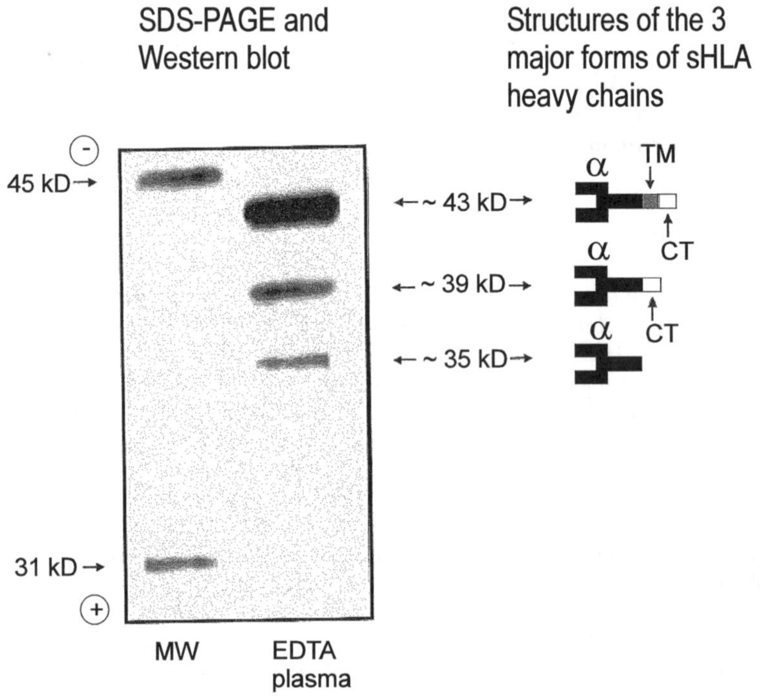

Figure 3.1. Molecular variants of sHLA class I molecules. Left panel: typical molecular weight variants of sHLA molecules obtained after SDS-PAGE analysis. Right panel: corresponding structures of the sHLA-I size variants. MW, molecular weight markers; TM, transmembrane domain; CT, cytoplasmic domain

The largest molecule is identical to membrane-anchored HLA class I antigens, thus representing the complete HLA-I heavy chain with a molecular size of 43 kD. It is thought that the 43 kD sHLA-I variant is the result of shedding processes. The smallest sHLA-I molecule, suggested to be a proteolytic cleavage product of membrane-anchored HLA-I, has a molecular weight of 35 kD and is identical in size to HLA molecules obtained after papain digestion of B lymphoblastoid cells. Since papain hydrolyses HLA-I molecules preferentially at amino acid position 271, the resulting molecules lack the transmembrane and cytoplasmic segments. This proteolytic cleavage product cannot be detected by immunoblotting with rabbit antiserum generated against a peptide corresponding to residues at amino acid position 328-338 within the cytoplasmic domain (Dobbe *et al.,* 1988). The intermediate sHLA-I variant has a molecular size of 39 kD. Krangel (1986) was the first to show that the 39 kD variant is synthesised from alternatively-spliced transcripts lacking exon 5, encoding the hydrophobic transmembrane anchor, and presents consequently as a secreted glycoprotein. Later studies using polymerase chain reaction and DNA sequencing from cellular RNA of peripheral blood mononuclear cells (Yang and Le 1994; Huang *et al.,* 1997) confirmed the earlier results by Krangel (1984). All three sHLA-I variants are found to be associated with β2m, since they can be immunoprecipitated with the monoclonal antibody (mAb) W6/32, a mAb recognising an HLA-I epitope within the α2-domain at residue 143 in association with β2m (Shields and Ribaudo 1998). In addition to β2m-associated sHLA-I, Pickl *et al* (1993) described sHLA-I molecules in supernatants of cell lines, and in human serum samples, which were not associated with β2m. In this study, the mAb LA-45 reacting with a linear epitope of the HLA class I α1-domain at residues 62 and 63 was used as detection reagent for β2m-free sHLA-I molecules. "Free" sHLA-I chains have a molecular weight of 35 kD and are proteolytic cleavage products of a metalloprotease (Demaria, 1992).

In addition to classical sHLA-I molecules, two HLA-G-specific transcripts have been described which lack exons 5 and 6 but retain the intron 4 sequence, resulting in a premature translation termination codon (Fujii *et al.,* 1994). One of the two transcripts also lacks exon 3, but both transcripts should be expressed as soluble HLA-G (sHLA-G) proteins since the transmembrane and intracellular domains were untranslated. In cell culture supernatants, the sHLA-G isoforms are found to display molecular weights of 35 kD and 27 kD. In amniotic fluids, however, sHLA-G are unusually glycosylated, leading to molecular sizes between 37 and 50 kD (McMaster, 1998).

Limited information is available on the molecular structures of soluble HLA class II (sHLA-II) antigens. sHLA-II should exist as a heterotrimer composed of the

Fluid	sHLA-I	sHLA-II
Plasma/Serum	+++	+++
Joint	+++	+++
Amnion	++	++
Urine	++	++
Bile	+	+
BAL	+	+
Cerebrospinal fluid	+	-
Sweat	+	?
Tears	+	?
Saliva	?	?

Table 3.1. Presence of sHLA molecules in body fluids.

class II α-chain, β-chain and peptide. It is likely that similar mechanisms are implicated for the production of sHLA-II molecules as for sHLA-I, i.e. shedding, proteolytic cleavage of membrane-anchored class II molecules, and alternative splicing yielding truncated soluble forms of class II molecules. With regard to the latter, alternatively spliced transcripts missing the transmembrane region have been described for certain HLA-DQB1 alleles, and their existence at the protein level in supernatants of homozygous B-lymphoblastoid cell lines (B-LCL) provide evidence for this (Briata *et al.,* 1989). In addition, alternatively spliced products for truncated cytoplasmic tails are reported for HLA-DR, DQ, and DP β-chains, but the respective soluble forms have not yet been found in body fluids (Auffray *et al.,* 1987; Tsukamoto *et al.,* 1987). Our own immunoprecipitation studies of plasma samples using polyclonal rabbit antiserum D77533 (anti HLA class II α-chain-specific) and C77532 (anti-HLA class II α,β-chain-specific) (Neefjes *et al.,* 1990) revealed 5 major sHLA class II variants in SDS-PAGE analysis (Figure 3.2).

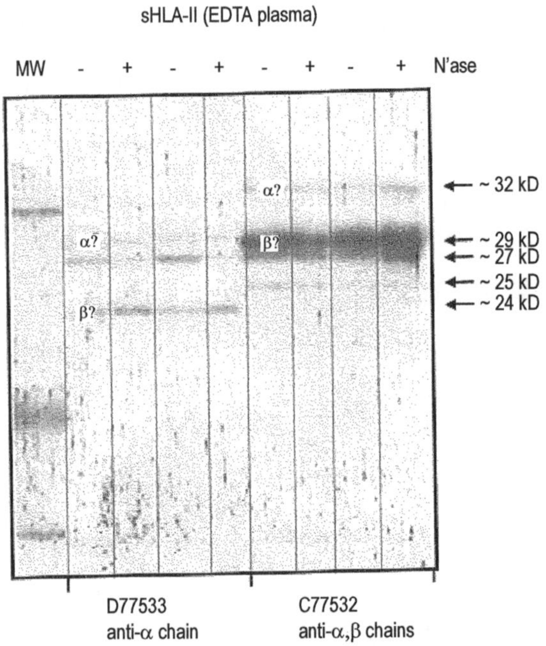

Figure 3.2. Molecular weight variants of sHLA-II molecules. The sHLA-II molecules from EDTA-plasma samples were immunoprecipitated either by the polyclonal antibody D77533 (specific for the α-chain of HLA class II) or by the polyclonal antibody C77532 (specific for the α- and β-chain of HLA class II). SDS-PAGE clearly reveals 5 different size variants of sHLA-II even after neuraminidase (N'ase) treatment.

Although the assessment of the sHLA-II variants observed to specific HLA class II isotypes (sHLA-DR, DQ, DP) remains to be further investigated, the data clearly demonstrate a high degree of heterogeneity of sHLA class II molecules in blood samples which might be released by different mechanisms. Furthermore we recently identified sHLA-DR molecules in the plasma which were complexed with the invariant chain (CD74), formerly thought only to be present in the cytoplasm or on the cell surface (Rebmann *et al.,* 1997).

Soluble HLA molecules in healthy individuals

Although the absolute amount of sHLA levels seems to be a matter of debate, there is an overall consensus in the following 3 areas:

1. sHLA molecules are present in the majority of body fluids, in which the highest relative levels are observed in plasma samples and the lowest in tears (Table 3.1)

2. The quantities of β2m-associated sHLA-I molecules in plasma or serum are significantly associated with certain HLA class I allotypes, indicating that the expression of sHLA-I molecules is under genetic control. As demonstrated in several population studies, HLA-A23 and A24 (Reisfeld *et al.,* 1976; Billing *et al.,* 1977; Kao *et al.,* 1988; Doxiadis *et al.,* 1989) and HLA-A29 and A33 (Adamashvili *et al.,* 1996) are associated with high sHLA-I levels; whereas HLA-A2 (Hagihara *et al.,* 1994) and HLA-A26 (Doxiadis *et al.,* 1989) are associated with low levels. The association of HLA-A9 with high sHLA-I levels is found in all subjects, but those of HLA-A29 and A33 differ with respect to the ethnic groups. HLA-A29 is associated with high sHLA-I levels primarily in Caucasians, and HLA-A33 primarily in African Americans (Adamashvili *et al.,* 1996). Besides this, in the Japanese population it has been found that donors which are negative for HLA-A2 but positive for HLA-A24 have significantly increased sHLA-I levels compared to donors which were positive for both allotypes HLA-A2 and HLA-A24 (Hagihara *et al.,* 1994). Therefore, HLA-A2 may have a suppressive effect on sHLA-I levels (Adamashvili *et al.,* 1996). For HLA-B allotypes there is evidence that high sHLA-I concentrations are associated with HLA-B14 and B62 (Zavazava *et al.,* 1990) and low levels with HLA-B47, B27, and B37 (Doxiadis *et al.,* 1989). However, the relationship of high and low sHLA-I levels to the above described HLA class I allotypes is not predictive of whether these HLA allotypes are present in high or low amount in the plasma, or whether all HLA allotypes demonstrate enhanced or repressed released. With regard to this, Kubens *et al.* analysed the presence of sHLA allotypes in plasma samples of 344 HLA class I-typed individuals by one dimensional isoelectric focusing of sHLA-I molecules immunoprecipitated with mAb W6/32 (Kubens *et al.,* 1994). It was found that sHLA-A24, B7, B18 and B62 were detectable in nearly all donors positive for these HLA allotypes, but sHLA-A26, B8 and B44 were rarely identified in the respective HLA allotypes. This observation supports the hypothesis that HLA class I genes can be divided in high secretor and low secretor status, where HLA-A24 and HLA-B62 belong to the high secretor, and HLA-A26 to the low secretor groups. The expression of at least two sHLA-I molecular weight variants seems also to be regulated. Dobbe *et al.,* (1988) were the first to show by SDS-PAGE analysis that an increased intensity of the 43 kD sHLA-I variant was associated

with the HLA-A24 allotype. One explanation for this enhanced shedding of HLA-A24 antigens might be the amino acid exchange of lysine for asparagine at residue 312 within the transmembrane domain (Aebi *et al.*, 1987) which may impair the anchoring of HLA-A24 molecules in the membrane. For the 39 kD variant, Haga *et al.*, (1991) reported that the lack of the 39 kD sHLA-I variant in plasma was associated with HLA-B7 and with female gender. These findings could not be confirmed by our group (Kubens *et al.*, 1994) but we were able to show in 12 families with 61 members, that absence or presence of the 39 kD variant was clearly inherited in linkage with HLA haplotypes. To date, few clear correlations between individual HLA-DR, DQ or DP allotypes and high or low amounts of sHLA-II have been described. However, an early report by Westhoff *et al.*, (1991) found an association between HLA-DR8 and low sHLA-II levels, but without reaching statistical significance. Another group reported an association between HLA-DR3 and high sHLA-II levels (Weyand *et al.*, 1991); and in the Japanese population an association between HLA-DR11 and high sHLA-II levels has been reported (Hagihara *et al.*, 1994).

3. Plasma release of sHLA-I (Doxiadis *et al.*, 1989), sHLA-II (Westhoff *et al.*, 1991), and sHLA-G (Rebmann *et al.*, 1999b) are constant over time in healthy subjects. However, sHLA-I and sHLA-II levels may be upregulated in vitro (Capobianchi *et al.*, 1985; Le *et al.*, 1995; Fellous *et al.*, 1982; Brieva *et al.*, 1990) and in vivo (Aulitzky *et al.*, 1991; Hillebrand *et al.*, 1994) by proinflammatory cytokines as TNFα, IL-2, and IFNα/γ. Interestingly, for fibrobast cells it has been shown that sHLA-I alternatively spliced transcripts are released in response of IFNγ and TNFα in a time and dose-dependent fashion (He and Le, 1995).

Clinical and biological relevance of sHLA

Infectious disease

Since sHLA levels increase in response to cytokines, it is not surprising that elevated sHLA levels have been observed during immunologically active periods, for example in infection diseases. Thus in patients suffering from varicella-zoster virus meningitis, high sHLA-I levels are observed in cerebrospinal fluid (CSF), associated with lymphocyte activation (Alvarez-Cermeno *et al.*, 1989). Little information is available on sHLA levels during bacterial infectious diseases. In a very recent report however, it has been demonstrated that low sHLA-DR plasma levels promote the development of sepsis in severely injured patients after polytrauma (Ditschkowski *et al.*, 1999).

Further, sHLA-I serum levels are significantly increased in patients with chronic hepatitis (Puppo *et al.*, 1995), in patients with active tuberculosis (Inostroza *et al.*, 1994), in patients with haemorrhagic fever with renal syndrome (Park *et al.*, 1997), and in children with atopic dermatitis (Moore *et al.*, 1997).

AIDS

In AIDS patients, elevated sHLA-I and sHLA-II levels are found in serum and in CSF (Alvarez-Cermeno *et al.,* 1990; Puppo *et al.,* 1990; Filaci *et al.,* 1995). It appears that the degree of sHLA-I increase correlates with the stage of the disease (Puppo *et al.,* 1990, 1994). It has been shown that serum sHLA-I molecules obtained from AIDS patients block specific cytotoxic T cells, suggesting that sHLA-I molecules or increased sHLA-I levels play a role in the suppression of immune response in AIDS patients (Puppo *et al.,* 1994).

Autoimmune disease

Levels of sHLA are also affected by autoimmune diseases such as rheumatoid arthritis (RA), systemic lupus erythematosis (SLE), and multiple sclerosis (MS). Elevated sHLA-I and sHLA-II levels have been found in serum and synovial fluid of RA patients (Weyand *et al.,* 1991; Stevenson *et al.,* 1990; Wolf *et al.,* 1998). However, differences of sHLA-I augmentation are observed among the ethnic groups of RA patients due to the different incidence of high secretor HLA class I alleles in some races e.g. HLA-A23 and A33 Black Americans (Adamashvili *et al.,* 1997). For SLE patients, a strong correlation between disease activity and high levels of β2m-associated as well as β2m-free sHLA-I molecules has been described (Bresciani *et al.,* 1998). The dominant appearance of the 43 kD sHLA-I variants in serum samples of SLE patients may reflect an increased shedding of these molecules from cell membranes. Controversial data on sHLA levels are reported for MS patients. Whereas Filaci *et al.* (1997) found increased sHLA-I and decreased sHLA-II levels in the plasma of MS-Patients, Ott *et al.* (1998) observed no differences in sHLA-I plasma levels between MS patients and controls, but significantly increased sHLA-II plasma levels. Conflicting results concerning sHLA-II levels in CSF were also reported by both groups. These discrepancies might be due to the different ELISA formats used and/or the small numbers of patients analysed.

An interesting finding was obtained from comparing sHLA-I levels in elderly subjects who respond to typhoid vaccinations, with those who did not respond (Saririan *et al.,* 1993). In the responders, sHLA-I levels detected before vaccination were higher than in non-responders. Furthermore, the sHLA-I levels increased after vaccination in responders whilst the sHLA-I levels remained low in non-responders, suggesting that sHLA-I plasma levels are associated with the capacity to generate an immune response.

Cancer

Relatively few studies have analysed sHLA levels in tumour patients. In patients with advanced gastric cancer, the total amount of sHLA-I in serum was found to be lower than in patients with earlier stages of disease (Shimura *et al.,* 1994). Lower sHLA-I levels were also observed in patients with malignant liver diseases compared to patients with other reasons for liver failure (McMillan *et al.,* 1997). In patients with acute lymphoblastoid leukemia, sHLA-II serum levels were significantly reduced compared to the sHLA-II levels of those with acute myeloid leukemia (Stevenson *et al.,* 1986).

Transplantation

Significantly increased sHLA-I serum levels have been observed during acute allograft rejection episodes in liver (Tilg *et al.,* 1992; Puppo *et al.,* 1994), heart (Zavazava *et al.,* 1993), kidney (Drouet *et al.,* 1995; Yang *et al.,* 1995), kidney/pancreas (Abendroth *et al.,* 1995), and lung transplant patients (DeVito-Haynes *et al.,* 1997). Furthermore, in body fluids closely related to the transplanted allograft, sHLA-I levels have also been found to be elevated during rejection episodes (Pollard *et al.,* 1989; DeVito-Haynes *et al.,* 1997). As the increased sHLA-I serum levels declined to normal values after the successful treatment of the rejection with immunosuppressive drugs, one can assume that the augmentation of sHLA-I is a result of immune activation induced by an in vivo antigenic challenge. This mechanism may also be responsible for the increase in sHLA-I during acute graft-versus-host disease (GvHD) in bone marrow recipients (Tsuji *et al.,* 1985; Westhoff *et al.,* 1989; Puppo *et al.,* 1996; Liem *et al.,* 1997). The clinical significance of these observations is still controversial. Puppo *et al.,* (1994, 1996) pointed out that an increase in sHLA-I predicts the onset of acute rejection and the onset of GvHD in liver and bone morrow recipients, respectively. Several other studies, however, have not confirmed these findings, since an augmentation of sHLA-I was also detected during episodes of viral and bacterial infection diseases (Tilg *et al.,* 1992; Liem *et al.,* 1997). Thus, monitoring of sHLA-I was found not to be a useful tool to distinguish between acute allogaft rejection episodes, acute GvHD, and other transplant-related complications. For liver recipients it has been shown that after transplantation, the contribution of sHLA-I size variants to total sHLA-I amounts changes drastically during immune activation, pointing to different mechanisms of sHLA-I release (Rebmann *et al.,* 1999a). During acute liver graft rejection, the 35 kD variant seems to be the most prominent sHLA-I molecule, indicating that the increase of total sHLA-I is due to an enhanced proteolytic cleavage of membrane-anchored HLA class I antigens. One study examined total sHLA-II in normal individuals and heart, liver, and kidney transplant patients. Here, there was no association either with rejection or with other transplant-related complications. Moreover in this study, the changes in sHLA-II levels did not appear with changes in sHLA-I levels (McDonald *et al.,* 1994). However, another study analysing sHLA-II levels in seven patients following bone marrow transplantation and five liver recipients, revealed that an augmentation of sHLA-II levels was associated with acute rejection and acute GvHD (Filaci *et al.,* 1995). Thus, although monitoring of total sHLA seems to be of doubtful use in the management of patient care, the monitoring of donor-derived sHLA molecules appears to be important as a non-invasive parameter for the recognition of acute rejection, since these sHLA-I molecules appear to reflect the status of the allograft. In addition to this, donor-derived sHLA molecules might be able to induce tolerance against the transplanted graft. This idea is generated from the observations that some liver transplants are tolerogenic; and that the liver is a major source for secreted sHLA-I molecules. Techniques such as one-dimensional isoelectric focusing (1D-IEF) or sHLA allotype-specific ELISA are necessary requirements for the differentiation of recipient- and donor-derived sHLA molecules. However, studies related to this topic are still very limited. The first relevant publication, from Sir Roy Calne and co-workers (Pollard *et al.*, 1990), showed that for three liver recipients, donor-specific sHLA-I allotypes occur in the peripheral blood and bile of patients immediately after implantation of the liver, and disappear when the liver is removed. Since recipient-derived sHLA-I allotypes were also detectable after liver transplantation, these authors concluded that cells other than those of the liver were able to release sHLA-I molecules. Meanwhile donor-derived sHLA-I allotypes have been identified in the plasma of patients following heart (Zavazava *et al.*, 1991; Koelman *et al.*, 1998), lung (DeVito-Haynes *et al.*, 1997), kidney (DeVito-Haynes *et al.*, 1994), and kidney/pancreas (DeVito-Haynes *et al.*, 1994) transplantation. Except for liver recipients, it seems that the occurrence of donor-derived sHLA-I allotypes is not continuous. Increasing amounts of donor-derived sHLA-I molecules have been observed during rejection episodes, but also during episodes of other clinical complications. From one study there is evidence that high and steady secretion of donor-derived sHLA-I allotypes favours stable graft function and survival (McDonald *et al.*, 1997). However, these data require further confirmation.

Studies which have analysed the relationship between sHLA, antibodies and antiidiotypic antibodies further support the thesis that sHLA may be related to tolerance or self-tolerance. King *et al.* (1989) first showed that the titers of alloantibodies in dialysis patients increase by the depletion of sHLA molecules. In renal and heart transplant patients, HLA antibodies and/or complex formation of sHLA-I with HLA antibodies may be associated with chronic rejection, whereas the appearance of antiidiotypic antibodies correlates with good long term graft function (Hardy *et al.*, 1991; Reed *et al.*, 1996; Suciu-Foca *et al.*, 1991). The purification of donor-specific sHLA-I molecules from liver recipients has revealed that a portion of donor sHLA-I molecules are complexed with IgM and IgG antibodies that could further be characterised as HLA antibodies (Mathew *et al.*, 1996). Furthermore these authors were able to show that donor sHLA-A3 molecules inhibit the cytolytic activity of an HLA-A3-restricted CD8+ T cell line. Both findings give hints to an important regulatory role of sHLA-I in the immune response to organ allografts in humans.

Pregnancy

From the immunological point of view, pregnancy can be considered as a successful transplantation of allogeneic paternal tissue to the mother. The role of sHLA molecules in pregnancy was first studied by Suciu-Foca and co-workers (Reed *et al.*, 1991). They found that antibodies against the mismatched alleles of the fetus, sHLA molecules derived from the fetus, and complex formation of both, can occur in the eighth week of pregnancy. Inostroza *et al.* reported elevated sHLA-I levels in the plasma of pregnant women during the first two trimesters, which reached normal values at the end of pregnancy (Inostroza *et al.*, 1997). The same observation was made by Russwurm *et al.*, (1998) for sHLA-II levels. Surprisingly, in cord blood samples sHLA-I levels seem to be lower than in corresponding blood samples from the mother (Inostroza *et al.*, 1997). However, it is quite questionable whether the changes in sHLA-I levels reflect simply hormonal and immune changes during pregnancy or whether they have an immunoregulatory effect. Studies which compare the sHLA levels of women with successful pregnancy with sHLA levels of women with fetal loss will be more helpful in clarifying these questions.

Immunoregulation

Studies using in-vitro cell culture systems provide strong evidence that the biological role of sHLA molecules suggested by the clinical studies are correct. A series of studies has revealed that peptides derived from HLA molecules down-regulate the immune response (Krensky *et al.,* 1994, 1995). Further, natural killer cells were inhibited by purified and recombinant sHLA-I molecules (Carbone *et al.,* 1996). Zavazava and co-workers were the first to show that detergent-solubilised HLA class I molecules inhibit the cytolytic activity of T cells by the induction of apoptosis (Zavazava and Kronke, 1996). For sHLA-II molecules it is reported that the one-way mixed lymphocyte culture is strongly inhibited by a preincubation of T cells with purified sHLA-II for 36 h (Smeraldi *et al.,* 1982). It has been shown that sHLA-II molecules obtained from the supernatants of monocyte cultures suppress the PHA response of mononuclear cells (Claus *et al.,* 1990). Lastly, there are hints that antigen-specific T cells can be selectively killed or anergized by sHLA-II molecules complexed with peptides (Nicolle *et al.,* 1994).

Methodology

Determination of sHLA concentration

In initial studies, the determination of sHLA-I antigens was assessed by radiolabelled reagents. In these assays either radiolabelled polyclonal anti-HLA antibodies or labelled HLA antigens obtained after papain digestion of cultured lymphoid cells were used in inhibition tests or radioimmunoassay formats. Nowadays, it is generally preferred that enzyme linked immunosorbant assay (ELISA) techniques are performed to determinate the sHLA concentration. For ELISA, monoclonal antibodies directed against a monomorphic or polymorphic epitope of HLA-I are coated on microtiter plates and after the incubation of the test sample, bound sHLA-I antigens are detected either by an anti-human β2m antibody or by an anti-human HLA-I antibody which binds to an epitope different from the coating antibody. Although the ELISA format may work consistently in individual laboratories and a high degree of interlaboratory correlation has been observed, there can be marked differences in absolute values of reported sHLA-I levels (Pouletty *et al.,* 1993). This might be due either to different standard reagents or to different monoclonal antibodies used for the ELISA. To overcome the problem of variation in sHLA-I standard reagents, all participants of the first international workshop on soluble HLA antigens accepted recombinant sHLA-B7 (rsHLA-B7) antigens (Grumet *et al.,* 1994), derived from a cell line transfected with human β2m and HLA-B7 genes, as the international standard reagent. However, in view of the high structural diversity of sHLA-I molecules, the application of a distinctive mAb may result in different absolute values for sHLA-I levels. The employment of an anti-human β2m antibody as a detection reagent permits the exclusive quantitation of β2m-associated sHLA-I molecules, whereas a combination of antibodies recognising different epitopes on HLA-I antigens will serve to measure both subsets of sHLA-I molecules, i.e. the β2m-associated and β2m-free forms. Moreover, a set of mAbs binding to different linear sequences of "denatured" HLA class I antigens offers the possibility to quantify β2m-free sHLA-I antigens. It is noteworthy that mAb W6/32 and TP25.99 differ in their ability to bind to certain HLA class I isotypes. Whereas mAb W6/32 binds to all HLA class I antigens including HLA-A, B, C, E and G, mAb TP25.99 binds to HLA-A, B, C and E but does not bind to HLA-G. This differential binding pattern was used to develop an assay for the detection of sHLA-G. In this two-step assay the samples were first immunodepleted of sHLA-A, B, C and E with mAb TP25.99, and the remaining sHLA-G molecules were then captured by mAb W6/32 and detected by an anti-human β2m antiserum (Rebmann *et al.,* 1999b).

Protocol for the determination of total β2m-associated sHLA-I

- Coat each well of the immunoadsorbent microtiter plates (Costar GmbH, Bodenheim, Germany) with 100 µl of mAb W6/32 (20 µg/ml in 0,05 M potassium carbonate buffer, pH 9.6) overnight at 4°C.
- Wash the plates three times with phosphate buffer saline (PBS) containing 0.05 % Tween 20 and block the remaining free binding sites with 1% bovine serum albumin (BSA) in PBS (pH 7.2) at room temperature (RT) for 30 min.
- After 3 washings add 100µl of sample to each well and incubate for 1 h at RT. Plasma samples are tested at dilutions of 1:26 and 1:51, whereas amniotic fluids are tested at a dilution of 1:10. Dilute the standard reagent rsHLA-B7 to concentrations of 2.5, 6.25, 25.0, 62.5, 125 ng/ml. (Using the indicated dilutions of the sera, all OD values obtained should be in the range of the calibration curve).
- Remove unbound molecules by three washing steps with PBS-Tween (0.05%).
- Bound sHLA-I associated with β2m are detected by incubation at RT for 1 h in peroxidase (POX)-labeled rabbit anti-human β2m antibody (Dakopatts, Hamburg, Germany) diluted to 1:1000 in PBS.
- After five further washes, add 100µl of substrate (0.075% H_2O_2, 0.1% ortho phenylenediamine in 0.035M citrate buffer, pH 5.0) to each well and incubate for 30 min at RT.
- Stop the reaction by adding 50µl of 3M H_2SO_4 and measure the OD at 490nm (Biotek Instruments, Winooski, Vt, USA).

Determination of sHLA allotypes

Using the principles described above, determination of sHLA class I allotypes is possible, e.g. sHLA-A2, A9, A3, B7. The specificities of these assays have been confirmed using either supernatants from B-lymphoblastoid cell line (B-LCL) reference cells from the 11th International Histocompatibility Workshop, or by a small number of plasma samples from HLA class I-typed healthy individuals. Normally, quantitative values for sHLA allotypes are given in relative units. For sHLA-A2 recombinant HLA-A2/Q10 human-mouse fusion protein, and for sHLA-B7 antigens, the international standard reagent rsHLA-B7 is available (Pouletty *et al.*, 1993). Although the monitoring of sHLA allotypes is of interest to distinguish between donor- and recipient-derived sHLA molecules after allografts, only a few studies on this topic have been published. This might reflect the difficulties in development of allotype-specific ELISA formats. From the practical standpoint, it is very important to capture high amounts of total sHLA molecules, as the individual proportions of specific sHLA allotypes is small. This means that microtiter plates with high binding capacity, and purified as well highly concentrated mAbs are absolutely necessary. Beside this, the most critical point is the specific detection of sHLA allotypes molecules with mAbs which were originally defined by cellular assays. As sHLA molecules can appear in different molecular structures or complex formation, it seems reasonable to expect that the binding affinitiy of mAbs to certain sHLA molecules will be lower than to their respective membrane-anchored molecules. Our own experiences have shown that only 2 out of 22 anti-human HLA-A2 mAbs work efficiently as capture reagents for sHLA-A2 molecules. However, these mAbs cross-react with sHLA-A9 molecules.

Protocol for the determination of sHLA-A2 molecules

- Coat each well of an immunoadsorbent microtiter plate (Costar GmbH, Bodenheim, Germany) with 100µl of a mixture of mAb 0397HA and mAb 0791HA (BMT Labor-Produkte, Krefeld, Germany) (1:200 dilution in PBS, pH 7.2) and incubate overnight at 4°C.
- Wash the plates three times with PBS-Tween 20 (0.05%) and block the remaining free binding sites with 1% BSA in PBS (pH 7.2) at RT for 30 min.
- After 3 washings, add 100µl of plasma samples diluted 1:2 in PBS to each well and incubate overnight at 4°C. As standard reagent, supernatant of an HLA-A2 homozygous cell line is used undiluted and in dilutions of 1:2, 1:4; 1:8, 1:16, 1:32. The OD value of the undiluted supernatant corresponds to 1000 Units of sHLA-A2.
- Remove unbound molecules by three washing steps with PBS-Tween 20 (0.05%).
- Bound β2m-associated sHLA-A2 molecules are detected by incubation for 1 h at 37°C in POX-labelled rabbit anti-human β2m antibodies (Dakopatts, Hamburg, Germany), diluted to 1:1000 in PBS.
- After five further washing steps, add 100µl of substrate (0.075% H_2O_2, 0.1% ortho phenylenediamine in 0.035 M citrate buffer, pH 5.0) to each well and incubate for 30 min at RT.

- Stop the reaction by adding 50µl of 3M H_2SO_4 and measure the OD at 490 nm (Biotek Instruments, Winooski, Vt, USA).

Determination of sHLA-II

Quantitation of sHLA-II molecules and their isotypes was first performed with xenoantisera produced in response to purified sHLA-II antigens. However, a variety of ELISA-based formats have since been described which utilise either monoclonal or polyclonal anti-human HLA class II antibodies, or a combination of both. Moreover, magnetic beads coated with anti-HLA class II antibodies have been used as a solid phase medium to capture sHLA-II molecules. Compared to sHLA-I, sHLA-II assays are much less reproducible between different laboratories, and are subject to dependence on standard reagents, antibodies, and assay sensitivity. To compound difficulties, sHLA-II standard reagents are less stable than those of sHLA-I (personal observations), and international standard reagents are as yet unavailable. The binding specificities of anti-human HLA class II mAbs must taken into account with respect to their ability to detect the α/β heterodimer complexed with peptides and to detect α/β heterodimers complexed with CD74. For example, mAb L243 recognises class II heterodimers exclusively with peptides, whereas the mAbs Tü36 and TAL1B5 detect sHLA-DR molecules either complexd with peptides or CD74 (Neefjes *et al.,* 1990).

Protocol for the determination of sHLA-DR α/β heterodimer complexed with peptides

- Coat each well of the immunoadsorbent microtiter plates (Costar GmbH, Bodenheim, Germany) with 100µl of mAb L243 (IgG2a, Becton Dickenson, Heidelberg) (0.025µg/ml in 0.05M potassium carbonate buffer, pH 9.6) overnight at 4°C.
- Wash the plates three times with PBS-Tween 20 (0.05%) and block the remaining free binding sites with 3% BSA in carbonate buffer (pH 9.6) at 37° C for 1 h.
- Wash the plates three times with PBS-Tween 20 (0.05%), add 100µl of undiluted EDTA plasma sample to each well, and incubated for 1.5 h at 37°C. Note: as a standard reagent, we used affinity-purified HLA-DR1, kindly provided by Dr. S. Jurcevic (Heart Science Centre, Transplant Immunology, Harefield Hospital, UK): this was used in concentrations of 0.2, 0.4, 0.65, 0.8 and 1.4 µg/ml.
- Remove unbound molecules by three washing steps with PBS-Tween 20 (0.05%).
- Detect bound sHLA-DR molecules by incubation for 1 h with mAb CR/43, specific for the β-chains of HLA class II molecules (IgG1, Boehringer, Heidelberg, Germany), diluted to 1:1.000 in PBS at 37°C.

- After three further washing steps, add 100µl of AP-conjugated goat anti-mouse IgG1 antibody (Serva, Heidelberg, Germany), diluted 1:1000, to each well and incubate for 1 h at 37°C.
- After three further washing steps, add 100µl of substrate (1nM 4-Methylumbelliferylphosphate in 1M diethanolamine and 0.5M $MgCl_2$) to each well. After 40 min stop the reaction by adding 50µl of 1M NaOH: measure the fluorescence intensities immediately (Ex 355nm / Em 460nm).

Biochemical analysis of sHLA molecules

The biochemical analysis of the heterogeneous composition of HLA-I molecules in plasma or body fluids is based on the immunoprecipitation of sHLA-I molecules. The most effective methodology for use with plasma samples is described by Kubens *et al.* (1994). The mAb W6/32 is coupled to immunomagnetic beads, coated with sheep anti-mouse Ig (Dynabeads M280, Dynal, Hamburg, Germany), and after an incubation with plasma samples, sHLA-I molecular weight variants are either analysed by SDS-PAGE or the sHLA-I allotypes are analysed by 1D-IEF as originally described by Neffjes *et al.*, (1986). Using 1D-IEF the sHLA-I molecules are separated according their isoelectric points (IP): this depends on the individual amino acid composition of the sHLA-I molecules. Since sHLA-I molecules exhibited identical IP to their respective membrane-anchored counterparts (Figure 3.3), it is unlikely that the presence or absence of transmembrane and cytoplasmic domains will influence the IP. This is supported by the fact that these domains are preferentially composed of uncharged amino acids and thus the total net charge should be equal for the three different sHLA-I variants. After separating sHLA-I molecules and Western blotting, the sHLA-I antigens are detected by antibodies able to bind to denatured molecules.

Protocol for SDS-PAGE and 1D-IEF analysis

Sample preparation

- Add 10µg of mAb W6/32 to 1ml of a suspension of 1 x 10^8 immunomagnetic beads coupled with sheep anti-mouse IgG (Dynabeads M280, Dynal, Hamburg, Germany). Incubate overnight at 4°C under rotation.
- Remove unbound antibody by three washing steps with PBS-Tween 20 (0.05%). The prepared bead suspension can be stored up to two weeks at 4°C.
- Add 0.25ml of EDTA plasma samples to 50µl of coupled beads and incubate overnight at 4°C under rotation.
- For SDS-PAGE analysis, heat the washed beads with 50µl SDS sample buffer (70mM Tris-HCl, 2% SDS, 10% glycerol, 150mM β-mercaptoethanol, pH 6.8) for 5 min at 95°C.

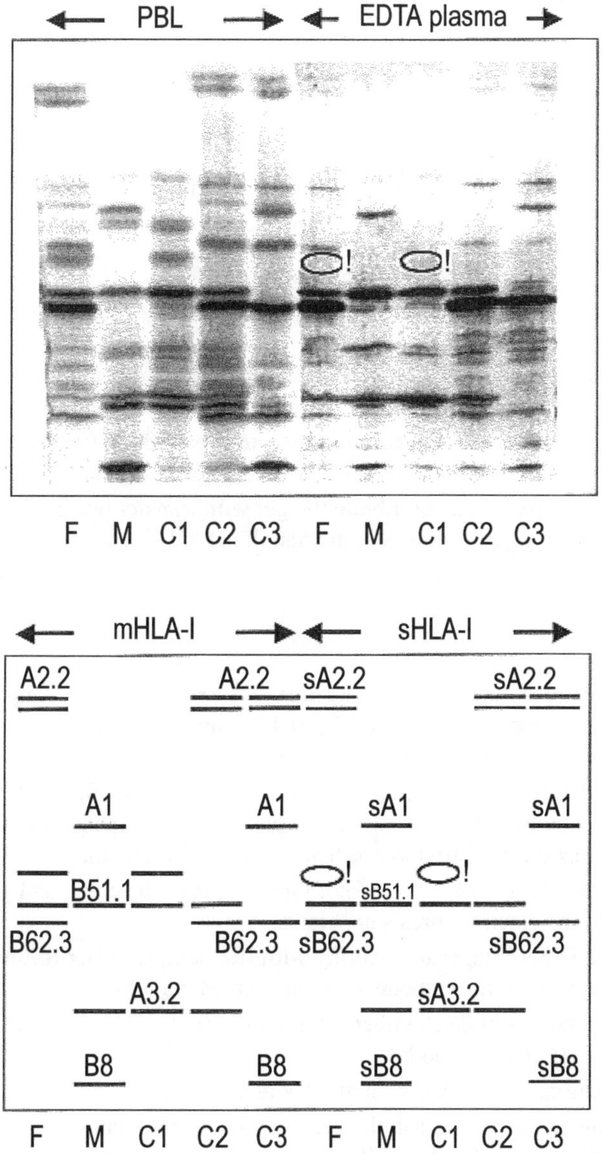

Figure 3.3. Biochemical segregation analysis of membrane-anchored and soluble HLA class I molecules. 1D-IEF analysis of a family with three members is shown. Left panel: isoelectric points of HLA class I antigens from peripheral blood lymphocytes (PBL) are identical to sHLA-I molecules from the corresponding EDTA plasma samples. Right panel: schematic drawing of relevant HLA class I antigen positions. Note that the sHLA-A31 molecules could not be detected by this method.

- For 1D-IEF analysis, incubate the washed beads with 0.2U neuraminidase type VIII (Sigma, München, Germany) in 50mM sodium acetate buffer (pH 5.0) containing 1mM $CaCl_2$ for 5 h at 37°C under rotation. Elute the sHLA-I molecules with 50μl of IEF sample buffer (8.5M urea, 2% Ampholyte pH 3.5 - 10, 2% Triton 100, and 150mM β-mercaptoethanol).
- Eluted sHLA-I molecules are subjected either to SDS-PAGE or to 1D-IEF, as appropriate.

SDS-PAGE

- SDS-PAGE is performed according to standard conditions, using gels consisting of 10% acrylamide and 0.54% bisacrylamide.
- Gels of dimensions 280mm (horizontal) x 180mm (vertical) x 1mm (thickness) are run at a constant voltage of 60V overnight.
- After separation, equilibrate the gel with transfer buffer (25mM Tris, 150mM glycine, and 20% methanol, pH 8.3).

1D-IEF

- Prepare the gel solution (9M urea, 2% Triton 100, 4% Ampholyte pH 5 - 7, 1% Ampholyte pH 3.5 - 10, 0.4% Ampholyte pH 7 - 9, 4.5% acrylamide, 0.26% bisacrylamide) 3 h before usage.
- Add 100μl of ammonium persulphate (10%) and 50μl TEMED to 50ml gel solution and pour into a gel chamber with dimensions of 280mm (horizontal) x 180 mm (vertical) x 1mm (thickness).
- Allow gel to polymerise for 45 min, remove the comb and place the gel into the electrophoresis apparatus.
- Load the samples and overlay with IEF sample buffer (diluted 1:4) followed by the cathode solution (50mM NaOH).
- Fill the electrode chambers: solutions are 50 mM NaOH (cathode) and 20 mM H_3PO_4 (anode).
- Electrophorese overnight at 12W and 1000V.
- After separation, wash the gels 5 times with a solution of 5mM Tris-HCl, 50% methanol and 1% SDS (pH 8.0) and then equilibrate with transfer buffer.

Western blotting

- Western blotting is performed according to Towbin *et al.,* (1979) using Immobilon PVDF membranes (Millipore GmbH, Neu-Isenburg, Germany).
- Block the free binding sites of the blotting membrane with 3% BSA in PBS-Tween 20 (0.1%).
- Bound sHLA-I molecules are detected by a polyclonal rabbit anti-human HLA class I heavy chain (Neefjes *et al.,* 1986). For this, incubate the blotting membrane overnight with antibody diluted to 1:10,000 in PBS-Tween 20 (0.05%).
- Remove unbound antibody by three washing steps with PBS-Tween 20 (0.05%).
- Detect bound antibody by incubating the blotting membrane with an AP-labelled goat anti-rabbit antiserum (1:1000) in PBS-Tween 20 (0.05%) for 1 h at RT.
- Develop the reaction with a solution containing nitro-tetrazolium (0.1mg/ml), 5-bromo-4-chloro-3-indolyl-phosphate (0.05 mg/ml), $MgCl_2$ (1mM) in Tris-HCl (0.1M, pH 9.6).

References

Abendroth, D, Storck, M, Techt, B and Zavazava, N. (1995). Analysis of the rejection markers tumor necrosis factor, ICAM-1, neopterin, interleukin-10, and soluble HLA in simultaneous pancreas and kidney transplantation with bladder drainage. *Transplant Proc*, **27**: 3114-3115

Adamashvili, IM, McDonald, JC, Fraser, PA, Milford, EL, Pressly, TA *et al.* (1995). Soluble class I HLA antigens in patients with rheumatoid arthritis and their families. *J Rheumatol*, **22**: 1025-1031

Adamashvili, IM, Fraser, PM and McDonald, JC. (1996). Association of serum concentrations of soluble class I HLA with HLA allotypes. *Transplantation,* **61:** 984-987

Alvarez-Cermeno, J, Echevarria, JM, Villar, LM, Lazaro, I, Bootello, A *et al.* (1989). Soluble class I antigens in serum and CSF of patients with varicella-zoster virus meningitis. *J Neurol Neurosurg Psychiatry*, **52**: 1194-1199

Alvarez-Cermeno, JC, Casado, C, Villar, LM, Ferreira, A, Varela, JM *et al.* (1990). Soluble class I antigens (sHLA) in CSF and serum of patients with HIV infection. *Acta Neurol Scand*, **82:** 14-17

Aebi, M, Hornig, H and Weissmann, C. (1987). 5' cleavage site in eukaryotic pre-mRNA splicing is determined by the overall 5' splice region, not by the conserved 5' GU. *Cell,* **50**: 237-246

Auffray, C, Lillie, JW, Korman, AJ, Boss, JM, Frechin, N *et al.* (1987). Structure and expression of HLA-DQ alpha and -DX alpha genes: interallelic alternat

Aulitzky, WE, Grosse-Wilde, H, Westhoff, U, Tilg, G, Aulitzky, W *et al.* (1991). Enhanced serum levels of soluble HLA class I molecules are induced by treatment with recombinant interferon-gamma (IFN-gamma). *Clin Exp Immunol*, **86:** 236-239

Billing, RJ, Safani, M and Peterson, P. (1977). Soluble HLA antigens present in normal human serum. *Tissue Antigens*, **10:** 75-82

Bresciani, A, Pirozzi, G, Spera, M, Lombardi, ML, Ambrosone, L *et al.* (1998). Increased level of serum HLA class I antigens in patients with systemic lupus erythematosus. Correlation with disease activity. *Tissue Antigens*, **52:** 44-50

Briata, P, Radka, SF, Sartoris, S and Lee, JS. (1989). Alternative splicing of HLA-DQ beta transcripts and secretion of HLA-DQ beta proteins: Allelic polymorphism in splicing and polyadenylation sites. *Proc Natl Acad Sci USA,* **86:** 1003-1007

Brieva, JA, Villar, LM, Leoro, G, Alvarez-Cermeno, JC, Roldan, E. *et al.* (1990). Soluble HLA class I antigen secretion by normal lymphocytes: relationship with cell activation and effect of interferon-gamma. *Clin Exp Immunol,* **82:** 390-395

Capobianchi, MR, Ameglio, F, Tosi, R and Dolei, A. (1985) Differences in the expression and release of DR, BR, and DQ molecules in human cells treated with recombinant interferon gamma: Comparison to other interferons. *Hum Immunol* **13:** 1-5

Charlton, RK and Zmijewski, CM. (1970). Soluble HL-A7 antigen: localization in the beta-lipoprotein fraction of human serum. *Science,* **170:** 636-637

Claus, R, Werner, H, Schulze, HA, Walzel, H and Friemel, H. (1990). Are soluble monocyte-derived HLA class II molecules candidates for immunosuppressive activity? *Immunol Lett*, **26**: 203-210

Carbone, E, Terrazzano, G, Colonna, M, Tuosto, L, Piccolella, E *et al.* (1996). Natural killer clones recognize specific soluble HLA class I molecules. *Eur J Immunol*, **26:** 683-689

Demaria, S, Schwab, R and Bushkin, Y. (1992). The origin and fate of β2m-free MHC class I molecules induced on activated T cells. *Cell Immunol,* **142**: 103-113

DeVito-Haynes, LD, Jankowska-Gan, E, Sollinger, HW, Knechtle, SJ and Burlingham, WJ. (1994). Monitoring of kidney and simultaneous pancreas-kidney transplantation rejection by release of donor-specific, soluble HLA class I. *Hum Immunol*, **40**: 191-201

DeVito-Haynes, LD, Jankowska-Gan, E, Heisey, DM, Cornwell, RD, Meyer, KC. *et al.* (1997). Soluble HLA class I in epithelial lining fluid of lung transplants: associations with graft outcome. *Hum Immunol*, **52:** 95-108

Ditschkowski, M, Kreuzfelder, E, Rebmann, V, Ferencik, S, Majetschak, M. *et al.* (1999). HLA-DR expression and soluble HLA-DR levels in septic patients after trauma. *Ann Surg,* (in press).

Dobbe, LM, Stam, NJ, Neefjes, JJ and Giphart, MJ. (1988). Biochemical complexity of serum HLA class I molecules. *Immunogenetics,* **27:** 203-210

Doxiadis, I, Westhoff, U and Grosse-Wilde, H. (1989). Quantification of soluble HLA class I gene products by an enzyme linked immunosorbent assay. *Blood*, **59:** 449-454.

Drouet, M, Petit, B, Peyronnet, P, Aussel, L, Venot, J. *et al.* (1995). Soluble HLA class I antigens in kidney allograft recipients. *Transplant Proc*, **27:** 1671

Fellous, M, Nir, U, Wallach, D, Merlin, G, Rubinstein, M. *et al.* (1982). Interferon-dependent induction of mRNA for the major histocompatibility antigens in human fibroblasts and lymphoblastoid cells. *Proc Natl Acad Sci USA*, **79:** 3082-3088

Filaci, G, Contini, P, Brenci, S, Gazzola, P, Lanza, L. *et al.* (1997). Soluble HLA class I and class II molecule levels in serum and cerebrospinal fluid of multiple sclerosis patients. *Hum Immunol*, **54:** 54-62

Filaci, G, Contini, P, Brenci, S, Lanza, L, Scudeletti, M. *et al.* (1995). Increased serum concentration of soluble HLA-DR antigens in HIV infection and following transplantation. *Tissue Antigens* **46**: 117-123

Fujii, T, Ishitani, A and Geragthy, DE (1994). A soluble form of the HLA-G antigen is encoded by a messenger ribonucleic acid containing intron 4. *J Immunol*: **153**: 5516-24

Grumet, FC, Buelow R, Kubens B, Grosse-Wilde H, Pouletty PJ. *et al.* (1994). Report of the second international soluble (sHLA) workshop. *Hum Immunol*, **40:** 153-165

Grumet, FC, Krishnaswamy, S, See-Tho, K, Filvaroff, E and Hiraki, DD. (1994). Soluble form of an HLA-B7 class I antigen specifically suppresses humoral alloimmunization. *Hum Immunol*, **40:** 235-246

Gussow, D and Ploegh, H. (1987). Soluble class I antigens: a conundrum with no solution? *Immunol Today,* **8:** 220-222

Hardy, MA, Suciu-Foca, N, Reed, E, Benvenisty, AL, Smith, C. *et al.* (1991). Immunomodulation of kidney and heart transplants by anti-idiotypic antibodies. *Ann Surg*, **214:** 528-530

Haga, JA, Riley, WJ and Kao, KJ. (1991). Effect of HLA phenotype and gender on expression of various forms of class I HLA in plasma. *Hum Immunol*, **32:** 79-84

Hagihara, M, Shimura, T, Yamamoto, K, Takebe, K. Munkhbat, B. *et al.* (1994). Soluble HLA class I and class II in Japanese. *Hum Immunol,* **40**: 171-173

He, X and Le, J. (1995). Alternative splicing of HLA class I transcripts induced by IFN-gamma and TNF in fibroblasts: release of soluble HLA class I heavy chain and an associate protein. *Cell Immunol*, **162**: 159-165

Hillebrand, K, Moritz, T, Westhoff, U, Niederle, N and Grosse-Wilde, H. (1994). Soluble HLA class I and beta-2-microglobulin plasma concentrations during interferon treatment of chronic myelogenous leukemia. *Vox Sang,* **67:** 310-314

Huang, F, Yamaguchi, A, Tsuchiya, N, Ikawa, T, Tamura, N. *et al.* (1997). Induction of alternative splicing of HLA-B27 by bacterial invasion. *Arthr Rheum,* **40:** 694-703

Kao, KJ, Scornik, JC, Riley, WJ and McQueen, CF. (1988). Association between HLA phenotype and HLA concentration in plasma or platelets. *Hum Immunol*, **21:** 115-124

King, DW, Reed, E and Suciu-Foca, N. (1989) Complexes of soluble HLA antigens and anti-HLA autoantibodies in human sera: possible role in maintenance of self-tolerance. *Immunol Res*, **8:** 249-262

Koelman CA, Mulder, A, Jutte, NM, Vaessen, LM, Balk, AH. *et al.* (1998). The application of human monoclonal antibodies for monitoring donor derived soluble HLA class I molecules in the serum of heart transplant recipients. *Hum Immunol*, **59**: 106-114

Krangel, MS, Pious, D and Strominger, JL. (1984). Characterization of a B lymphoblastoid cell line mutant that secretes HLA-A2. *J Immunol*, **132**: 2984-2991

Krangel, MS. (1985). Unusual RNA splicing generates a secreted form of HLA-A2 in a mutagenized B lymphoblastoid cell line. *EMBO J,* **4:** 1205-1210

Krangel, MS. (1986). Secretion of HLA-A and -B antigens via an alternative RNA splicing pathway. *J Exp Med,* **163:** 1173-1190

Krangel, MS. (1987). Two forms of HLA class I molecules in human plasma. *Hum Immunol*, **20**: 155-165

Krensky, AM and Clayberger, C. (1995). HLA-derived peptides as novel immunotherapeutics. *Clin Immunol Immunopathol,* **75:** 112-116.

Krensky, AM and Clayberger, C. (1995). Human leukocyte antigen derived peptides as novel immunosuppressives. *Proc Assoc Am Physicians*, **107**: 81-85

Kubens, BS, Päßler, M and Grosse-Wilde, H. (1994). Detection efficacy of soluble HLA-A, B antigens using 1D-IEF. *Eur. J. Immunogenetics,* **21**: 469-477

Kubens, BS, Päßler, M and Grosse-Wilde, H. (1994). Segregation study of soluble 39 kD HLA class I heavy chain. *Hum Immunol,* **40**: 247-252

Le, J and Hua, JC. (1995). Production of soluble HLA-class-I molecules by IFN-gamma-induced colon-adenocarcinoma cells. *Int J Cancer,* **60:** 576-581

Inostroza, J, Munoz, P, Espinoza, R, Millaqueo, L, Diaz, P. *et al.* (1994). Quantitation of soluble HLA class I heterodimers and beta 2-microglobulin in patients with active pulmonary tuberculosis. *Hum Immunol*, **40**: 179-182

Inostroza, J, Ferrada, J, Navarrete, C and Sorensen, R. U. (1997). Soluble histocompatibility class I antigens and beta 2-microglobulin in pregnant females and cord blood samples. *Hum Immunol*, **54:** 63-68

Liem, LM, Koelman, CA, Doxiadis, I, van Houwelingen, JC, Goulmy, E. *et al.* (1997). Elevated serum HLA class I levels coincide with acute and chronic graft-versus-host disease. *Bone Marrow Transplant* **20:** 227-234

Mathew, JM, Shenoy, S, Phelan, D, Lowell, J, Howard, T. *et al.* (1996). Biochemical and immunological evaluation of donor-specific soluble HLA in the circulation of liver transplant recipients. *Transplantation*, **62:** 217-223

McDonald, JC, Adamashvili, I, Hayes, JM, Aultman, DF, Rhynes, VK. *et al.* (1994). Soluble HLA class II concentrations in normal individuals and transplant recipients. Comparison with soluble HLA class I concentrations. *Transplantation*, **58:** 1268-1272

McDonald, JC, Adamashvili, I, Zibari, GB, Aultmn, DF, Mancini, MC. *et al.* (1997). Serologic allogeneic chimerism. *Transplantation*, **64:** 865-871

McMaster, M, Zhou, Y, Shorter, S, Kapasi, K, Geraghty, DE. *et al.* (1998). HLA-G isoforms produced by placental cytotrophoblasts and found in amniotic fluid are due to unusual glycosylation. *J Immunol,* **160**: 5922-5928

McMillan, RM, Gelder, FB, Zibari, GB, Aultman, DF, Adamashvili, I. *et al.* (1997). Soluble fraction of class I human histocompatibility leukocyte antigens in the serum of liver transplant recipients. *Clin Transplant*, **11:** 98-103

Moore, C, Ehlayel, M, Inostroza, J, Leiva, LE and Sorensen, RU. (1997). Elevated levels of soluble HLA class I (sHLA-I) in children with severe atopic dermatitis. *Ann Allergy, Asthma, Immunol* **79**: 113-118

Neefjes, JJ, Doxiadis, I, Stam, NJ, Beckers, CJ and Ploegh, HL (1986). An analysis of HLA class I antigens of man and other species by one-dimensional IEF and immunoblotting. *Immunogenetics* **23**: 164-169

Neefjes, JJ, Stollorz, V, Perters, PJ, Geuze, HJ and Ploegh, HL. (1990). The biosynthetic pathway of MHC class II but not class I molecules intersects the endocytic route. *Cell,* **61:** 171-183

Nicolle, MW, Nag, B, Sharma, SD, Willcox, N, Vincent, A. *et al.* (1994). Specific tolerance to an acetylcholine receptor epitope induced in vitro in myasthenia gravis CD4+ lymphocytes by soluble major histocompatibility complex class II-peptide complexes. *J Clin Invest*, **93:** 1361-1369

Park, CW, Yun, SN, Yang, CW, Kim, TG, Han, H. *et al.* (1997). Serum and urine soluble HLA class I antigen concentrations are increased in patients with hemorrhagic fever with renal syndrome. *Korean J Inter Med*, **12:** 52-55

Ott, M, Seidl, C, Westhoff, U, Stecker, K, Seifried, E. *et al.* (1998). Soluble HLA class I and class II antigens in patients with multiple sclerosis. *Tissue Antigens*, **51**: 301-304

Pickl, WF, Majdic, 0, Faé, I, Reuschel, R, Holter, W. *et al.* (1993). The soluble pool of beta 2-microglobulin free HLA class I alpha-chains. Qualitative and quantitative characterization. *J Immunol*, **151:** 2613-2622

Pollard, SG, Davies, HS and Calne, RY. (1989). Soluble class I antigen in human bile. *Transplantation* **48**: 712-713

Pollard, SG, Davies, HF and Calne, RY. (1990). Preoperative appearance of serum class I antigen during liver transplantation. *Transplantation*, **49:** 659-662

Pouletty, PJ, Ferrone, S, Amesland, F, Cohen, N, Westhoff, U. *et al.* (1993). Summary report from the first international workshop on soluble HLA-antigens. *Tissue Antigens,* **42:** 45-54

Puppo, F, Orlandini, A, Ruzzenenti, R, Comuzio, S, Salamito, A. *et al.* (1990). HLA class I soluble antigen serum levels in HIV-positive subjects - correlation with cellular and serological parameters. *Cancer Detect Prevent,* **14:** 321-323

Puppo, F, Ruzzenenti, R, Brenci, S, Lanza, L, Scudeletti, M. *et al.* (1991). Major histocompatibility gene products and human immunodeficiency virus infection. *J Lab Clin Med,* **117:** 91-100

Puppo, F, Brenci, S, Lanza, L, Bosco, O, Imro, MA. *et al.* (1994). Increased level of serum HLA class I antigens in HIV infection. Correlation with disease progression. *Hum Immunol* **40:** 259-263

Puppo, F, Pellicci, R, Brenci, S, Nocera, A, Morelli, N. *et al.* (1994). HLA class-l-soluble antigen serum levels in liver transplantation. A predictor marker of acute rejection. *Hum Immunol,* **40:** 166-170

Puppo, F, Brenci, S, Montinaro, E, Lanza, L, Contini, P. *et al.* (1994). Inhibition of alloreactive cytotoxic T cell activity by HIV-positive sera: Potential role of circulating soluble HLA class I molecules. *AIDS Res Hum Retroviruses,* **10:** 1061-1064

Puppo, F, Picciotto, A, Brenc, S, Varagona, G, Scudeletti, M. *et al.* (1995). Behaviour of soluble HLA class I antigens in patients with chronic hepatitis C during interferon therapy: an early predictor marker of response? *J Clin Immunol,* **15**: 179-184

Puppo, F, Brenci, S, Ghio, M, Bignardi, D, Contini, P. *et al.* (1996). Serum HLA class I antigen levels in allogeneic bone marrow transplantation: A possible marker of acute GVHD. *Bone Marrow Transplantation,* **17:** 753-756

Puppo, F, Indiveri, F, Scudeletti, M and Ferrone, S. (1997). Soluble antigens: new roles and uses. *Immunol Today,* **18:** 154-155

Rebmann, V, Dornmair, K and Grosse-Wilde, H. (1997). Biochemical analysis of plasma-soluble invariant chains and their complex formation with soluble HLA-DR. *Tissue Antigens,* **49**: 438-443

Rebmann, V, Päßler, M, Erhard, J, Lange, R, Eigler, FW. *et al.* (1999a). Monitoring of soluble HLA class I size variants after liver transplantation. *Hum Immunol* (in press).

Rebmann, V, Pfeiffer, K, Päßler, M., Maier, S, Ferrone, S. *et al.* (1999b). Detection of soluble HLA-G and HLA class I molecules in plasma and amniotic fluids. *Tissue Antigens* (in press).

Reed, EF, Hong, B, Ho, E, Harris, PE, Weinberger, J. *et al.* (1996). Monitoring of soluble HLA alloantigens and anti-HLA antibodies identifies heart allograft recipients at risk of transplant-associated coronary artery disease. *Transplantation*, **61:** 366-372

Reed, E, Beet, AE, Hutcherson, H, King, DW and Suciu-Foca, N. (1991). The alloantibody response of pregnant women and its suppression by soluble HLA antigens and anti-idiotypic antibodies. *J Reprod Immunol*, **20**: 115-128

Reisfeld, RA, Allison, JP, Ferrone, S, Pellegrino, MA and Poulik, MD. (1976). HL-A antigens in serum and urine: isolation, characterization, and immunogenic properties. *Transplant Proc*, 8: 173-178

Russwurm, GP, Mackler, AM, Fagoaga, OR, Brown, WS, Sakala, EP. *et al.* (1998). Soluble human leukocyte antigens, interleukin-6, and interferon-gamma during pregnancy. *Am J Reprod Immunol*, **38:** 256-262

Saririan, K, Wali, A, Almeida, RP and Russo, C. (1993). Increased serum HLA class I molecule levels in elderly human responders to influenza vaccination. *Tissue Antigens*, **42:** 54-61

Shields, MJ and Ribaudo, RK. (1998). Mapping of monoclonal antibody W6/32: Sensitivity to the amino terminus of β2-microglobulin. *Tissue Antigens*, **51:** 567-570

Shimura, T, Hagihara, M, Yamamoto, K, Takebe, K, Munkhbat, B. *et al.* (1994). Quantification of serum-soluble HLA class I antigens in patients with gastric cancer. *Hum Immunol*, **40:** 183-186

Smeraldi, RS, Fabio, G, Bonara, P, Villa, MG, Vanoli, M. *et al.* (1982). MLC-specific suppressor T lymphocytes in man. I. Their induction in vitro by soluble HLA-DR antigens. *J Immunol,* **128:** 1394-1398

Stevenson, FK, George, AJ, Walters, MT and Hamblin, TJ. (1986). Analysis of soluble HLA class II antigenic material in patients with immunological diseases using monoclonal antibodies. *J Immunol Methods* **86:** 187-190

Stevenson, FK, Douglass, WA, Spellerberg, MB, Walters, MT and Cawley, MI. (1990). Soluble histocompatibility antigens in synovial fluids of patients with rheumatoid arthritis. *Clin Exp Immunol*, **80**: 32-37

Suciu-Foca, N, Reed, E, Ho, E, Cohen, DJ, Benvenisty, AL. *et al.* (1991). Soluble HLA antigens, anti-HLA antibodies, and anti-idiotypic antibodies in the circulation of renal transplant recipients. *Transplantation* **51:** 593-601

Suciu-Foca, N, Ho, E, King, DW, Yu, YP, Yu-Kai, S. *et al.* (1991). Soluble HLA and anti-idiotypic antibodies in transplantation: Modulation of anti-HLA antibodies by soluble HLA antigens from the graft and anti-idiotypic antibodies in renal and cardiac allograft recipients. *Transplant Proc*, **23:** 295-296

Tilg, H, Westhoff, U, Vogel, W, Aulitzky, WE, Herold, M. *et al.* (1992). Soluble HLA class I serum concentrations increase with transplant-related complications after liver transplantation. *J Hepatol,* **14**: 417-419

Towbin, H, Staehelin, T and Gorden, J (1979). Electrophoretic transfer of proteins from polyacrylamide gels to nitrocellulose sheets: procedure and some applications. *Proc Natl Acad Sci USA* **76**: 4350-4354

Tsuji, K, Kusama, M, Nakatsuji, T and Kato, S. (1985). Biological significance of Ss (serum soluble) HLA-class I antigens in bone marrow transplantation. *Tokai J Exp Clin Med*, **10**: 169-174

Tsukamoto, K, Yasunami, M, Kimura, A, Inoko, H, Ando, A. *et al.* (1987). DQ1β gene from HLA-DR2-Dw12 consists of six exons and expresses multiple DQw1β polypeptides through alternative splicing. *Immunogenetics,* **25:** 343-356

Van Rood, JJ, van Leeuwan, A and van Santen, MCT. (1970). Anti HL-A2 inhibitor in normal human sera. *Nature,* 226: 366-371

Vincent, C, Revillard, JP and Betuel, H. (1976). Purification of HLA antigens from urine. *Transplantation,* **22:** 500-507

Westhoff, U, Doxiadis, I, Beelen, DW, Schaefer, UW and Grosse-Wilde, H. (1989). Soluble HLA class I concentrations and GVHD after allogeneic marrow transplantation. *Transplantation*, **48:** 891-893

Westhoff, U, Thinnes, FP, Gotz, H and Grosse-Wilde, H. (1991). Quantitation of soluble HLA class II molecules by an enzyme-linked immunosorbent assay. *Vox Sang,* **61:** 106-110

Weyand, CM, Jendro, M and Goronzy, JJ. (1991). Soluble HLA-DR molecules in patients with HLA class II versus class I associated disorders. *Autoimmunity* **8:** 281-285

Wolf, R, Adamashvili, IM, Gelder, FB, Hall, VC, Fraser PA. *et al.* (1998). Soluble HLA-I in rheumatic diseases. *Hum Immunol*, **59**: 644-649

Yang, D and Le, J. (1994): Targeted amplification of alternatively spliced transcripts of major histocompatibility complex class I heavy chain. *J Immunol Methods,* **176:** 265-270

CHAPTER 4

CROSSMATCHING BY LYMPHOCYTOTOXICITY AND FLOW CYTOMETRY

S. Martin
Transplantation Laboratory
Manchester Royal Infirmary
Oxford Road
Manchester M13 9WL

A. Harmer
Tissue Typing Laboratory
Guy's Hospital
London SE1 9RT

Introduction

In the early days of transplantation it was recognised that pre-formed antibodies present in recipient serum at the time of renal transplantation and directed against donor HLA antigens caused hyperacute rejection (Kissmeyer-Nielsen, 1966) . It has since become universally accepted that a positive complement dependent lymphocytotoxic (CDC) crossmatch due to HLA specific antibodies in a current patient serum sample is a contraindication to transplantation. The CDC crossmatch is thus firmly established as an essential pre-transplant test.

In a crossmatch test, sera from the recipient are incubated with lymphocytes from the potential organ donor. When donor reactive antibodies are present, the addition of rabbit complement to the test results in cell killing ie. a positive test result and the transplant does not proceed. However, despite its wide usage there is not complete standardisation between laboratories in the way the test is performed.

The standards issued by both the American Society for Histocompatibility and Immunogenetics (ASHI) and by the European Federation for Immunogenetics (EFI) demand that a technique more sensitive than the standard microlymphocytotoxicity assay should be used and in the US the antihuman globulin (AHG) assay is widely adopted (Fuller *et al*, 1997). In a recent publication, Zachary *et al.*, (1995) examined modifications of the CDC test and assessed the effect of varying several components on test outcome. They observed that while the AHG method increased test sensitivity, a similar level of sensitivity could be achieved by substituting B cells for T cells or doubling either the serum or complement incubation times. In the UK the AHG assay is seldom employed but extended incubation times for the CDC crossmatch are often used to increase the sensitivity of the test.

The first study of flow cytometric crossmatching by Garovy *et al.,* in 1983 showed the method to be more sensitive than conventional CDC crossmatches for the detection of antibody. The greater sensitivity of flow cytometry and an association between a positive flow crossmatch and graft rejection was confirmed by Chapman *et al.,* (1985). Thistlethwaite *et al.,* (1986) showed the technique to be more sensitive than the AHG augmented CDC crossmatch as well as the standard method. Rodey *et al.,* (1987) demonstrated that extra reactivities detected by flow cytometry could be attributed to definable HLA specificities, supporting the possibility that positive flow cytometry crossmatches may be of clinical significance.

Clinical relevance

Although it is a well established pre-transplant test, there can still be debate on the clinical relevance of a positive CDC crossmatch. A positive crossmatch result *per se* need not be a contraindication to transplantation. The crucial factors determining clinical significance are the specificity and immunoglobulin class of the antibodies causing the positive result. Therefore, it is not only the sensitivity but also the specificity of the crossmatch test that is important. Transplantation must not be denied on the basis of antibodies that will not affect transplant outcome.

It is generally accepted for renal and thoracic organ transplantation that IgG antibodies directed against donor HLA-A or -B specificities and present at the time of transplant will cause hyperacute rejection (Chapman *et al.,* 1986a; Fenoglio *et al.,* 1989; *Smith et al.,* 1993). Although less data are available, donor HLA-DR specific antibodies present in the recipient may also result in rejection (Mohanakumar 1981). The outcome will differ between individuals and between organs depending on antibody titre and level of expression of HLA-DR on the donor organ. Normal hearts do not constitutively express HLA-DR so it will not appear until after transplantation as a result of ischaemic or immunological injury. Kidneys however, with inter-individual variation (Fuggle *et al.,* 1983; Evans *et al.,* 1984), do express HLA-DR so that donor HLA-DR specific antibodies could have an early effect on transplant outcome.

IgM autoreactive antibodies react with autologous as well as allogeneic lymphocytes in the CDC crossmatch test and have been shown to be irrelevant to transplant outcome (Ting & Morris 1983). They therefore give rise to false positive results. IgM antibodies can be digested with dithiothreitol (DTT) and when used in the crossmatch test it abrogates positive results due to IgM. That will remove not only the autoantibodies but also IgM alloantibodies that could be detrimental to transplant outcome.

The clinical relevance of antibodies in non-current sera is also a point of debate. There have been reports of successful renal transplantation with a "peak positive, current negative" crossmatch (Cardella *et al.,* 1985) but again it is the specificity of the antibodies that is the crucial factor. IgG HLA-A or B specific antibodies present in historic sera are associated with accelerated rejection (Chapman *et al.*, 1986a). It has been suggested that the earlier antibody response might be associated with T cell activation which then later mediates acute graft rejection (Roelen *et al.*, 1994). However, rejection could also be antibody mediated as there has been a report of a renal transplant following a "peak positive, current negative" crossmatch due to an IgM alloantibody which resulted in a secondary antibody response within 5 days post-transplant, vascular rejection and transplant failure (Worthington *et al.*, 1998a).

There is little information on the role of antibodies to HLA-Cw or HLA-DQ specificities in transplant failure. Renal transplant failure in a patient who had antibodies to HLA-Cw5 present in the donor has been reported (Chapman *et al.*, 1986b). If patients have antibodies to HLA-Cw or HLA-DQ, many centres now consider it advisable to avoid organ donors with those specificities as they would when a patient has antibodies to HLA-A, B and DR.

Crossmatch results can only be reliably interpreted in the context of a comprehensive antibody screening programme (Rodey *et al.*, 1997; Worthington *et al.*, 1998b). If sera are carefully screened during patient work-up for transplantation then HLA specific antibodies can be defined and hence a patient's crossmatch reactivity against a particular donor of known HLA type predicted. This avoids unnecessary crossmatching and facilitates interpretation of positive results. Similarly, the presence of autoantibodies can be identified in advance through antibody screening and autocrossmatching and false positive crossmatch results avoided. Antibody definition pre-transplant is particularly important for patients awaiting thoracic organ transplantation when only limited time is available for pre-transplant crossmatching.

In relation to flow cytometry crossmatching (FCXM), which groups of potential recipients require the use of this more sensitive crossmatch test pre-transplant is a matter on which centres differ. In 1987 Cook *et al.* found a clear association between a positive flow crossmatch and graft failure in CDC crossmatch negative renal allograft recipients. This association was significant only in sensitised recipients (those with previous failed grafts or with panel reactive antibodies). Other studies have demonstrated associations between positive FCXMs and complications in both first and re-grafts (Lazda *et al.*, 1988; Talbot *et al.*, 1990). In one of the largest studies of FCXM and primary kidney transplantation there was a significant association between a positive T cell FCXM and reduced graft survival at one year (Ogura *et al.*, 1993). In contrast other studies have not found a significant association between a positive FCXM and graft function (Horsburgh *et al.*, 1992; Evans *et al.*, 1992) although the latter study did show a non-significant trend towards poor graft survival in the small number of regrafts studied. Many centres have adopted the use of the FCXM for regrafts and/or patients with high levels of panel reactive antibodies but not for unsensitised patients whilst others use the FCXM for all potential transplant recipients irrespective of their sensitisation status.

All the studies described above have focused on the T cell FCXM. B cell FCXMs are also performed by increasing numbers of laboratories. Martin *et al.*, (1993) describe a significant association between positive T and B cell FCXMs and graft failure. The demonstration of antibody binding to both T and B cells suggests the antibody detected is likely to be directed at the HLA class I antigens. A T cell positive FCXM where there is no antibody binding with B cells suggests that the antibody may not be HLA specific. B cell positive FCXMs may occur when the T cell FCXM is negative. Lazda (1994) found that a strongly positive B cell FCXM was significantly associated with poorer graft survival at one year compared with those where negative, or weakly positive, B cell FCXMs occurred. This association was found only in those patients receiving allografts mismatched for at least one HLA-DR antigen suggesting that the antibody detected may be specific for HLA class II.

Sumitran-Karuppan (1992) found that the FCXM could be used to great advantage in determining the likely outcome of renal allografts where the specificity of the antibody could be clearly defined. This study demonstrated that in the cases where a positive FCXM could be attributed to HLA specific antibodies there was an increased risk of rejection episodes, even when the CDC crossmatch was negative. These studies emphasise that, as in CDC crossmatching, it is of great importance to understand the antibody profile of the patient serum samples when interpreting the results of FCXMs.

Methods

1. Preparation of lymphocytes

1a. Preparation of lymphocytes from whole blood

Peripheral blood lymphocytes (PBL) are used for prospective crossmatching of living organ donor/recipient pairs and recipients of thoracic organ transplants when a result must be obtained prior to organ retrieval.

PBL are usually obtained from peripheral blood by discontinuous density gradient centrifugation using a Ficoll/sodium metrizoate solution at a density of 1.077 at 18-22°C. Diluted blood is layered on to the separation medium and the density is such that during centrifugation red cells and granulocytes pass through the medium while platelets, lymphocytes and monocytes remain above with the mononuclear cells at the interface. The platelets are then removed from the mononuclear cells by differential washing.

☑ anticoagulated peripheral blood

☑ Ficoll/sodium metrizoate lymphocyte separation medium (LSM), density 1.077 at 18-22°C (available from several commercial sources e.g. Nycomed, Lymphoprep)

1. Dilute blood with equal volume of balanced salt solution/culture medium (eg. Hanks' Balanced Salt Solution (HBSS), Gibco)

2. Carefully layer the diluted blood over half its volume of LSM: avoid mixing.

3. Centrifuge at 800*g* for 20 min at 18-22°C. Avoid mixing during centrifugation by ensuring there is no braking.

4. Carefully remove cells from the plasma/LSM interface

5. Resuspend cells in HBSS and centrifuge at 500*g* for 5 min

6. Repeat wash step 5 twice

7. Resuspend cells in culture medium (eg. RPMI, Gibco) for standardisation

Troubleshooting

Low cell yields and/or inadequate lymphocyte purity are the most common problems with density gradient separation. These can be caused by:

- Mixing of the blood or cell suspension with the LSM. Care should be taken during layering and centrifugation to avoid cell/LSM mixing.
- Overloading the gradient. The blood or cell suspension should be adequately diluted before layering on to the LSM.

1b. Lymphocyte preparation from spleen

1. Place a piece of spleen approximately 1.0cm^2 in a Petri dish containing HBSS and cut into fragments using a scalpel. Firmly squeeze each fragment with forceps to tease out the cells.

2. Transfer the cell suspension to a plastic tube.

3. Wash the spleen fragments in fresh HBSS to ensure that all cells are harvested and transfer the cell suspension to the tube.

4. Separate lymphocytes using LSM as in *Protocol 1a.*

To help remove phagocytic cells from the spleen cell suspension, the spleen cell suspension can be incubated with carbonyl iron prior to layering on LSM (0.2g / 50ml cell suspension, 30 min, 37°C. Phagocytic cells and carbonyl iron can then be drawn to the side of the tube with a magnet while non-phagocytic cells are carefully removed.

1c. Lymphocyte preparation from lymph node

1. Trim excess fatty tissue from the lymph node and place lymph node in a petri dish containing HBSS.

2. Slice the lymph node with a scalpel and squeeze with forceps to expel the lymphocytes.

3. Transfer cell suspension to a plastic tube and allow any tissue debris / cell aggregates to settle to the bottom.

4. Transfer the supernatant cell suspension to a clean tube, top up with HBSS and centrifuge at 500*g* for 5 min.

5. Decant supernatant, resuspend the cells in HBSS and centrifuge as in step 4.

6. Resuspend cells in culture medium for standardisation.

2. Separation of T and B cells

Preparations of isolated T cells or B cells can be obtained using immunomagentic beads. For example T cells can be isolated using Class I Dynabeads which bind CD8+ cells (Dynal 210.02) and B cells by using Class II Dynabeads which bind a non-polymorphic epitope of the class II beta chain (Dynal 210.04). Immunomagnetic beads are also available from One Lambda and Biotest.

- ☑ Complement fixation test (CFT) diluent (ICN Flow 28-101-05) 1 tablet dissolved in 100ml distilled water.
- ☑ Class I Dynabeads (Dynal 210.02)
- ☑ Class II Dynabeads (Dynal 210.04)

1. Transfer 1ml of isolated lymphocytes at a concentration of $5x10^6$/ml into a 13ml tube with cap.

2. Add 15µl of Class I or Class II Dynabeads. Incubate on melting ice for 5 min, mixing by inverting the tube at regular intervals.

3. Place tube in the Magnetic Particle Concentrator (MPC, Dynal 120.02) and leave for 2 min.

4. Remove solution using a pastette taking care not to disturb the beads against the magnet.

5. Remove the tube from the MPC. Add 3ml of cold saline/CFT, cap the tube and mix by inverting gently.

6. Place tube on MPC and leave for 2 minutes.

7. Repeat steps 4-6.

8. Pipette off solution and remove tube from MPC

9. Resuspend the bead/cell rosettes in 75µl HBSS/CFT

This provides sufficient cells for one Terasaki plate

Troubleshooting

The most common problems are inadequate cell yield and/or purity. These can be caused by:

- Reagents being insufficiently cold. All reagents must be kept and used at 4°C and incubation steps carried out on ice.
- Destruction of cell/bead rosettes. Care must be taken when washing and pipetting the rosettes.
- Knocking beads off the side of the tube while aspirating the supernatant.

3. Collection and storage of sera for crossmatching

Serum samples should be obtained regularly from patients awaiting transplantation. Ideally 5 -10 ml clotted blood samples should be collected on a monthly basis. Samples should also be obtained 10-14 days after a blood transfusion. The serum should be decanted and stored below -20°C to be used for crossmatching as required. If samples are likely to be used frequently for crossmatching with multiple potential donors it may be desirable to store small aliquots of serum to avoid repeated freeze/thawing. Some centres may require a fresh serum sample to be obtained at the time of crossmatching, in which case the sample should be separated, frozen and then thawed before use to ensure that the new sample has been treated in the same way as the other stored samples which are to be used in the crossmatch. The frequency of sample collection and requirements for samples used for crossmatching are procedures which should be agreed by consultation between the laboratory, medical staff and clinics.

4. Complement dependent cytotoxicity (CDC) crossmatch

The CDC crossmatch may be performed using unseparated, isolated PBLs or spleen cells or with separated T cells and/or B cells. Splenic lymphocytes will usually comprise at least 60% B cells so that when they can be used for crossmatching it is possible to detect antibodies to HLA-DR and -DQ in addition to antibodies to HLA-A, -B, -Cw without further B cell separation. However, when PBL are the target separated B cell crossmatches are required to detect HLA-DR and -DQ specific antibodies.

The incubation times used in the CDC crossmatch vary between different laboratories. The second incubation following the addition of complement is usually twice the length of the first incubation of cells with serum. Commonly used incubation times are 30 + 60 min, 45 + 90 min, 60 + 120 min. In general the longer the incubation times the greater the sensitivity of the test and increased sensitivity is recommended for crossmatching.

4a. CDC crossmatch

☑ Complement fixation test (CFT) diluent (ICN Flow 28-101-05) 1 tablet dissolved in 100ml distilled water.

☑ Lyophilised rabbit complement (each batch of complement should be tested by checkerboard titration prior to use to evaluate activity)

☑ Ethidium bromide/acridine orange stain. 0.2mg/ml acridine orange (Sigma E8751), 0.1mg/ml ethidium bromide (BDH CI 46005), 15% w/v bovine haemoglobin (Sigma H2625), 2.5% w/v sodium EDTA (BDH AnalaR 10093) in PBS. Store in 2ml aliquots at -30°C.

☑ Black calligraphy ink (10%) can be used as a quenching agent in place of bovine haemoglobin

☑ Terasaki trays

All CDC crossmatch tests should be set up in triplicate.

1. Dispense 1µl of each serum into the wells of an oiled Terasaki tray. Every plate should contain at least 1 negative and 1 positive control serum sample.

2. Add 1µl of lymphocytes at 2 x 10^6 / ml to each well and incubate for 45 min at 22°C.

3. Immediately prior to use reconstitute lyophilised rabbit complement with distilled/sterile water.

4. Add 5µl complement to each well

5. Incubate for 90 min at 22°C

6. Thaw ethidium bromide/acridine orange stain prior to use and add 1µl stain to each well.

7. Read plates using an inverted microscope with a UV light source.

8. Score according to percentage of viable cells present in each well. Viable cells are stained green, dead cells are stained red.

Scores are given as shown in Table 4.1

% cell death	Score	Interpretation
0 - 10	1	Negative
11 - 20	2	Probably negative
21 - 50	4	Weak positive
51 - 80	6	Positive
81 - 100	8	Strong positive
	0	Invalid result

Table 4.1. International Histocompatibility Workshop Scoring System

4b. DTT modification of the CDC crossmatch

The addition of DTT to sera will abolish any reactivity due to IgM antibodies. Each serum sample is tested with and without the addition of DTT to determine whether reactivity is due to IgG or IgM antibodies. This modification to the CDC assay is used to reduce IgM autoreactive antibodies that are irrelevant to transplant outcome. As it will also reduce IgM alloantibodies that may adversely effect transplant function it is recommended that the DTT crossmatch is only used for patients known to have IgM autoantibodies and without IgM alloantibodies unless the specificity is clearly defined.

☑ 0.1M dithiothreitol (DTT) (stored frozen in 100µl aliquots) (Sigma D0632)

☑ 0.1M Cystine (Sigma C8630)

DTT treated serum and untreated serum should be tested in parallel.

1. Prepare crossmatch trays for untreated sera as in Protocol 4a including IgG and IgM controls.

2. Transfer 36µl of each serum sample to a Beckman tube.

3. Add 4µl 0.1M DTT, mix thoroughly.

4. Add 1µl DTT treated serum to the wells of a Terasaki tray. Every plate should contain a negative control sample, an IgG positive control sample and an IgM positive control sample.

5. Add 1µl of lymphocytes to each well of the tray and incubate for 45 min at 22°C.

6. Immediately prior to use reconstitute lyophilised complement with sterile water. Transfer 1ml complement to a separate container and add 25µl of cystine, mix well.

7. Add 5µl of cystine free complement to the trays containing untreated sera. Add 5µl cystine treated complement to the trays containing DTT treated sera.

8. Proceed as in CDC crossmatch *Protocol 4a.*

9. Interpretation of positive results: for the DTT crossmatch results to be valid, the IgG control must be unaffected by DTT treatment and the IgM control activity must be abolished. Total reduction of cytotoxicity in treated wells indicates original reaction was due to IgM antibodies. No reduction of cytotoxicity indicates that original reaction was due to IgG antibodies. Partial reduction of cytotoxicity indicates a mixture of IgG and IgM antibodies.

An alternative approach is to prepare replicate sets of crossmatch trays. For one set, the untreated sera, proceed as in *Protocol 4a.* For the other set, the DTT crossmatch:

1. Resuspend the lymphocytes at 2×10^6 / ml in culture medium containing 0.01M DTT (ie. 0.1ml 0.1M DTT plus 0.9ml medium)

2. Proceed from step 5 of *Protocol 4b.*

4c. Quality Control

It is essential that each crossmatch tray includes a negative control serum to check cell viability and a positive control serum to check both complement activity and the expression of cell surface HLA.

- *Negative control:* the most commonly used negative control is a pool of human blood group AB sera or a single human AB serum that have been extensively tested by CDC to ensure no reactivity with lymphocytes. If human AB serum is not available then extensively tested negative sera from untransfused males is acceptable.
- *Positive controls:* the monoclonal antibody W6/32 recognises an epitope shared by HLA-A, -B, -C molecules and is commonly used as a positive control to check complement activity and the presence of cells expressing those molecules. When B cell crossmatches are being performed a control is required to determine the percentage of B cells present. The monoclonal antibody L243 which recognises an epitope on HLA-DR, -DQ, -DP molecules is suitable.
- *DTT controls:* for DTT crossmatches the activity of the DTT must be checked using a serum known to contain IgG antibodies and one known to contain IgM antibodies. A pool of alloantisera from highly sensitised patients can be used as the IgG control. The IgM control can be a serum or pool of sera from patients known to have IgM autoreactive lymphocytotoxic antibodies. Alternatively, a commercially available IgM monoclonal antibody can be used (Serotec MCA349)

- *Replicates:* All crossmatch tests should be performed in at least duplicate and preferably triplicate. In order to control for tray related anomalies the replicates should be on separate trays.

4d. Troubleshooting

When a syringe dispenser is used to dispense cells into a Terasaki tray with sera in the wells it is possible to transfer serum from one well to the next on the tip of the syringe. This can be avoided by:

- A 'shooting' technique whereby the syringe dispenser is held vertically over the well ensuring the needle is not in contact with the serum and operating the button firmly. To ensure the cells and serum are adequately mixed trays should be centrifuged at 120*g* for 30 sec.
- Using an automated cell dispenser (Biotest). This can be used to dispense cell suspension and also complement. Trays should be centrifuged as above to ensure adequate mixing.

5. Standardisation of the flow cytometer

It is important that daily procedures should be in place to ensure that the machine is performing within acceptable standards. This is normally achieved by the use of one or more of a variety of beads. The machine manufacturers market beads which can be used to check the basic alignment of the machine is within acceptable standards (CaliBRITE beads - Becton Dickinson, Flow Check fluorospheres - Coulter). A daily log of the results of running beads, including details of the machine settings should be kept. Variation in performance should be noted and may indicate that the machine requires servicing.

If the results of tests performed at different times are to be directly compared a further level of standardisation will be necessary. Beads which give number of peaks of fluorescence which correspond to a known number of molecular equivalents of soluble fluorescence (MESF, MEF) can be used (eg. Quantum beads - Flow Cytometry Standards Corporation, Fluorospheres - Dako). A linear regression line can then be drawn and the MEF of each sample can be calculated.

6. Flow cytometry crossmatch

6a. 2-colour flow cytometry crossmatch

The 2-colour FCXM is used to determine IgG binding to a cell population of interest. A fluorescein isothiocyante (FITC) conjugated anti-human IgG antibody is used to identify antibody binding along with a phycoerythrin (RPE) conjugated monoclonal antibody to either CD3 to identify T cells or CD19 or CD20 to identify B cells. Antibodies for flow cytometry are available from a number of sources including Becton Dickinson, Coulter, Dako, Harlan Seralab, Serotec, Sigma and Stratech Scientific.

A saline solution containing 0.1% bovine serum albumin or other protein agent to block non-specific background binding should be used for all washing steps in the procedure and for resuspending isolated lymphocytes. The saline solution may also contain sodium azide at a concentration of 0.1% to prevent capping of receptors.

The volume of serum, number of cells, dilutions of polyclonal and monoclonal antibodies, incubation times and temperatures and wash volumes used in the FCXM vary between laboratories. These variables should be established by the individual laboratory, this will be discussed in greater detail in *Protocol 6c.* The protocol given below is for example only. All crossmatches should be set up in at least duplicate.

1. Prepare lymphocytes as described in Section 1 and resuspend in PBS/0.1% BSA/0.1% azide at 5 x 10^6 / ml.

2. Add 20μl serum to tubes. A negative and a positive control must be included.

3. Add 2x10^5 cells to each tube and mix well.

4. Incubate for 30 min at 22°C

5. Wash by adding 2ml saline solution to each tube and centrifuge at 400*g* for 5 mins.

6. Repeat wash step.

7. Decant supernatant.

8. Resuspend cells in 50μl saline solution.

9. Add 5μl IgG/FITC (Dako F056)

10. Add 5μl CD3/RPE (Dako R810) or CD19/RPE (Dako R808)

11. Incubate for 30 min at 4°C

12. Wash twice as in step 5

13. Resuspend cells in 500μl saline solution

14. Run samples on flow cytometer

15.Collect data on 10,000 lymphocytes (20,000 if B cells from PBL are to be analysed). The lymphocyte population can be identified by forward and side scatter properties.

16. Analyse the IgG binding for each sample by gating the FL2 positive cell population (CD3 or CD19 cells) and drawing the FL1 histogram for the gated cells. The mean or median channel number can be obtained from the histogram statistics.

6b. 3- colour flow cytometry crossmatch

This method identifies T and B cell populations in a lymphocyte sample and analyses each for binding of alloantibodies (Robson & Martin, 1996).

All crossmatches should be set up in at least duplicate.

1. Wash lymphocytes 3 times in PBS/0.1% BSA/0.01% azide and resuspend at 5 x 10^6 / ml.

2. Add 20µl of test serum to the tubes. A negative and positive control must be included.

3. Add 30µl of cell suspension to each tube and mix by vortexing.

4. Incubate for 1 h at 22°C.

5. Wash samples twice in 5ml PBS/0.1% BSA/0.01% azide at 22°C by centrifuging at 300*g* for 5 min.

6. Decant supernatant and resuspend cells in residual PBS by vortexing.

7. Dilute FITC-conjugated anti-human IgG (Dako F056) antibody 1:1 with PBS/0.1% BSA/0.01% azide and add 3µl to each tube. Vortex the tubes.

8. Incubate at 4°C for 20 min in the dark.

9. Wash twice with cold PBS/0.1% BSA/0.01% azide at 300*g* for 5 min.

10. Repeat step 6.

11. Add 4µl RPE-CY5 conjugated anti-CD3 (Dako C7067) and 3ul RPE conjugated anti-CD19 (Dako R808)

12. Vortex mix the tubes.

13. Incubate at 4°C for 30 min.

14. Wash in PBS/0.1% BSA/0.01% azide.

15. Resuspend to a final volume of 500µl.

16. Run samples on flow cytometer.

17. Collect data on 1000 B cells. The lymphocyte population can be defined by forward and side scatter.

18. FITC/IgG binding to T cells can be analysed by gating the RPE-CY5/CD3 positive population and to B cells by gating the RPE/CD19 population.

6c. Optimisation of FCXM assays

There are a number of variables within the FCXM method which should be investigated by the individual laboratory in order to optimise the assay.

1. Cell/serum ratio: This may be investigated by using known positive and negative samples with cells as appropriate. The number of cells should be sufficient to allow counting of 5,000 - 20,000 events per sample. The cell/serum ratio should be determined such that known positives are detected but the serum volume should not be so great that there is a 'prozone' effect causing loss of a positive signal with increasing quantities of serum.

2. Wash volumes/wash numbers: The number of wash steps and volume of wash solution used should be sufficient to remove any unbound human antibody following the first incubation. Any unbound antibody which remains after the wash steps may bind the IgG/FITC preventing it from binding to the human antibody bound to the cell surface and thus reducing the sensitivity of the assay.

3. Polyclonal/monoclonal antibodies: These should be used according to the manufacturers instructions and should be titrated using known positive and negative cell serum combinations in order to maximise the difference in fluorescence between positive and negative samples. Some combinations of FITC/RPE conjugated antibodies, when added together, interact which can cause skewing of the FL1/FL2 signal. This can lead to incorrect results being obtained. Combinations of antibodies should be checked for this interaction and if found to be present the IgG/FITC should be added and incubated without the CD/RPE. A wash step should then be performed before addition of the CD/RPE antibody and a further incubation step.

6d. Interpretation of Results

Interpretation of results can lead to differences between centres in the results obtained for the same tests (Harmer 1996, Shenton 1997). A number of different methods are commonly used, all rely on a comparison of the test sample with the negative control.

1. Channel shift: This is the difference between the mean or median channel number of the test samples and that of the negative control. Some centres take an

absolute value for channel shift as a positive cut off e.g. 10, 20 or 40 channels. Other centres calculate the mean and standard deviation of the mean or median channel for 3 or more replicates of the negative control and then class a positive sample as one where the mean channel value is a given number (e.g. 2 or 3) of standard deviations greater than that of the negative control.

2. Relative fluorescence: The relative mean or median fluorescence (RMF) is calculated by dividing the mean or median channel number of the test by that of the negative control. This gives a measure of the relative fluorescence of the test compared to the control irrespective of the mean or median channel of the negative control. A cut-off value can then be established for positivity (e.g. RMF = 1.5, 2, 2.5)

3. Molecules of Fluorescence: If calibration beads are used at the time of the crossmatch test the number of molecular equivalents of soluble fluorescence (MEF) can be calculated for each sample. These can be used to calculate either the difference in MEF or the relative MEF of test and negative control.

Each laboratory should establish their own cut-off for positivity whichever method they choose to use. This may be determined by a retrospective study to investigate the clinical relevance of a given level of positivity in the transplant population or by titering of known HLA specific antibodies to the required level of detection (e.g. a given number of doubling dilutions beyond the cut off for detection by cytotoxicity).

6e. Quality Control

The most commonly used negative control is pooled human AB serum (see Section 4c). It is essential that all control sera to be used for flow cytometry crossmatching should be individually screened by flow cytometry prior to pooling to ensure that the sera do not contain any IgG autoantibodies which can be detected by flow cytometry.

A positive control comprising pooled serum from highly sensitised recipients known to have HLA specific IgG antibodies is commonly used. The pooled serum should contain antibodies which react with all HLA class I specificities. It may be desirable to include a weak positive control which is a dilution of the positive control such that the fluorescent signal is just above the positive cut-off which is used.

7. Crossmatching by ELISA

Commercially available ELISA based techniques are becoming increasingly used for the detection and definition of HLA specific antibodies in patients awaiting transplantation and also for monitoring antibody production following transplantation (Worthington *et al.*, 1998b). A number of studies have shown an association between antibodies detected by ELISA but not CDC with transplant outcome, although the majority of the currently available ELISA assays do not detect IgM alloantibodies which can be associated with transplant failure (Worthington *et al.,* 1998a). One major advantage of the ELISA tests is that they only detect HLA specific antibodies and not non-HLA and autoreactive antibodies that are irrelevant to transplant outcome.

As the ELISA techniques become more widely used for antibody screening it is logical that they should also be considered for crossmatching. The technique would invlove purification and capture on to ELISA trays the donor HLA molecules to be used as targets in the test. Currently one ELISA crossmatch kit is available commercially (CrossStat, SangStat) that detects antibodies to donor HLA-A, -B and Cw antigens but not HLA-DR, -DQ. Large studies are required to establish the role of ELISA crossmatch techniques in donor/recipient pre-transplant crossmatching as were carried out before the clinical application of flow cytometry crossmatching.

8. External Quality Assurance

It is a requirement for laboratory accreditation (Clinical Pathology Accreditation (UK) Ltd, EFI, ASHI) that laboratories participate in external quality assurance (EQA) schemes relevant for the services they provide. Within the United States EQA schemes for histocompatibility are provided under the auspices of ASHI and there are a number of schemes within Europe.

In the UK there is a UK NEQAS for H & I which, amongst others, has a scheme for crossmatching by cytotoxicity and one for crossmatching by flow cytometry. These schemes involve the distribution of blood samples of known but not revealed HLA phenotype and sera containing antibodies of known but not revealed specificity along with hidden negative sera. Once the relevant crossmatches have been completed and results returned the phenotypes and specificities are revealed and the results scored on the basis of consensus. Points are awarded for accuracy and reproducibility. While the EQA schemes cannot exactly mirror the acute donor/recipient crossmatch they provide an essential yardstick for laboratory performance compared with the H & I community as a whole and enable the identification of laboratories whose performance is unacceptable.

Adequate performance is essential for laboratory accreditation and to ensure that transplant programmes are supported by high quality H & I services. The quality of antibody identification, definition and crossmatching is one of the key factors that can influence transplant outcome.

References

Cardella, CJ, Falk, JA, Halloran, P, Robinette, M, Arbus, G, *et al.* (1985) Renal transplantation in patients with a positive crossmatch on non-current sera: long term follow-up. *Transplant Proc* **17**: 626-627

Chapman, JR, Deierhoi, MH, Carter, NP, Ting, A, Morris, PJ. (1985) Analysis of flow cytometry and cytotoxicity crossmatches in renal transplantation. *Transplant Proc* **17**: 2480-2481

Chapman, JR, Taylor, C, Ting, A, Morris, PJ. (1986a). Immunoglobulin class and specificity of antibodies causing positive T cell crossmatches: relationship with renal transplant outcome. *Transplantation* **42**: 608-613

Chapman, JR, Taylor, C, Ting, A, Morris, PJ. (1986b). Hyperacute rejection of a renal allograft in the presence of anti-HLA-Cw5 antibody. *Transplantation* **42**: 91-93

Cook, DJ, Terasaki, PI, Iwaki, Y, Terashita, GY, Lau, M. (1987) An approach to reducing early kidney transplant failure by flow cytometry crossmatching. *Clinical Transplantation* **1**: 253-256

Evans, PR, Lane, AC, Lambert, CM, Reynolds, WM, Wilson, PJ, *et al.* (1992). Lack of correlation between IgG T-lymphocyte flow cytometric crossmatches with primary renal allograft outcome. *Transplant International* **5**: S609-S612

Evans, PR, Trickett, P, Smith JL, Maciver, AG, Tate, D, *et al.* (1984). Variable expression of HLA-DR antigens in the human kidney. *Disease Markers* **2**: 251-253

Fenoglio, J, Ho, E, Reed, E, Rose, E, Smith, C, *et al.* (1989). Anti-HLA antibodies and heart allograft survival. *Transplant Proc* **21**: 807-809

Fuggle, SV, Errasti, P, Daar, AS. (1983). Localisation of MHC (HLA-ABC and DR) antigens in 46 kidneys. Differences in HLA-DR staining of tubules between kidneys. *Transplantation* **35**: 385-390

Fuller, TC, Fuller AA, Golden, M, Rodey, GE. (1997). HLA alloantibodies and the mechanism of the antiglobulin-augmented lymphocytotoxicity procedure. *Human Immunology* **56**: 94-105

Garovoy, MR, Rheinschmidt, MA, Bigos, M, Perkins, H, Colombe, B. (1983) Flow cytometry analysis: a high technology crossmatch technique facilitating transplantation. *Transplant Proc* **15**: 1939-1944

Harmer, AW, Garner, S, Bell, AE, Anyanwu, C, Cavanagh, G, *et al.* (1996) Evaluation of the flow cytometric crossmatch. Preliminary results of a multicentre study. *Transplantation* **61**: 1108-1111

Horsburgh, T, Mistry, N, Weston, S, Morgan, J, Donnelly, PK, *et al.*(1992) Relevance of positive crossmatches in renal transplantation. *Transplant Proc* **24**: 2508-2509

Kissmeyer-Nielsen, F, Olsen, S, Petersen, VP, Fjeldborg, O. (1966). Hyperacute rejection of kidney allografts associates with pre-existing humoural antibodies against donor cells. *Lancet* **1**: 662

Lazda, VA, Pollak, R, Mozes, MF, Joasson, O. (1988) The relationship between flow cytometer crossmatch results and subsequent rejection episodes in cadaver renal allograft recipients. *Transplantation* **45**: 562-565

Lazda, VA. (1994) Identification of patients at risk for inferior renal allograft outcome by a strongly positive B cell flow cytometry crossmatch. *Transplantation* **57**: 964-969

Martin, S, Liggett, H, Robson, A, Connolly, J, Johnson, RWG. (1993) The association between a positive T and B cell flow cytometry crossmatch and renal transplant failure. *Transplant Immunol* **1**: 270-276

Mohanakumar, T, Rhodes, C, Mendez-Picon, G, Goldman, M, Moncure, C, *et al.* (1981). Renal allograft rejection associated with presensitization to HLA-DR antigens. *Transplantation* **31**: 93-95

Ogura, K, Terasaki, PI, Johnson, C, Mendaz, R, Rosentahl, JT, *et al.* (1993) The significance of a positive flow cytometric crossmatch test in primary kidney transplantation. *Transplantation* **56**: 294-298

Robson, A, Martin, S (1996). T and B cell crossmatching using three-colour flow cytometry. *Transplant Immunol* **4**: 203-208

Rodey G, Bollig B, Oldfather J, Schutte L, Flye W, Phelan D. (1987) Extra reactivities detected in flow-cytometry-positive CDC-negative crossmatches are definable HLA specificities. *Transplant Proc* **19**: 778-779

Rodey, GE, Revels, K, Fuller, TC (1997). Epitope specificity of HLA class I alloantibodies. Stability of cross-reactive group patterns over extended time periods. *Transplantation* **63**: 885-893

Roelen, DL, van Bree, FPMJ, Witvliet, MD. (1994). IgG antibodies against HLA antigen are associated with activated cytotoxic T cells against this antigen. IgM are not. *Transplantation* **57**: 1388-1392

Shenton, BK, Bell, AE, Harmer, AW, Boyce, M, Briggs, D, *et al.* (1997) Improtance of methodology in the flow cytometric crossmatch: a multicentre study. *Transplant Proc* **29**: 1454-1455

Smith, JD, Danskine, AJ, Laylor, RM, Rose, ML, Yacoub, MH. (1993). The effect of panel reactive antibodies and the donor specific crossmatch on graft survival after heart and heart-lung transplantation. *Transplant Immunology* **1**: 60-65

Sumitran-Karuppan, S, Ohlman, S, Moller, E. (1992) The occurrence of cytotoxic and non-complement fixing antibodies in the crossmatch serum of patients with early acute rejection episodes. *Transplantation* **54**: 839-843

Talbot, D, Givan, AL, Shenton, BK, Stratton, A, Coates, E, *et al.* (1990) The prospective value of the preoperative flow cytometric crossmatch assay in renal transplantation. *Transplantation* **49**: 809-810

Thistlethwaite, JR, Buckingham, MR, Stuart, JK, Stuart, FP. (1986) Detection of presensitisation in renal allograft recipients using a flow cytoemtric immunofluorescence crossmatch. *Transplant Proc* **18**: 676-679

Ting, A and Morris, PJ. (1983). Successful transplantation with a positive T and B cell crossmatch due to autoreactive antibodies. *Tissue Antigens* **21**: 219-226

Worthington, JE. *et al.,* (1998a). The detection of HLA specific antibodies by PRA-STAT and their association with transplant outcome. *Transplantation* **65**: 121-125

Worthington, JE, (1998b). A novel strategy for the detection and definition of HLA specific antibodies in patients awaiting renal transplantation. *Transplant Int* **11 (Suppl 1):** S372-S376

Zachary, AA, Klingman, L, Thorne, N, Smerglia, AR, Teresi, GA. (1995). Variations of the lymphocytotoxicity test. *Transplantation* **60**: 498-503

PART 2

DNA-BASED HISTOCOMPATIBILITY TESTING

PART 2 OVERVIEW

DNA-BASED HISTOCOMPATIBILITY TESTING

J. L. Bidwell
University of Bristol
Department of Pathology and Microbiology
Homoeopathic Hospital Site
Cotham, Bristol BS6 6JU, England

Correlation between DNA polymorphism and HLA phenotypes was first revealed using restriction fragment length polymorphism (RFLP) analysis in the early to mid-1980s. The RFLP method was based on hybridisation of a radiolabelled cDNA probe to genomic DNA restriction fragments, previously separated by electrophoresis and transferred to a support membrane by traditional Southern blotting. Sceptics of molecular biology methods in HLA became convinced that DNA typing was an important development, when it was shown conclusively in 1993 that donor-recipient HLA-DR/DQ matching by RFLP analysis improved allograft survival (Opelz *et al.,* 1993). RFLP had its limitations, however, particularly in typing of HLA class I alleles, and it was eventually phased out in favour of the newer, polymerase chain reaction (PCR)-based techniques. These are able to define allelic specificity, if not always at the individual allele level, then at least at the allelic group or subgroup level.

The extreme polymorphism of HLA genes, and the patchwork nature of their DNA sequence motifs, represent enormous challenges for molecular biologists. In the last 10 years, a multiplicity of techniques has been developed, or applied from related molecular diagnostic disciplines, in response to these challenges. Some of these may be classified as follows (for a review see Bidwell, 1994):

Probe-hybridisation techniques:

- **PCR-SSO (sequence-specific oligonucleotides): dot-blot** and reverse dot-blot
- PCR-oligocapture sandwich assay
- PCR-dual-phase oligocapture
- PCR-HPA (hybridisation protection assay)

Electrophoresis-based techniques:

- **PCR-SSP (sequence-specific primers)**
- PCR-RFLP (restriction fragment length polymorphism)
- **PCR-SBT (sequencing-based typing)**

DNA conformational analysis techniques:

- PCR-SSCP (single stranded conformational polymorphism)
- PCR-HA (heteroduplex analysis)
- PCR-UHG (heteroduplex analysis with a universal heteroduplex generator)
- **PCR-RSCA (reference strand-mediated conformational analysis)**

Of the above, those highlighted in bold typeface are covered by this volume, since they represent the principal contemporary techniques in routine use in the majority of histocompatibility laboratories. Despite the undoubted advantages and disadvantages of certain methods, a single method has still not been universally adopted. This is perhaps understandable, since the adoption of a method is influenced by factors which are of differing priorities within individual laboratories. These factors may include cost of synthesising or purchasing reagent kits, cost and complexity of instrumentation, labour and staff skills required, sample throughput requirements and the potential for automation, precision and reproducibility of the method, and the clinical urgency to obtain results.

Apart from the principal DNA-based histocompatibility testing methods detailed in chapters 5 to 8, Part 2 of this volume contains two further chapters of importance and relevance: Chapter 9 reviews the subject of microsatellite loci within the human MHC, their clinical relevance and DNA-based methods of analysis; and Chapter 10 reviews on-line HLA sequence databases and alignments, with World Wide Web site listings and details of available computer software packages.

References

Bidwell, J (1994) Advances in DNA-based HLA-typing methods. *Immunol Today* **15**: 303-307

Opelz, G, Mytilineos, J, Scherer, S, Dunckley, H, Trejaut, J et al. (1993) Analysis of HLA-DR matching in DNA-typed cadaver kidney transplants. *Transplantation* **55**: 782-785

CHAPTER 5

PCR-SSP TYPING

M. Bunce
Transplantation Immunology
Nuffield Department of Surgery
Oxford Transplant Centre
Churchill Hospital
Oxford, OX3 7LJ, England

Introduction

The use of molecular typing methods for defining HLA class I and class II alleles is now commonplace. Molecular methods offer flexibility of resolution, improved reproducibility and greater accuracy compared to traditional serological methods (Bunce *et al.*, 1996; Jordan *et al.*, 1995; Lorentzen *et al.*, 1997; Mytilineos *et al.*, 1997; Yu *et al.*, 1997). The advantages of PCR-based methods of typing has led to the widespread use of molecular typing methods even to the extent where they have totally replaced serological methods in some centres. This chapter describes a PCR-based HLA typing method utilising sequence-specific primers (PCR-SSP) which is applicable to the identification of all HLA class I and class II alleles, as well as alleles from non-HLA loci (Fanning *et al.*, 1997; Procter *et al.*, 1996).

Most PCR-SSP systems features multiple small volume PCR reactions where each reaction is specific for an allele, or more commonly a group of alleles which correspond to a serologically defined antigen. PCR-SSP specificity is derived from matching the terminal 3'- nucleotide of the primers with the target DNA sequence. *Taq* polymerase can extend 3'-matched primers but not 3'-mismatched primers, consequently only target DNA complementary to both primers is efficiently amplified. PCR-SSP works because *Taq* polymerase lacks 3' to 5'-exonucleolytic proofreading activity (Chien *et al.*, 1976; Tindall and Kunkel, 1988). Such an activity would correct the mismatched terminal base of an SSP primer in a mismatched primer-template complex and subsequently permit efficient priming with the "repaired" primer. Thus the 3'-mismatch principle can be used to identify virtually any single point mutation within one or two PCR-SSP reactions (Newton *et al.*, 1989; Wu *et al.*, 1989). The theoretical specificity of a PCR-SSP primer mix is derived from the intersection of both primers' specificities. Thus, if sense primer matches HLA-A*0101 and A*0102 and the antisense primer matches HLA-A*0101 and A*0103 then if PCR stringency is maintained that primer mix will be specific for HLA-A*0101. To type an individual completely at any given locus multiple PCR-SSP reactions are set up and subjected to PCR under identical conditions. The presence or absence of PCR amplification is detected in gel electrophoresis step with visualisation by ethidium bromide incorporation (see Figure 5.1). An important feature of SSP is that each individual reaction contains primers to amplify a so called "housekeeping" gene (Olerup and Zetterquist, 1992) which detects possible PCR inhibition and thus acts as a positive control. Without this positive control it would be difficult to discriminate between a failed PCR reaction and a negative PCR reaction, and hence all homozygous results would be questionable.

PCR-SSP was predicted to be applicable to HLA analysis in 1989 (Wu *et al.*, 1989) and was first applied in a limited fashion to HLA typing DPB in 1990 (Fugger *et al.*, 1990), whilst Lanchbury *et al* utilised the 3'-mismatch concept to obtain DR4 group-specific amplification prior to DR4 SSOP subtyping (Lanchbury *et al.*, 1990). The first comprehensive PCR-SSP HLA typing system was described in 1992 by Olerup and Zetterquist for low resolution HLA-DRB1 typing, including group-specific detection of DRB3 and DRB4 using 19 PCR-SSP reactions (Olerup and Zetterquist, 1992). PCR-SSP was soon applied to detect polymorphisms in other class II loci such as HLA-DQB1 (Bunce *et al.*, 1993; Olerup *et al.*, 1993) HLA-DQA1 (Olerup *et al.*, 1993) and DPB1(Knipper *et al.*, 1994). Identification of class I alleles by PCR-SSP was first reported by Browning *et al* (Browning *et al.*, 1993) who described low resolution typing of HLA-A. Thereafter, medium resolution PCR-SSP systems were rapidly described for HLA-C (Bunce *et al.*, 1994; Bunce and Welsh, 1994) and HLA-B (Bunce *et al.*, 1995a) with low resolution HLA-B typing systems also being described (Sadler *et al.*, 1994). Phototyping was the first PCR-SSP system to allow the simultaneous detection of HLA-A, B, C, DRB1, DRB3, DRB4, DRB5, and DQB1 alleles (Bunce *et al.*, 1995b). This method has a resolution and accuracy far greater than average serology, and only takes 3 h to complete, making it suitable for genotyping cadaver donors. The development of automatic dispensing equipment and better electrophoresis equipment has facilitated the use of Phototyping in many laboratories and in some laboratories, including our own (since Sept 1994), it has completely replaced serology. An example of genotyping using the Phototyping method is shown in Figure 5.1.

Published PCR-SSP methods generally define a single locus (Browning *et al.*, 1993; Bunce *et al.*, 1994; Bunce *et al.*, 1996; Bunce *et al.*, 1995a; Bunce *et al.*, 1993; Bunce and Welsh, 1994; Gilchrist *et al.*, 1998; Knipper *et al.*, 1994; Krausa *et al.*, 1993; Krausa and Browning, 1996; Olerup *et al.*, 1993; Olerup and Zetterquist, 1992; Sadler *et al.*, 1994; Savelkoul *et al.*, 1995) or they may be, as described here, a combination of loci known as Phototyping (Bunce *et al.*, 1995b). The methods in this chapter are designed for medium resolution typing of HLA-A, B, C, DRB1, DRB3, DRB4, DRB5 and DQB1 which is updated from our previous publications (Bunce *et al.*, 1995b). The reactions described can be used as a whole set, or they can be broken up into various locus-specific units. For all our different typing sets we use a single PCR-SSP protocol utilising one PCR program which enables us to rapidly incorporate new PCR-SSP reactions into our system without changing any protocols or parameters. Adopting this philosophy gives any PCR-SSP system tremendous flexibility and greatly facilitates routine use of all our PCR-SSP systems for HLA and non-HLA genes.

An advantage of PCR-SSP over PCR-SSOP methods (see chapter 6) is that PCR-SSP detects polymorphisms linked on an individual chromosome (*cis*) whereas PCR-SSOP detects polymorphisms on both DNA chromosomes (*cis* or *trans*). Thus, PCR-SSP has greater power for discriminating between heterozygosity involving two closely related alleles. In addition, the nucleic acid substitutions present on novel unsequenced allelic variants can be identified by PCR-mapping. In this technique, a potential new allele is mapped by using a sense primer that recognises the allelic variant (normally from the initial molecular typing) in combination with multiple antisense primers in multiple reactions. The positive and negative reactions with these primer mixes can then be used to map out many of the allelic variants polymorphisms. Whilst this approach is certainly no substitute for sequencing, it has been used to successfully identify many new class I alleles (Bunce *et al.*, 1994; Bunce *et al.*, 1995a; Bunce *et al.*, 1995b; Bunce and Welsh, 1994; Krausa *et al.*, 1995) and class II alleles (Aldener and Olerup, 1993; Poli *et al.*, 1996); which were subsequently proved correct by sequencing.

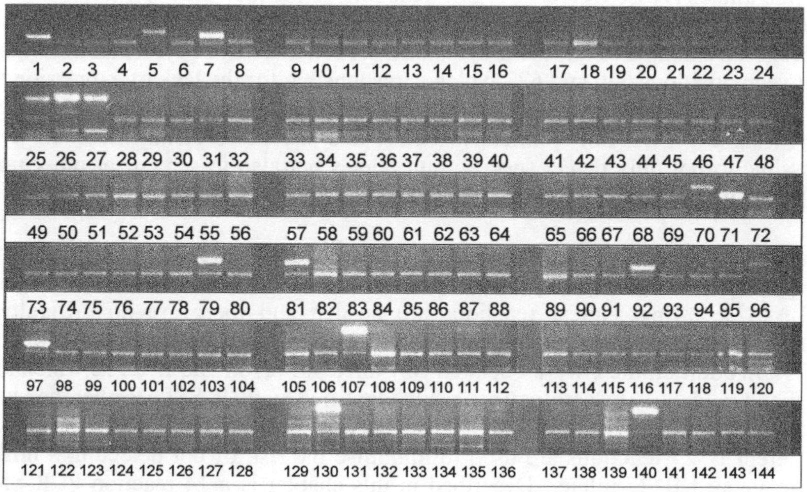

Figure 5.1 Phototyping
This Phototype was produced using the primer mixes shown in Tables 5.3a-d. The cathode end of the gel is at the top.

Alleles identified	**Positive lane numbers**
A*0101-4N	1, 25
A*2402-14 (excludes A*2406/8/13/03v)	5, 7
Bw4	26
Bw6	27
B*52011/2	79, 81
B*1529	70, 71
Cw*0704	92
Cw*1202	96, 97
DRB1*1501-6/8	107
DRB5*01/02	130
DQB1*0602/10/13	140

One disadvantage of solely using molecular typing methods based on existing sequence information is that new allelic variants may not be detected at all, or they may not be discriminated from a known allele. To avoid missing new allelic variants when using just PCR-SSP or SSOP, a policy of using large numbers of primers or probes can be adopted which has the dual advantage of potentially detecting novel alleles and enhancing the resolution of the typing system. However even extensive SSP or SSOP typing systems cannot on their own discriminate between normally expressed alleles and expression variants unless the novel mutation by chance disrupts the annealing of a primer or probe to target DNA. Thus, null alleles and low expressed alleles are normally only detected by a combination of serological and molecular methods. Once the mutation giving rise to null alleles is discovered PCR-SSP reactions to identify the polymorphism can be devised. Some mutations giving rise to null alleles are likely recur in other alleles: an example of this is the cytosine insertion in a row of cytosines anywhere between positions 620 and 627 which is responsible for the lack of expression of A*2411N (Magor *et al.*, 1997), A*01014N (Laforet *et al.*, 1997) and B*5111N. By designing PCR-SSP primers to detect this site of recurring mutation it is possible to not only detect specific null alleles but also to screen for other null alleles with this insertion (Bunce *et al.*, manuscript submitted).

One of the most frequently requested HLA tests is for HLA-B27 testing as an aid to diagnosis of various spondyloarthropathies. PCR-SSP is extremely suitable for HLA-B27 testing as few reactions are needed and there are no difficulties discriminating between serologically crossreactive antigens such as B7, B40 and B73. In addition the Bw6-associated B27 alleles B*2708 and B*2712 which are difficult to identify by serology are easily identified by PCR-SSP. Rather than just using a single pan-B*27 PCR-SSP reaction it is recommended that at least two different B*27 reactions are used to minimise the risk of not detecting a novel unsequenced B*27 allele. Described in this chapter is a 14-reaction PCR-SSP typing for B*27 detection and allele-specific typing so that alleles that may not predispose to spondyloarthropathy can be distinguished from those that do (Lopez-Larrea *et al.*, 1995).

Clinical relevance

There are many reasons for tissue typing: matching for solid and bone marrow transplantation, anthropological studies, disease association studies, forensic studies and to facilitate investigations into T-cell mediated immunity. The tissue typing method most suited to each application is a balance of resolution, sample numbers, time, money, sample material and the expertise of the individuals performing the typing.

Serological typing methods are traditionally used to define HLA antigens at the cell surface level. However discrepancies between serological methods and recently developed PCR-DNA-based methods of HLA typing have shown that molecular methods frequently offer superior resolution and accuracy over serological methods (Bunce *et al.*, 1996; Jordan *et al.*, 1995; Lorentzen *et al.*,

1997; Otten *et al.*, 1995; Yu *et al.*, 1997) which is reflected in many disease and transplantation studies (Barnardo *et al.*, 1996; Charron *et al.*, 1997; Mallon *et al.*, 1996; Mignot *et al.*, 1997; Mytilineos *et al.*, 1997; Opelz *et al.*, 1997; Speiser *et al.*, 1996; Tonks *et al.*, 1997; Young *et al.*, 1997).

The hallmark of virtually all PCR-based typing systems is that the resolution is flexible from very low resolution to high resolution depending on the number of primers or probes used. Allele-specific typing by any molecular method presents the researcher with a powerful analysis tool. In disease studies a weak association with serological antigens may become crystal clear when individual amino acids are taken into account. In transplantation, the analysis of immunodominant epitopes present on multiple alleles can only really be investigated by high-resolution typing of all donors and recipients. These applications of high-resolution typing will also need a different breed of computer analysis. Instead of correlating disease or rejection with a list of antigens the computer programs of the future will be required to correlate disease or rejection with linear and conformational epitopes (Barnardo *et al.*, 1997). It is also expected that computer programs will be required to correlate disease/rejection with peptide presentation in either class I or class II molecules. Ultimately this may lead to the discovery that certain combinations of class I and class II antigens present within an individual will predispose that individual to disease or rejection given exposure to certain pathogens or transplanted antigens.

In bone marrow transplantation a beneficial effect of matching has been shown with serological techniques (Anasetti *et al.*, 1989; Atkinson *et al.*, 1982; Beatty, 1992). However, serologically defined antigens often encompass multiple alleles (Bodmer *et al.*, 1995), many of which are relevant. Recently class I and class II molecular typing has been applied to bone marrow transplantation which has shown a high degree of mismatching at the allelic level, especially for HLA-C (Barnardo *et al.*, 1996; Petersdorf *et al.*, 1994b) and DP (Santamaria *et al.*, 1994; Speiser *et al.*, 1996) but also at other loci (Speiser *et al.*, 1996). Defining mismatches at the allelic level appeared to correlate with high MLC responses (Baxter-Lowe *et al.*, 1992) and high donor anti-recipient CTLp responses (Barnardo *et al.*, 1996; Speiser *et al.*, 1996). Speiser *et al* concluded that HLA class I and class II allele mismatches between unrelated phenotypically matched pairs were frequent and associated with increased incidence of post-transplant complications and morbidity (Speiser *et al.*, 1996). These findings would indicate that molecular typing is extremely desirable for unrelated bone marrow transplantation and that the higher the resolution the better.

In renal transplantation, virtually all matching studies have confirmed the original findings by Ting and Morris that DR matching is more beneficial than class I matching in renal transplantation (Ting and Morris, 1978). Subsequently, kidneys were exchanged between transplant centres on the basis of DR compatibility using low resolution serological methods that divided the DR antigens into the broad groups DR1-DR10. When molecular typing became available for class II it was applied to transplant pairs to identify whether fine specificities or allelic typing improved the DR matching effect or indeed whether inaccurate serological typing was compromising the observed DR matching effect. The first application of molecular techniques was applied by Opelz *et al* in the Collaborative Transplant Study (Opelz *et al.*, 1991). This study retrospectively used restriction fragment length polymorphisms (RFLP) and identified a better graft survival rate for RFLP compatible grafts versus serologically typed grafts. This study gave much impetus to the notion that molecular typing was necessary for accurate class II typing as up to 25% of all serological donor types were found to be incorrect. Recently Opelz *et al* have correlated matching the DR subgroups DR1-DR18 with improved graft survival compared to matching for broad DR specificities DR1-10 (Opelz *et al.*, 1997) therefore accurate typing and matching of donors and recipients is required for optimal graft survival. PCR-SSP typing of cadaver donors offers real advances over serological methods in terms of accuracy of the typing, especially for class II (Otten *et al.*, 1995), the rapid availability of results and the fact that the typing can be performed on small amounts of cadaver donor blood prior to the cessation of life support systems. The fact that SSP typing can be used on cadaver donor blood samples before the donated organs are removed means that cold ischaemia damage can be minimised and hence graft survival may be enhanced. Although class I matching in renal transplantation is secondary to class II matching the benefits of using class I PCR-SSP for donors is much the same as for class II, i.e. better accuracy and greater resolution. No large studies have yet been reported on the effects of class I allele matching in renal transplantation although it is clear that even minor mismatches can result in graft loss (Baan *et al.*, 1993; Chapman *et al.*, 1986). Molecular typing also benefits transplantation in that the HLA antigens present on lymphocytes used for antibody screening will be better characterised. This in turn allows greater characterisation of anti-HLA antibodies in patients awaiting transplantation which allows better definition of acceptable mismatches.

Molecular methods such as PCR-SSP offer a great advantage over serological techniques in that they have almost total flexibility to deal with the ever increasing number of HLA alleles (compare allele numbers between 1989 and 1996 for instance (Bodmer *et al.*, 1990; Bodmer *et al.*, 1997)). If a new allele is described that is not detected or masks an existing allele using PCR-SSP systems a new PCR reaction to identify the allele can be readily devised. By comparison, it is more difficult to predict the reactivity of a new antigen by serological means. Another drawback of serology (with the exception of monoclonal antibodies) is that even if a laboratory does have alloantisera to discriminate between antigenic splits sooner or later these rare alloantisera run out whereas molecular reagents can just be re-synthesised.

It is now clear that maximum allelic compatibility at all HLA loci is desirable for successful bone marrow transplantation and therefore the most accurate techniques should be used wherever possible (Petersdorf *et al.*, 1994a). This is not to say there is no place for serological methods: it is frequently easier and cheaper for laboratories with an extensive serological set up to do all the preliminary typing using serological methods and to perform final selection of donors by using high resolution molecular methods. If you are applying high resolution typing to all loci in unrelated bone marrow transplantation the chances of finding an exact HLA match are greatly diminished (Schipper *et al.*, 1996; Speiser *et al.*, 1994). The solution is then to develop strategies for identifying which mismatches matter and which do not. This may depend on identifying cytotoxic cell precursor frequencies (Barnardo *et al.*, 1996; Speiser *et al.*, 1996) or one may rely on the use of computer programs (Barnardo *et al.*, 1997) to identify which mismatches theoretically matter and which do not.

For the majority of research applications a medium resolution method is the best place to start. It allows the researcher to quickly focus on candidate loci, antigens or alleles which can then be further defined by higher resolution techniques. In most cases it does not matter which medium resolution technique is used, so long as it is performed accurately. Perhaps the best general purpose method for typing all HLA loci to a medium resolution is the PCR-SSP method. It has the advantage of flexible resolution coupled with ease of interpretation and speed of result. The speed of result can be important in the tissue typing of cadaver donors for solid organ transplantation. The perceived drawback of PCR-SSP for many is the large number of individual PCR required. However, this is no longer a disadvantage since there are now various technical innovations which have greatly simplified the use of multiple small volume PCR. For instance it is now possible to dispense PCR mixtures and primer mixes entirely with multichannel automatic dispensing pipettes or dedicated dispensing machines, and gel electrophoresis equipment has been manufactured to allow direct loading from 96 well formats. Eventually the electrophoresis step is likely to be eradicated completely as ELISA-based detection systems become commonplace.

Methods

Any typing method based on known sequences is always out of date by the time the method is published. The alleles recognised at the time of manuscript preparation are shown in Table 5.1. It should be noted that allelic sequences may be deleted or corrected over time and these changes can influence the expected results of your typing system. It is therefore recommended that a relevant internet database such as the HLA Informatics Site **http://www.anthonynolan.com/HIG/data.html** is frequently consulted for information on additions and changes.

The methods described here were initially described for Phototyping (Bunce *et al.*, 1995b). For efficient SSP amplification without false positive amplifications the conditions need to be highly stringent as it is theoretically possible for 3'-mismatch extension (Kwok *et al.*, 1990; Newton *et al.*, 1989; Wu *et al.*, 1989). SSP stringency is multifactorial, relying on the concentration of all the PCR constituents such as target DNA, *Taq*, dNTPs, Tris and free magnesium. PCR stringency kinetics also relies on individual primer factors such as primer sequence, length and type of primer-template mismatches. The following methods should provide you with enough information to efficiently test and set up and the PCR-SSP system of your choice.

Design of PCR primers and PCR primer mixes.

Consistent design of PCR primers along with use of the most up-to-date sequence alignments are key features of successful and accurate PCR-SSP HLA typing. All primers are initially designed to have a primer-template annealing temperature of

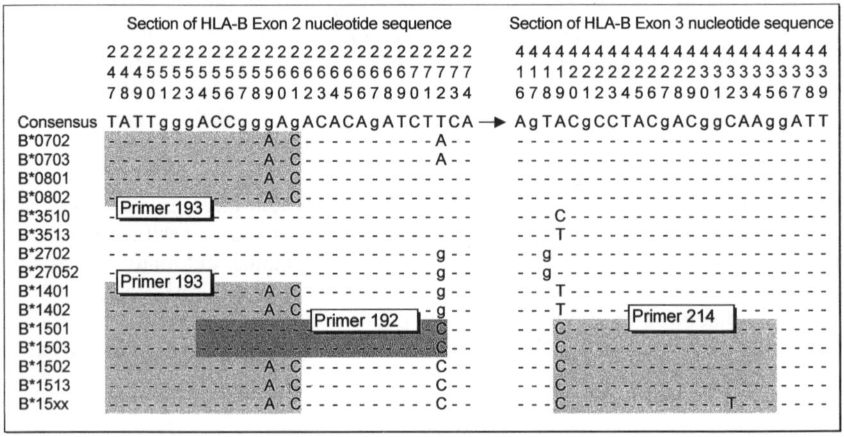

Figure 5.2. PCR-SSP primer design concepts

There are seven different HLA-B sequences found between positions 259 and 272: all four bases can be found at position 272 coupled with a dimorphic motif at nucleotides 259 and 261. Primer mix 73 uses a combination of primer 192 and 214 to identify many B*15 alleles, but it is mainly used for discriminating between the B*1501-like group of alleles and the B*1502 and B*1513 alleles. The mismatches at position 12 and 14 of primer 192 are sufficient to destabilise primer-template annealing in B*1502 and B*1503-positive individuals and thus allow discrimination between B*1501/3 and B*1502/13 groups. Single template-primer mismatches further along a primer may or may not have an adverse effect on primer specificity. For example the antisense primer 214 has a single mismatch at position 14 from the 3-prime end with the fictitional allele B*15xx. If primer 214 was used in conjunction with primer 193 it is likely that the B*15xx amplification would be only slightly weaker than that seen for, say B*1513. Primers that utilise internal mismatches for their specificity must be carefully titrated and properly tested before use to prevent false-positive amplification of closely related alleles. Primer 193 is extremely reliable for identification of the matching alleles as not only does it possess the necessary terminal 3'-mismatch but it has an additional mismatch at the third base. This is an ideal PCR-SSP primer.

HLA-A		HLA-B				HLA-Cw	HLA-DRB1/3/4/5				HLA-DQB1
*0101	*2608	*07021	*1802	*4003	*5504	*0102	*0101	*0810	*1309	*1506	*0201
*0102	*2609	*07022	*1803	*4004	*5505	*0103	*01021	*0811	*1310	*1507	*0202
*0103	*2611N	*07023	*1804	*4005	*5506	*02021	*01022	*0812	*1311	*1508	*0203
*0104N	*2901	*0703	*1805	*4006	*5601	*02022	*0103	*0813	*1312	*16011	*03011
*0201	*2902	*0704	*2701	*4007	*5602	*02023	*0104	*0814	*1313	*16012	*03012
*0202	*2903	*0705	*2702	*4008	*5603	*02024	*03011	*0815	*1314	*16021	*0302
*0203	*3001	*0706	*2703	*4009	*5604	*0203	*03012	*0816	*1315	*16022	*03032
*0204	*3002	*0707	*2704	*4010	*5701	*0302	*03021	*0817	*1316	*1603	*0304
*0205	*3003	*0708	*27052	*4011	*5702	*03031	*03022	*0818	*1317	*1604	*0305
*0206	*3004	*0709	*27053	*4012	*5703	*03032	*0303	*0819	*1318	*1605	*0306
*0207	*3006	*0801	*2706	*4014	*5704	*03041	*0304	*09012	*1319	*1607	*0307
*0208	*31012	*0802	*2707	*4015	*5801	*03042	*0305	*1001	*1320	*1608	*0308
*0209	*31012v	*0803	*2708	*4016	*5802	*0305	*0306	*11011	*1321		*0401
*0210	*3201	*0804	*2709	*4017	*5901	*0306	*0307	*11012	*1322	DRB3	*0402
*0211	*3202	*0805	*2710	*4018	*67011	*0308	*0308	*11013	*1323	*01011	*0501
*0212	*3301	*1301	*2711	*4101	*67012	*0309	*0309	*1102	*1324	*01012	*0502
*0213	*3303	*1302	*2712	*4102	*7301	*04011	*0310	*1103	*1325	*01013	*05031
*0214	*3401	*1303	*3501	*4103	*7801	*04012	*0311	*11041	*1326	*01014	*05032
*0215N	*3402	*1304	*3502	*4201	*78021	*0402	*04011	*11042	*1327	*0102	*0504
*0216	*3601	*1401	*3503	*4202	*78022	*0403	*04012	*1105	*1328	*0103	*06011
*02171	*4301	*1402	*3504	*4402	*8101	*0404	*0402	*1106	*1329	*0104	*06012
*02172	*6601	*1403	*3505	*44031	*8201	*0405	*0403	*1107	*1330	*0201	*06013
*0218	*6602	*1404	*3506	*44032		*0501	*0404	*11081	*1331	*0202	*0602
*0219	*6603	*1405	*3507	*4404		*0502	*04051	*11082	*1332	*0203	*0603
*0220	*68011	*1501	*3508	*4405		*0602	*04052	*1109	*1333	*0204	*0604
*0221	*68012	*1502	*35091	*4406		*0603	*0406	*1110	*1401	*0205	*06051
*0222	*6802	*1503	*35092	*4407		*0604	*0407	*1111	*1402	*0206	*06052
*0224	*68031	*1504	*3510	*4408		*0701	*0408	*1112	*1403	*0207	*0606
*0225	*68032	*1505	*3511	*4409		*0702	*0409	*1113	*1404	*0208	*0607
*0226	*6804	*1506	*3512	*4410		*0703	*0410	*1114	*1405	*0301	*0608
*0227	*6805	*1507	*3513	*4501		*0704	*0411	*1115	*1406	*0302	*0609
*0301	*6806	*1508	*3515	*4601		*0705	*0412	*1116	*1407	*0303	*0610
*0302	*6808	*1509	*3516	*4701		*0706	*0413	*1117	*1408		*0611
*0303N	*6901	*1510	*3517	*4702		*0707	*0414	*1118	*1409	DRB4	*0612
*0304	*7401	*1511	*3518	*4703		*0708	*0415	*1119	*1410	*01011	*0613
*1101	*7402	*1512	*3519	*4801		*0710	*0416	*1120	*1411	*0102	*0614
*1102	*7403	*1513	*3520	*4802		*0801	*0417	*1121	*1412	*0103	
*1103	*8001	*1514	*3521	*4803		*0802	*0418	*1122	*1413	*0104	
*1104		*1515	*3522	*4804		*0803	*0419	*1123	*1414	*0105	
*2301		*1516	*3523	*4901		*0804	*0420	*1124	*1415	*0201N	
*2402		*1517	*3524	*5001		*12021	*0421	*1125	*1416	*0301N	
*2402102L		*1518	*3701	*5002		*12022	*0422	*1126	*1417		
*2402v		*1519	*3702	*51011		*1203	*0423	*1127	*1418	DRB5	
*2403		*1520	*3801	*51012		*12041	*0424	*1128	*1419	*01011	
*2403v		*1521	*38021	*51021		*12042	*0425	*1129	*1420	*01012	
*2404		*1522	*38022	*51022		*1205	*0426	*1130	*1421	*0102	
*2405		*1523	*39011	*5103		*1206	*0427	*1131	*1422	*0103	
*2406		*1524	*39013	*5104		*1301	*0428	*1132	*1423	*0104	
*2407		*1525	*39021	*5105		*14021	*0429	*1201	*1424	*0105	
*2408		*1526N	*39022	*5106		*14022	*0701	*12021	*1425	*0106	
*2409N		*1527	*3903	*5107		*1403	*0703	*12022	*1426	*0107	
*2410		*1528	*3904	*5108		*1502	*0704	*12032	*1427	*0108N	
*2411N		*1529	*3905	*5109		*1503	*0801	*1204	*1428	*0109	
*2413		*1530	*39061	*5110		*1504	*08021	*1205	*1429	*0201	
*2414		*1531	*39062	*5111N		*15051	*08022	*1301	*1430	*0202	
*2501		*1532	*3907	*5113		*15052	*08032	*1302	*1431	*0203	
*2502		*1533	*3908	*52011		*1506	*08041	*13031	*15011	*0204	
*2601		*1534	*3909	*52012		*1601	*08042	*13032	*15012		
*2602		*1535	*3910	*5301		*1602	*08043	*1304	*15021		
*2603		*1537	*3911	*5302		*16041	*0805	*1305	*15022		
*2604		*1538	*3912	*5401		*1701	*0806	*1306	*15023		
*2605		*1539	*40011	*5501		*1702	*0807	*13071	*1503		
*2606		*1540	*40012	*5502		*1801	*0808	*13072	*1504		
*2607		*1801	*4002	*5503		*1802	*0809	*1308	*1505		

Table 5.1. List of alleles considered for PCR-SSP. See Table 5.3 for information on primer mixes and alleles amplified. Note that A*31012v, A*2402v and A*2403v have now been officially named as A*3103, A*2417 and A*2418, respectively.

Sense orientation primers

No.	Position	Sequence 5'-3'
36	22-43	TTgTggCAgCTTAAgTTTgAAT
41	20-38	TCCTgTggCAgCCTAAgAg
44	88-109	TACTTCCATAACCAggAggAgA
46	60-77	gACggAgCgggTgCggTA
47	17-38	gTTTCTTggAgCAggTTAAACA
48	21-40	CCTgTggCAgggTAAgTATA
50	26-46	AgTACTCTACgggTgAgTgTT
52	17-39	gTTTCTTgAAgCAggATAAgTTT
53	73-91	CggTTgCTggAAAgACgCg
61	17-38	gTTTCTTgCAgCAggATAAgTA
68	17-38	gTTTCTTggAgTACTCTACgTC
69	18-38	TTTCTTggAgCTgCgTAAgTC
70	17-38	gTTTCTTggAgCTgCTTAAgTC
76	135-152	ggAgTACCgggCggTgAg
77	44-63	gCTACTTCACCAACgggACC
79	61-77	ACggAgCgCgTgCgggg
82	70-89	gTgCgTCTTgTgAgCAgAAg
181	60-77	gACggAgCgCgTgCgTTA
263	75-94	gTTCCTggACAgATACTTCC
264	75-94	gTTCCTggAgAgATACTTCC
270	-20 to +1	gATCgTTCgTgTCCCCACAA
273	19-38	TTCTTggAgTACTCTACggg
283	-20 to +1	gATCgTTCgTgTCCCCACAg
347	18-38	TTTCgTgCTCCAgTTTAAggC
348	127-144	gACgTggggg TgTACCgC
349	63-81	ggAgCgCgTgCgTCTTgTA
353	70-89	gTgCgTCTTgTgACCAgATA
1465	59-77	ggACggAgCgCgTgCgTCT
1630	158-174	TggggCggCCTgATgAg
1631	154-170	gAgCTggggCggCCTgC
1634	81-102	ggACAgATACTTCTATAACCAA
1674	14-32	CACgTTTCTTggAgCTgTg

Antisense orientation primers

No.	Position	Sequence 5'-3'
37	257-276	CTgCACTgTgAAgCTCTCAC
38	257-276	CTgCACTgTgAAgCTCTCCA
39	199-216	CCgCCTCTgCTCCAggAg
40	199-217	CCCgCTCgTCTTCCAggAT
49	232-252	CCCgTAgTTgTgTCTgCACAC
51	220-239	CTgCAgTAggTgTCCACCAg
54	173-192	CTggCTgTTCCAgTACTCCT
58	221-240	TCTgCAATAggTgTCCACCT
78	231-251	TggTAgTTgTgTCTgCATACg
102	169-187	TgTTCCAgTACTCggCgCT
104	199-217	CCCgCCTgTCTTCCAggAA
107	170-188	CTgTTCCAgTgCTCCgCAg
111	250-266	CCgCggAACgCCACCTC
112	250-267	CgTgCggAgCTCCAACTg
151	231-251	CCgTAgTTgTgTCTgCAgTAA
152	250-267	CCCgCggTACgCCACCTC
252	211-226	CCACCgCggCCCgCgC
255	212-228	gTCCACCCggCCCCgCT
256	170-188	CTgTTCCAggACTCggCgA
258	208-224	ACCgCggCCCgCCTgTC
259	211-227	TCCACCgCggCCCgCTC
261	169-188	CTgTTCCAgTACTCggCATC
268	220-239	CTgCAgTAATTgTCCACCCg
314	126-144	CTggTACTCCCCCAggTCA
350	220-238	TgCACACCgTgTCCAACTC
351	221-238	TgCACACCCTgTCCACCg
354	170-188	CTgTTCCAgTACTCggCgg
485	211-227	TCCACCgCggCCCgCTT
491	140-156	CTCCgTCACCgCCCggT
492	171-189	gCTgTTCCAgTACTCAgCg
866	130-147	CgCCTggTACTCCCCCAg
1466	170-189	gCTgTTCCAgTACTCggCgT
1635	199-217	CCCgCCTgTCTTCCAggAT

Table 5.2a. HLA Class II primers. The No. column is the primer identification number. The position column refers to the annealing position of the primer according to the numbering system of Mason and Parham (1998) and Marsh (1998)

60°C or 62°C based on the popular formula 2X (number of A and T bases) + 4X (number of G and C bases) = annealing temperature in °C. Generally the higher the annealing temperature the less specific the primer is likely to be. Ideally primers should have an even ratio of G/C to A/T bases but this is not always possible to achieve, and in fact some primers work well in PCR-SSP with 100% G/C content. Where possible primers are designed with the specificity-dependent nucleotide on the terminal 3'- nucleotide but internal mismatches in a primer may also significantly contribute to a primer's specificity as shown in Figure 5.2.

The primers described here for the updated Phototyping set and the B*27 subtyping are shown in Table 5.2. Purchase or synthesis primers as desalted oligonucleotides (Cruachem, Glasgow) on a 25OD (approx 0.2mM) scale and are resuspended in ddH_20 at a concentration of 2000mg/ml and stored frozen until required. Generally, primers can also be left at 4°C for long periods. The primer combinations giving rise to the primer mixes are shown in Tables 5.3-5.4.

Sense orientation primers

No.	Position	Sequence 5'-3'	No.	Position	Sequence 5'-3'
4	284-302	CACAggCTgACCgAgTgAg	272	189-206	CgCCACgAgTCCgAggAA
130	402-419	CCgCgggTATgACCAgTC	278	300-317	gAgCCTgCggACCCTgCT
159	325-343	TACAACCAgAgCgAggCCA	280	149-167	gCTACgTggACgACACgCT
160	326-343	ACAACCAgAgCgAggCCg	284	247-265	TATTgggACgAggAgACAg
165	158-176	ACgACACgCAgTTCgTgCA	286	186-203	CgACgCCgCgAgCCAgAA
173	78-98	CCACTCCATgAggTATTTCTT	288	283-302	TCACAgACTgACCgAgCgAA
174	241-259	CCggAgTATTgggACCTgC	290	264-282	ACggAATgTgAAggCCCAg
187	217-234	gCgCCgTggATAgAgCAA	291	184-200	AgCgACgCCgCgAgCCA
188	190-206	gCCgCgAgTCCgAggAC	292	239-257	ggCCggAgTATTgggACgA
189	254-272	ACCggAACACACAgATCTg	294	283-302	TCACAgACTgACCgAgAgAg
191	255-272	CCgggAgACACAgATCTg	294	283-302	TCACAgACTgACCgAgAgAg
192	254-272	ACCgggAgACACAgATCTC	295	110-126	CCCggCCCggCAgTggA
193	243-261	ggAgTATTgggACCggAAC	296	222-240	gTggATAgAgCAggAgggT
194	268-285	AACATgAAggCCTCCgCg	312	262-282	ACACAgATCTACAAgACCAAC
195	253-272	gACCggAACACACAgATCTT	313	252-270	ggACCgggAgACACAgAAC
197	230-246	AgCAggAggggCCggAA	366	294-312	CCgAgTgAACCTgCggAAA
198	78-97	CCACTCCATgAggTATTTCg	367	322-341	TACTACAACCAgAgCgAggA
202	124-141	ggggAgCCCCgCTTCATT	368	284-302	CACAgACTgACCgAgTgAg
203	265-283	CAgATCTACAAggCCCAgg	369	196-213	AgTCCAAgAggggAgCCg
205	83-103	CCATgAggTATTTCTACACCg	371	78-98	CCACTCCATgAggTATTTCTC
206	253-272	gACCggAACACACAgATCTA	395	190-206	gCCgCgAgTTCgAgAgg
207	294-311	CCgAgAgAgCCTgCggAA	402	275-292	AggCCCACTCACAgACTC
207	294-311	CCgAgAgAgCCTgCggAA	433	344-363	ggTCTCACACCCTCCAgAAT
208	293-311	ACCgAgAgAACCTgCggAT	434	78-98	CCACTCCATgAggTATTTCAC
208	293-311	ACCgAgAgAACCTgCggAT	435	303-319	CCTgCgCACCgCgCTCC
209	189-206	CgCCgCgAgTCCgAgAgA	451	406-423	gggTACCggCAggACgCT
239	406-423	gggTACCAgCAggACgCT	475	264-282	ACggAAAgTgAAggCCCAg
240	259-278	gAgACACAgAAgTACAAgCg	572	273-292	CAAggCCAAggCACAgACTT
242	295-312	CgAgAgAgCCTgCggAAC	573	297-314	AgAgAACCTgCggATCgC
243	192-209	CgCgAgTCCgAggATggC	574	284-301	CACAgACTgACCgAgAgg
246	78-97	CCACTCCATgAggTATTTCC	575	231-247	gCAggAggggCCggAgT
251	300-317	ggACCTgCggACCCTgCT	1605	342-361	CAggTCTCACACCCTCCAgT
271	125-142	gggAgCCCCgCTTCATCT	1719	Int 143-60	gCGAggggACCgCAggC

Table 5.2b. HLA Class I primers (sense orientation). See Table 5.2a legend for explanatory notes. Antisense orientation primers are detailed on continuation sheet.

Antisense orientation primers

No.	Position	Sequence 5'-3'	No.	Position	Sequence 5'-3'
126	477-494	TgAgCCgCCgTgTCCgCA	244	571-588	CAggTATCTgCggAgCCC
127	361-379	ggTCgCAgCCATACATCCA	247	463-479	gCggCggTCCAggAgCg
143	368-385	gCCCCAggTCgCAgCCAA	249	538-556	CCTCCAggTAggCTCTCAA
145	559-576	gAgCCACTCCACgCACTC	250	299-316	gCAggTTCCgCAggCTCT
146	539-557	CCCTCCAggTAggCTCTCT	276	499-515	TCCCACTTgCgCTgggT
157	474-490	CCgCCgTgTCCgCggCA	277	387-403	ggAggAAgCgCCCgTCg
166	302-318	gCgCAggTTCCgCAggC	280	149-167	gCTACgTggACgACACgCT
167	559-576	gAgCCACTCCACgCACCg	281	280-298	CTCggTCAgTCTgTgCCTT
168	559-576	gAgCCACTCCACgCACgT	282	280-299	TCTCggTAAgTCTgTgCCTT
170	538-556	CCTCCAggTAggCTCTCTg	285	412-430	CgTCgTAggCgTACTggTC
171	391-407	CCgCggAggAAgCgCCA	287	559-576	gAgCCCgTCCACgCACTC
183	368-384	CCCCAggTCgCAgCCAg	294	283-302	TCACAgACTgACCgAgAgAg
184	512-528	CgCACgggCCgCCTCCA	298	423-443	ATgTAATCCTTgCCgTCgTAA
191	255-272	CCgggAgACACAgATCTg	299	555-572	CACTCCACgCACgTgCCA
207	294-311	CCgAgAgAgCCTgCggAA	300	448-466	AgCgCAggTCCTCgTTCAA
208	293-311	ACCgAgAgAACCTgCggAT	301	414-431	CCgTCgTAggCgTgCTgT
212	538-556	CCTCCAggTAggCTCTgTC	302	453-471	CCAAgAgCgCAggTCCTCT
213	387-402	gAggAggCgCCCgTCg	315	368-384	CCCCAggTCgCAgCCAC
214	419-435	CTTgCCgTCgTAggCgg	317	526-543	TCTCAgCTgCTCCgCCgT
215	420-438	ATCCTTgCCgTCgTAggCT	377	538-556	CCTCCAggTAggCTCTCCA
216	435-454	CgTTCAgggCgATgTAATCT	378	853-870	CAgCCCCTCgTgCTgCAT
217	544-561	CgTgCCCTCCAggTAggT	379	601-618	CgCgCgCTgCAgCgTCTT
218	559-576	gAgCCACTCCACgCACTC	382	538-556	CCTCCAggTAggCTCTCAg
219	572-589	CCAggTATCTgCggAgCg	388	361-379	ggTCgCAgCCAAACATCCA
220	603-619	CCgCgCgCTCCAgCgTg	389	589-608	AgCgTCTCCTTCCCATTCTT
221	605-622	TACCAgCgCgCTCCAgCT	392	419-436	CCTTgCCgTCgTAggCgA
223	353-372	gCCATACATCCTCTggATgA	393	412-429	gTCgTAggCgTCCTggTC
224	361-379	CgTCgCAgCCATACATCAC	394	363-382	CCACgTCgCAgCCATACATT
225	527-544	CTCTCAgCTgCTCCgCCT	425	412-430	CgTCgTAggCgTACTggTT
227	369-385	gCCCCACgTCgCAgCCg	429	259-278	gCCTTCACATTCCgTgTgTT
228	411-428	TCgTAggCgTCCTggTgg	431	559-575	AgCCCgTCCACgCACCg
229	499-516	CTCCAACTTgCgCTgggA	433	344-363	ggTCTCACACCCTCCAgAAT
232	246-265	gTgTgTTCCggTCCCAATAT	438	317-335	CTCTggTTgTAgTAgCggA
234	319-337	CgCTCTggTTgTAgTAgCg	486	257-276	CTTCACATTCCgTgTCTCCT
235	787-806	gCCCACTTCTggAAggTTCT	572	273-292	CAAggCCAAggCACAgACTT
236	354-371	CCATACATCgTCTgCCAA	573	297-314	AgAgAACCTgCggATCgC
237	302-318	gCgCAggTTCCgCAggC	574	284-301	CACAgACTgACCgAgAgg
238	559-576	gAgCCACTCCACgCACAg	575	231-247	gCAggAggggCCggAgT
241	463-479	gCCgCggTCCAggAgCT	818	485-502	gggTgATCTgAgCCgCCT

Table 5.2b (continued). HLA Class I primers (antisense orientation).

Lane	PM No	Sense primer	Sense conc. †	Anti-sense primer	Anti-sense conc.	Amplicon size	Locus	Alleles amplified
1	151	286	5	431	5	629	A	*0101 *0102 *0103 *0104N
2	3	296	5	302	5	489	A	*0201-22/25-27
3	4	291	7	299	7	628	A	*0301 *0302 *0303N *0304 *2403v
4	2	286	3	168	3	630	A	*3601
5	5	284	10	302	10	464	A	*2301 *2402 *2402102L *2402v *2403 *2403v *2404 *2405 *2406 *2407 *2409N *2410 *2411N *2413 *2414
6	6	292	10	249	10	557	A	*2301 *2403v *2413
7	7	292	10	170	10	557	A	*2402 *2402102L *2402v *2403 *2404 *2405 *2407 *2409N *2410 *2411N *2414
8	8	239	4	167	4	170	A	*2501 *2502 *2601 *2603 *2605 *2607 *2608 *2611N *4301 *6601
8	8	239		145	4	170	A	*6602 *6603
9	9	193	10	298	10	440	A	*2501 *2502 *2601 *2602 *2603 *2604 *2605 *2606 *2608 *2609 *2611N *3401 *3402 *6601 *6602 *6603
10	10	294	10	298	10	400	A	*2501 *2502
11	11	288	10	298	10	400	A	*2601 *2602 *2604 *2607 *2608 *2609 *2611N *4301
12	12	174	10	298	10	442	A	*4301
13	13	239	10	168	10	170	A	*2609 *3401
13	13	451	10	168		170	A	*31012v *3402
14	14	290	5	298	5	419	A	*2502 *3402 *6601 *6602
14	14	475	5	298		419	A	*3401
15	15	290	3	167	5	552	A	*1101 *1102 *1103 *2502 *6601
16	152	174	5	300	5	465	A	*2901 *2902 *2903
17	18	295	5	301	5	561	A	*3001 *3002 *3003 *3004 *3006
18	184	434	5	486	5	198	A	*31012 *31012v
19	153	173	10	234	10	259	A	*3201 *3202
20	154	434	10	429	10	200	A	*3301 *3303
21	22	173	15	300	15	628	A	*3201 *3202 *7401 *7402 *7403
22	23	290	3	302	10	447	A	*68011 *68012 *6802 *6806 *6808 *6901
23	24	290	3	171	10	383	A	*6901
24	25	367	10	287	10	494	A	*8001
25	112	367	10	394	10	300	A	*0101 *0102 *0104N *1101 *1102 *1103 *1104 *31012v *3402 *3601 *8001
26	165	435	5	235	10	1331	B	*0802,*1301,*1302,*1303,*1304,*2701,*38021,*38022,*4402,*44031,*44032,*4404,*4405,*4407,*4408,*4410,
26	165	208	5	235		1341	B	*0803,*1513/16-17/23/24,*2702,*3801,*4406,*4901,*51011-11N/13,*52011/2,*5301/2,*5701-04,*5801-2,*5901
26	165	251	5	235		1334	B	*2703,*2704,*27052,*27053,*2706,*2707,*2709,*2710,*2711,*3701,*3702,*4701,
26	165	278	5	235		1334	B	*2703,*2704,*27052,*27053,*2706,*2707,*2709,*2710,*2711,*3701,*3702,*4701,
27	31	242	10	235	10	1339	B	*07021-9,*0801/4/5,*1401/5,*150-512/14/15/18-22/25-40,*1801-5,*2708/12,*3501-24,*39011-12,*40011-18,*4101-3, (cont'd on next line)
								*4201/2,*4409,*4501,*4601,*4702/3,*4801-4,*5001/2,*5401,*5501-6,*5601-4,*67011-12,*7801-2,*8101,*8201
28	34	193	10	221	10	619	B	*07021 *07022 *07023 *0703 *0704 *0705 *0706 *0707 *0708 *0709 *8101
29	35	312	10	221	10	600	B	*0703
30	36	195	10	212	10	543	B	*0801 *0802 *0803 *4406 *5108
31	155	195	10	220	10	606	B	*0801 *0802 *0803
32	37	280	10	225	10	635	B	*2704 *2706 *2710 *4005 *4015 *4016 *4017 *4901 *5001 *5002
33	38	208	10	215	10	385	B	*4901 *5901
34	39	246	10	215	10	600	B	*4501 *4901 *5001 *5002
35	40	207	5	219	10	535	B	*1514 *4409 *4501 *5002 *8201
36	160	202	10	285	10	546	B	*1804
36	160	202		393	10	545	B	*4406
36	160	272	10	285		481	B	*3519 *4003 *4009 *4018 *4405
36	160	272		393		480	B	*4402 *44031 *44032 *4404 *4407 *4409

Table 5.3a. Primer mix information for reactions 1-36

† μl of primer per ml of control solution (see notes on testing control solutions). Stock primer concentration is 2000μg/ml.

Lane	PM No	Sense primer	Sense conc. †	Anti-sense primer	Anti-sense conc.	Amplicon size	Locus	Alleles amplified
37	42	192	4	220	10	605	B	*4101 *4102 *4103
38	43	272	10	276	10	566	B	*3519 *4002-6/8/9/11/14-18 *4101-3 *4402-5/7/9/10 *4501 *4701-3 *4901 *5001/2
39	44	192	4	247	10	465	B	*1533 *40011-6/9-12/14-18 *4101-3 *4801-4
40	45	272	10	218	10	627	B	*40011 *40012 *4002 *4003 *4004 *4006 *4007 *4008 *4009 *4010 *4011 *4014 *4016 *4017 *4018 *4701-3
41	46	280	10	229	10	607	B	*40011 *40012 *4007
42	47	243	10	215	10	486	B	*1301 *1302 *1303
43	48	197	10	127	10	389	B	*1401 *1402 *1403 *1404
44	49	205	10	232	10	182	B	*1402 *1403 *1405 *3904
45	50	207	10	217	10	507	B	*39011 *39013 *39021 *39022 *3903 *3904 *3905 *39061 *39062 *3907 *3908 *3909 *3910 *3911 *3912 *67011 *67012
46	51	206	4	217	10	548	B	*3910 *67011 *67012
47	172	208	10	217	10	508	B	*3801
47	172	435	10	217		498	B	*38021 *38022
48	53	209	10	217	10	612	B	*3801-02 *3901-12 *67011 *67012
49	54	208	10	223	10	319	B	*1513 *4406 *5104 *5301 *5302 *5801
50	56	194	10	213	10	374	B	*5801 *5802
51	55	194	6	224	6	351	B	*5701 *5702 *5703 *5704
52	166	243	10	438	10	143	B	*1301 *1302 *1303 *1304 *1513 *1516 *1517 *1524 *4408 *5701 *5702 *5703 *5704
53	57	187	10	214	10	458	B	*1801 *1802 *1803 *1804 *1805
54	58	209	10	236	10	422	B	*39061 *39062 *5501 *5502 *5503 *5505 *5601 *5901 *7301
55	59	242	10	215	10	383	B	*4501 *5001 *5002 *5401 *5501 *5502 *5503 *5505 *5601 *5602 *5604 *8201
56	60	203	10	238	10	551	B	*5601 *5602 *5603 *5604
57	61	395	10	236	10	421	B	*5401
58	62	280	10	281	5	149	B	*2702 *2703 *2704 *27052 *27053 *2706 *2707 *2708 *2709 *2710 *2711
58	62	280		282	5	150	B	*2701
59	63	188	10	212	10	606	B	*3701 *4406 *5108
60	64	192		392	10	422	B	*3701 *39021 *39022 *3908
61	65	192		228	10	414	B	*3702 *4701 *4702 *4703
62	66	367	10	236	10	289	B	*7301
63	67	203	10	220	10	594	B	*4201 *4202
64	68	209	8	229	8	567	B	*4012 *4801 *4803 *4804 *8101
65	69	194	10	225	10	516	B	*1516 *1517
66	70	240	10	241	10	460	B	*4601
67	72	243	10	250	10	124	B	*1501/2/4-8/11/12/14/15/19-21/25-18/30-35/38-40
68	73	192	4	214	10	421	B	*1304 *1501/3-7/12/14/19/20/24-27/32-35/38-40 *4003 *4802
69	156	271	10	223	10	487	B	*4802 Cw*0710
70	74	209	10	214	10	486	B	*0709 *1503 *1518 *1523 *1529 *3907 *4802 *5603
71	75	271	10	238	10	691	B&C	*1503 *1509 *1510 *1518 *1523 *1529 *1537 *4802 Cw*0703
72	76	189	4	238	10	562	B	*1509 *1510 *1518 *1521 *1523 *1537

Table 5.3b. Primer mix information for reactions 37-72

† µl of primer per ml of control solution (see notes on testing control solutions). Stock primer concentration is 2000µg/ml.

Lane	PM No	Sense primer	Sense conc. †	Anti-sense primer	Anti-sense conc.	Amplicon size	Locus	Alleles amplified
73	77	243	5	219	5	637	B	*1514 *4408
73	77	243		244	5	636	B	*1512 *1519
74	78	193	5	377	5	553	A&B	A*2501/2 A*2601-6/9/11N A*3401A*6601-3 A*6801-6 *1508 *1511 *1515 *1522 *5603
75	79	193	10	223	10	369	B	*1502/13/21 *3501-9/11/12/15/18-21/23/24 *4406 *5104 *5301 *5302
76	80	188	10	237	10	128	B	*1522 *1801-5 *3501-13/1518/20-24 *7801 *78021 *78022
77	81	195	10	213	10	389	B	*3501/3-9/11/15/17-19/21/23/24 *5301 *5302
77	81	195		277	10	390	B	*3502
78	82	207	10	216	10	400	B	*1509 *7801 *78021 *78022
79	83	208	10	216	10	401	B	*51011 *51012 *51021 *51022 *5103 *5104 *5105 *5106 *5107 *5108 *5109 *5111N *52011 *52012
80	84	193	5	216	5	451	B	*1509 *51011 *51012 *51021 *51022 *5103 *5104 *5105 *5106 *5107 *5108 *5109 *5111N *7801 *78021*78022
81	85	192	5	216	7	440	B	*52011 *52012
82	86	368	2	315	1	340	Cw	*0102 *0103
83	87	366	10	145	10	522	Cw	*02021 *02022 *02023 *02024 *0203 *1701 *1702
84	88	368	7	389	7	564	Cw	*0302 *03031 *03032 *03041 *03042 *0305 *0306 *0308 *0309
85	89	366	7	143	7	331	Cw	*04011 *04012 *0402 *0403 *0404 *0405 *1801 *1802
86	90	366	10	379	10	564	Cw	*0501
87	91	367	10	127	10	297	Cw	*0602 *0603 *0604
88	92	130	10	378	10	1056	Cw	*0701 *0702 *0703 *0706 *0707 *0708 *0710
89	93	313	3	184	3	516	Cw	*0701 *0706 *0707
90	94	367	5	183	5	302	Cw	*0702 *0703 *0710
91	95	367	10	238	10	494	Cw	A*2604 *0703
92	96	367	5	379	5	536	Cw	*0704
93	182	165	5	166	5	160	Cw	*0801 *0802 *0803 *0804
93	182	165		317	5	625	Cw	*0801 *0803
94	99	159	3	389	3	523	Cw	*03031 *03032
95	100	160	10	389	10	522	Cw	*0302 *03041 *03042 *0305 *0306 *0308 *0309
96	101	368	15	126	10	450	Cw	*12021 *12022 *1301
97	102	369	15	126	10	538	Cw	*12021 *12022
98	103	368	15	157	15	446	Cw	*1203 *1206
99	104	371	15	388	15	541	Cw	*14021 *14022 *1403
100	106	366	10	223	10	318	Cw	*1502 *1503 *1504 *15051 *15052 *1506
101	107	366	10	382	10	502	Cw	*0203 *0404 *0604 *0707 *1502 *1503 *1504 *15051 *15052 *1506 *1701 *1702
102	109	368	4	146	4	513	Cw	*1601
103	110	366	4	146	4	503	Cw	*1602
104	111	366	10	377	10	502	Cw	*02021 *02022 *02023 *02024 *0602 *0603 *12041 *12042 *1205
105	113	36	10	39	10	194	DRB1	*0101 *01021 *01022 *0104
106	114	36	10	40	10	195	DRB1	*0103
107	115	41	10	252	10	206	DRB1	*15011 *15012 *15021 *15022 *15023 *1503 *1504 *1505 *1506 *1507 *1508
108	185	41	10	491	10	136	DRB1	*1507 *16011 *16012 *16021 *16022 *1603 *1604 *1605 *1607 *1608

Table 5.3c. Primer mix information for reactions 73-108

† μl of primer per ml of control solution (see notes on testing control solutions). Stock primer concentration is 2000μg/ml.

Lane	PM No	Sense primer	Sense conc. †	Anti-sense primer	Anti-sense conc.	Amplicon size	Locus	Alleles amplified
109	162	68	10	255	10	211	DRB1	*03011 *03012 *03021 *03022 *0303 *0304 *0305 *0306 *0307 *0308 *0309 *0310 *0311 *1107
110	118	46	10	38	10	216	DRB1	*03011 *03012 *0304 *0306 *0308 *0310 *0311 *1327
111	119	44	10	37	10	188	DRB1/3	*0302/5 *1109/20 *1302/5/26/29/31 *1402/3/9/13/19/24/27/30 *1608 DRB3*0206
112	120	47	10	37	10	259	DRB1	*0401/5/7-9/14/16/17/19-21/24/26/28/29 *1122
112	120	47		38	10	259	DRB1	*0402 *0403 *0404 *0406 *0410 *0411 *0412 *0413 *0415 *0418 *0422 *0425 *0427 *1410
113	121	48	10	49	10	231	DRB1	*0701 *0703
114	122	50	10	51	10	213	DRB1	*0801/2/032/4/6-13/15-17/19 *1415
114	122	50	10	102	10	161	DRB1	*0801 *08032 *0805 *0806 *0810 *0812 *0816 *0817 *0818
115	123	52	10	49	10	235	DRB1	*09012
116	124	53	10	37	10	203	DRB1	*1001
117	125	68	10	54	10	175	DRB1	*0308 *1101-4/6-21/23-29/32
117	125	273	10	54		173	DRB1	*1105 *1204 *1411
118	126	50	15	256	15	162	DRB1	*1201 *12021 *12022 *12032 *1205
119	183	68	10	259	10	210	DRB1	*1102/3/11/14/16/20/21 *1301/2/4/8/15/16/19/20/22-24/27-29/31/32 *1416
119	183	273	10	259		208	DRB1	*1317
120	127	263	10	259	10	152	DRB1	*1116 *1120 *1301 *1302 *1308 *1316 *1320 *1327 *1328 *1329 *1331 *1332 *1416
120	127	263		252	10	151	DRB1	*1309
121	168	44	10	40	10	129	DRB1	*1116 *1120 *1301 *1302 *1306 *1310 *1315 *1316 *1327 *1328 *1331 *1332
121	168	44		485		139	DRB1	*1310 *1419 *1421
122	169	44		258	10	136	DRB1	*1109 *1305 *1306 *1318 *1326 *1403 *1412 *1427 *1608
122	169	44		485		139	DRB1	*1310 *1419 *1421
123	167	68	10	485	10	210	DRB1	*13031 *13032 *1310 *1333 *1419 *1421
124	170	68	10	102	10	170	DRB1	*13031 *13032 *1304 *1312 *1313 *1321 *1330 *1332 *1333 *1413
125	131	68	10	104	10	200	DRB1	*1101/4/6/9/-12/15/23-25/27-29/32 *1305 *13071 *13072 *1311 *1314 *1318 *1321 *1324 *1326 *1422 *1425 *1427
126	132	68	10	261	10	171	DRB1	*0301-7/9/11 *1301/2/5-071/8-11/14-16/18-20/22-25/27-29 *1402/3/6/9/12/14/17/19-21/23/24/27/29/30
127	171	263	10	58	10	165	DRB1	*1117 *1401 *1404 *1405 *1407 *1408 *1410 *1411 *1414 *1423 *1426 *1428
127	171	263		51	10	164	DRB1	*0809 *1318 *1415
127	171	264	10	58		165	DRB1	*1418
127	171	264		51		164	DRB1	*1403 *1412 *1427
128	134	68	10	107	10	171	DRB1	*0310 *1401 *1407 *1416 *1422 *1425 *1426
129	135	44	10	51	5	151	DRB1/3	*1318 *1403 *1412 *1427
129	135	44		39	5	128	DRB1	*0301-3/5-8/10/11 *1402 *1406 *1409 *1413 *1417 *1418 *1419 *1421 *1429 *1430 DRB3*0206
130	186	61	10	492	10	172	DRB5	*01011 *01012 *0102 *0103 *0104 *0105 *0106 *0107 *0108N *0109 *0201 *0202 *0203 *0204
131	164	69	10	268	10	221	DRB3	*01011 *01012 *01013 *01014 *0103 *0104
132	138	76	10	151	10	116	DRB3	*0201 *0202 *0203 *0205 *0206 *0207 *0208
133	139	70	10	38	10	259	DRB3	*0201 *0204 *0301 *0302
134	140	283	5	314	5	151	DRB4	*0101 *0102 *0103101 *0104 *0105 *0201N
135	1054	270	5	866	5	167	DRB4	*0103102N
136	142	77	10	350	10	194	DQB1	*0305
137	143	82	10	112	10	197	DQB1	*0201 *0202 *0203
138	144	77	20	78	20	207	DQB1	*0401 *0402
139	145	79	10	152	10	206	DQB1	*0501 *0502 *05031 *05032 *0504
140	146	347	10	111	10	248	DRB1	*06011 *06012 *06013
140	146	348	10	111		139	DQB1	*0602 *0603 *0610 *0611 *0613 *0614
141	147	349	10	350	10	175	DQB1	*0603 *0604 *06051 *06052 *0607 *0608 *0609 *0612 *0614
141	147	349		351	10	175	DRB1	*0606
142	148	181	20	112	20	207	DQB1	*03011 *03012 *0304
143	149	353	20	354	20	118	DQB1	*0302 *0307 *0308
144	150	1465	2	1466	2	130	DQB1	*0203 *03032 *0306

Table 5.3d. Primer mix information for reactions 109-144

† μl of primer per ml of control solution (see notes on testing control solutions). Stock primer concentration is 2000μg/ml.

PM No	Sense primer	Sense conc. †	Anti-sense primer	Anti-sense conc.	Amplicon size	Locus	Alleles amplified
1048	402	10	249	10	521	A	*0201 *0204 *0206 *0207 *0209 *0210 *0214 *0215N *0216 *02171 *02172 *0218 *0220 *0221 *0224 *0225 *0226
945	208	10	146	10	504	A	*2402 *24021 *2402v *2403 *2405 *2407 *2408 *2409N *2410 *2411N *2414
1005	198	10	227	10	547	B	*0801 *0802 *0803 *0804 *0805 *3912
360	242	10	220	10	564	B	*0801 *0804 *0805 *4101 *4102 *4103 *4201 *4202
1112	1719	10	438	10	348	B	Bw4
1113	1719	5	237	5	331	B	Bw6 (not B*4018) *4703
263	294	10	228	10	385	B	*2704 *2708 *2712
1064	208	10	218	10	523	B	*2702 *5110
307	195	10	392	10	423	B	*3503 *3506 *5113
1055	202	10	236	10	487	B	*51011 *51021 *5103 *5107 *5108 *5109 *5110 *5111N *5113 *52012 *7801 *78022
977	203	10	168	10	551	B	*4201 *4202 *5401 *5501 *5502 *5503 *5504 *5505 *67011 *67012
960	206	10	425	10	417	B	*0705 *0706 *3910 *4201 *4202 *5401 *5501-6 *5601 *5602 *5604 *67011 *67012 *8101 *8201
1016	240	15	818	15	483	Cw	*0501 *0502 *0802 *0804
1075	4	5	184	5	484	Cw	*0701 *0702 *0704 *0705 *0706 *0708 *0710
1076	1605	10	377	10	214	Cw	*0602 *0603 *1203 *12041 *12042 *1205 *1206 *16041
1017	368	10	127	10	335	Cw	*0102 *0103 *1203 *1206 *14021 *14022 *1403 *1601 *16041
1053	47	10	261	10	171	DRB1	*0401-4/6-8/13/14/18-23/25/27
	48	10	258	10	203	DRB1	*0701 *0703 *0704
1051	1634	10	1635	10	136	DRB1	*08032/10/12/14/15/18/19 *1102/14/18/19/21/31 *13031 *13032 *1304 *1312 *1313 *1317 *1322 *1323 *1330 *1333
1052	1630	10	37	10	118	DRB1	*1101-5/8-15/19/20/22-32
1151	1631	10	38	10	122	DRB1	*0310 *1401 *1404 *1410 *1416 *1426 *1428 *1431
1079	1674	10	255	10	214	DRB3	*0102
1082	70	7	256	7	171	DRB3	*0301 *0302 *0303

Table 5.3e. Primer mix information for supplementary reactions

† μl of primer per ml of control solution (see notes on testing control solutions). Stock primer concentration is 2000μg/ml.

Lane	PM No	Sense primer	Sense conc. †	Anti-sense primer	Anti-sense conc.	Amplicon size	Alleles amplified
1	255	575	10	228	10	437	B*1517 B*2701 B*2702 B*2704 B*27052 B*27053 B*2708 B*2710 B*2712 B*3702 B*4701 B*4702 B*4703
2	897	574	10	515	10	500	B*2703 B*27052 B*27053 B*2707 B*2709
3	257	574	10	400	10	391	B*2703 B*27052 B*27053 B*2710
4	258	280	10	430	10	115	B*2703
5	259	208	10	228	10	375	B*1517 B*2702
6	260	572	10	228	10	395	B*2701
7	261	573	10	228	10	371	B*1517 B*2702
8	262	433	10	225	10	200	B*2704 B*2706 B*2710
9	263	294	10	228	10	385	B*2704 B*2708 B*2712
10	264	191	10	285	10	415	B*2706
11	265	191	10	425	10	415	B*2707 B*2711
12	266	207	10	228	10	374	B*2708 B*2712 B*4702 B*4703
13	873	191	10	1519	10	420	B*2709
14	62	280	10	281	5	149	B*2702 B*2703 B*2704 B*27052 B*27053 B*2706 B*2707 B*2708 B*2709 B*2710 B*2711
14	62	280	10	282	5	150	B*2701

Table 5.4. Primer mix information for HLA-B*27 subtyping

† µl of primer per ml of control solution (see notes on testing control solutions). Stock primer concentration is 2000µg/ml.

General information on PCR-SSP using Phototyping methods.

The basic tenet of the Phototyping method is that multiple primer mixes consisting of water, cresol red allele-specific and control-specific primers are synthesised, tested and stored in 1ml primer mix volumes. A typing set collected from these stored primer mixes is dispensed in 5ml volumes under mineral oil in 96-well PCR plates. Separate from the primer mixes a PCR buffer (called TDMH) containing all the other ingredients of PCR is made up and stored frozen in aliquots awaiting the addition of DNA and *Taq* polymerase. DNA is then added to a predetermined volume of the TDMH and 8ml of this mixture is added to each well of the PCR plate prior to PCR amplification and agarose gel electrophoresis. This method allows extreme flexibility in the design and incorporation of any new primer mixes.

One of the key factors in maintaining PCR stringency is the concentration of the primers used: the concentrations given in Table 5.3 are to be used as a guide only as the optimal concentrations should be determined empirically within individual laboratories.

Good quality DNA is paramount for successful PCR-SSP. Sodium citrate or EDTA anticoagulated blood is preferred to heparinised blood as heparin is a severe inhibitor of PCR and especially PCR-SSP (Satsangi *et al*., 1994). If heparinised blood is the only source then the DNA extraction protocol described below should allow for satisfactory typing.

DNA extraction

This method is modification of Miller's salting-out procedure (Miller *et al*., 1988) in which the use of proteinase K is omitted and an organic solvent extraction phase is added. This yields large quantities of good quality DNA in less than 30 min which is suitable for PCR-SSP.

Centrifuge 5ml of EDTA or trisodium citrate anticoagulated blood and aspirate Buffy coat into a 15ml polypropylene tube (Alpha, LW3075). Add 10ml of RCLB, invert several times and leave to stand for 5 min. Centrifuge at 1000*g* for 5 min. Pour off supernatant and gently rinse pellet in 2ml of RCLB. The pellet should be white with a pink halo. If there is too much haemoglobin resuspend the pellet in RCLB, agitate and centrifuge. When the pellet is homogeneously white it can be stored at -70°C or you can continue to the next step. Resuspend pellet in 3ml of NLB+SDS (warm NLB+SDS if precipitate visible). Add 1 ml of 6M NaCl, vortex (precipitate should be visible). Add 2ml of chloroform and shake until homogenous milky solution is seen. Centrifuge for 10 min at 1000*g*. Aspirate the DNA (top phase) into a 20ml tube. If the DNA phase is not clear in appearance transfer to a clean polypropylene tube and repeat the chloroform extraction step. Do not suck up any protein from the interface. Add two volumes of 95% ethanol, gently rock until all of the DNA is precipitated. Centrifuge for 5 min at 700*g* and resuspend in 70% ethanol, centrifuge and repeat this washing step. Transfer the

DNA precipitate into a sterile 0.5ml microcentrifuge tube, pellet the DNA, and remove the excess ethanol either by centrifugal evaporation, lyophilisation or allowing it to dry on the bench. Resuspend the DNA in 300μl of sterile ddH_2O. From 5ml of blood you can expect to obtain DNA concentrations in the range of 0.2 to 1.0mg/ml.

Dispensing primer mixes.

Tested primer mixes (see under Notes, below) should be dispensed in 1ml volumes in 1ml straight tubes (Integra Biosciences, 8110-00) which are suitable for placing in standard 96-well format in a 96-well rack (Integra Biosciences, 8100-00). These tubes and racks are suitable for use both with 8/12 channel hand-held electronic multi-dispensing pipettes (Anachem, EP-M8-250 or Alpha, 710-310) and also with 96-well robotic dispensers such as the Robbins Hydra (Robbins Scientific). Using a 12 channel electronic dispensing pipette add 10ml of mineral oil (Sigma, M8662) to 96 well PCR plates (Advanced Biotechnology, AB-0600). Dispense 5 ml of each primer mix into the appropriate wells of the PCR plates using the Robbins Hydra dispenser. Completed trays may be stored for 6-12 months at -30°C, preferably in sealed bags or with individual plate sealers (Costar, 6524).

Setting up PCR-SSP using TDMH buffer:

Thaw out plate(s) containing the primer mixes. Thaw out a 13.3ml aliquot of TDMH and add 64ml of 5unilts/ml *Taq* polymerase (Bioline). This mixture will keep at 4°C for at least one week. Count how many individual PCR-SSP reactions is required for each individual DNA sample (protocol given here is for 144 reactions). For each 5ml primer mix 8ml of TDMH/DNA/*Taq* mixture is added. It is important for maintenance of the $MgCl_2$ concentration that the ratio of TDMH to all other PCR ingredients is 1:0.6. Thus, for 144 reactions add 16ml of DNA to 1416ml of TDMH/*Taq* mix. Vortex briefly and pour mixture into a disposable trough (Saxon Europe). Place six 250ml tips on an 8-channel electronic multidispenser and draw up an appropriate volume. Dispense 8 ml of DNA/TDMH/*Taq* mixture to 6 wells at a time; keep the tip at the top edge of the mineral oil meniscus and allow the mixture to roll of the tip and through the mineral oil. On no account allow the tips to touch the primer mix otherwise carry-over, and consequently false-positive amplifications may occur. On addition of the TDMH mixture to the primer mixes the cresol red will change colour from yellow to purple. When the tray is complete, seal with a fresh tray sealer, centrifuge briefly (200g for 5 sec) to ensure all PCR reactions are mixed and submerged below the oil (vortexing completed plates is not recommended).

Setting up PCR-SSP using heparin-contaminated DNA.

Make a 0.2unit/μl solution of heparinase II (Sigma, H6512) by adding 50μl of ddH_2O to a 10 unit vial. Add 5μl heparinase per 15μl DNA, agitate and incubate for 90 min at 37°C. Add to TDMH mixture as above. Heparinase activity is destroyed by freeze-thawing.

PCR amplification program.

This program is suitable for Perkin Elmer 9600 (Cetus), MJR PTC100 or PTC 200 machines (MJR). 96°C for 60 sec, 5 cycles of: 96°C for 20 sec, 70°C for 45 sec and 72°C for 25 sec; 21 cycles of : 96°C for 25 sec, 65°C for 50 sec, 72°C for 30 sec; 4 cycles of: 96°C for 30 sec, 55°C for 60 sec, 72°C for 90 sec. Cool by ramping to 20°C for 30 sec prior to termination of the program. The program takes approximately 1.5 h to run.

Some thermoplastics used for PCR are not an exact fit for every PCR machine and consequently accurate heat transfer to the PCR reaction may be affected. To ensure correct thermodynamics, we dip the PCR vessels into a little light paraffin oil, and blot excess on tissues before placing in PCR machines.

Apply firm and even pressure to the top surface PCR vessels during thermocycling. Preferably use a heated lid.

Electrophoresis.

Use large electrophoresis tanks (Flowgen, G3-0416) utilising gel trays accommodating gel combs (Flowgen, G3-0416) with teeth spatially separated for use with multichannel pipettes. Pour 400mls of 1% agarose into the taped off gel tray and insert the combs, allow 20 min to set. Fill electrophoresis tank with 2.2L of 0.5x TBE (can be left in tank and reused at least 15 times). Remove tape and combs and submerge gel tray in tank. Using a multichannel repeating syringe (Robbins Scientific, 1021-03-5) add 5ml of orange G loading buffer. Using a multichannel pipette load 18ml of 8 or 12 PCR reactions at a time to the gel (depending on tray layout). Electrophorese for 20 min at 200V or until the orange G can be seen to have travelled 3cm.

Gel photography.

Visualise the PCR amplicons using 312nm UV transillumination. Record results by gel photography using either Polaroid photography in conjunction with Wratten 22 and 2a filters or any other suitable imaging system. Two rapid exposures with a shutter speed of 4 and aperture of *f*5.6 are recommended.

To facilitate identification of positive PCR reactions it is recommended that the electrophoresis lanes are labelled by using an overhead projector acetate with the lane numbers printed in the correct spatial orientation. The OHP acetate is laid over the gel in the correct position prior to photography. It is recommended that the OHP is laminated (to prevent wear) and that windows between one row of number and another (where the PCR amplicons appear) are cut out to reduce interference from the plastic fluorescing in UV light.

Interpretation of results.

PCR-SSP interpretation of HLA genotypes is relatively easy, and generally results can be interpreted with little or no prior experience. Each PCR-SSP reaction is deemed to have worked if the control amplification is present. The control amplicon in all reactions, except primer mixes 165 and 31, is a 796 base pair fragment from the third intron of DRB1 as previously used by Olerup and Zetterquist (Olerup and Zetterquist, 1992) whereas the 256bp control amplicon in the primer mix 165 and 31 reactions is from exon 15 of the adenomatous polyposis coli gene as previously used by Sadler *et al* (Sadler *et al.*, 1994). Positive allele-specific amplifications are identified by the presence of a correct sized PCR allele-specific amplicon, whereas absence of an allele-specific amplicon implies absence of the alleles identified in a given primer mix. If a reaction has neither control or allele-specific amplicons the reaction has failed and is deemed "not tested". The alleles that would have been amplified in this reaction are therefore also not tested. Fortunately, many alleles are amplified in more than one reaction so sporadic PCR failures do not often affect full assignation of a genotype. If all of the reactions have failed then the whole result is not tested and must be repeated (see trouble shooting in the notes section). Alleles are assigned by identifying the pattern of positive and negative reactions and interpreting these with reference to the information given in Table 5.3

Notes

Testing control solutions.

Getting the right concentration of control primers in the stock control solutions is of vital importance as these solutions are the basis for all the primer mixes. The concentration of primers must be not so high that the allele-specific amplicon is out-competed by the controls. On the other hand, if the concentration of control primers are too low then the control amplicon will be difficult or impossible to visualise and many primer mixes may appear to be not tested. To establish a good working concentration titrate the control primers (suggested titration: 5, 2.5, 1.25µl/ml) in the presence of a constant concentration of a pair of allele-specific primers. Test this titration against some DNA samples of varying quality and of varying genotype (some positive and some negative for the allele-specific primers). The optimal concentration of control primers is found when the control amplicon does not out compete the allele-specific amplicon in HLA allele-positive reactions and yet is present in all allele-negative samples.

Testing allele-specific primers.

The majority of primer mixes will function well using the recommended concentrations given in Table 5.3. However there is some variability in amplification efficiencies between batches of oligonucleotides and primer mixes so that every new synthesis of primer mixes must be properly tested as optimal primer concentrations will fluctuate from batch to batch. If a large volume (20-50ml) of primer mixes are being synthesised for the first time it is advisable to test the recommended concentrations first by making up 0.5ml and testing on appropriate control samples. An ideal primer mix should produce allele-specific amplicons that are easily visible in all expected positive samples and clearly negative in expected negative samples: if possible test some DNA of poor quality as well as normal DNA to ensure a robust primer mix is obtained. If a primer mix is weak or negative with expected positive DNA samples increasing the concentration of primers seldom fails to improve results. Similarly, false-positive amplifications can be removed by titrating either both primers or one of the primers (asymmetric titration). Sense primers with the 3'- end at position 272 (for example primer 192) all utilise internal mismatches at positions 12 and 14 of the primer. Primer mixes involving these primers require careful testing and subsequent titration of the sense primer to avoid weak amplification of similar sequences. For example primer mix 73 is designed to amplify B*1501 and some other B*15 alleles but not B*1502. Because the primer 192 is only mismatched internally between B*1501 and B*1502 it is possible B*1502 might be amplified in this mix therefore this mix must be tested with B*1502 as well as B*1501 before being put into general use.

Initially, some primer mixes (especially primer mixes 152 and 76) fail to produce allele-specific and control-specific amplicons, instead producing primer-dimer. These primers also need careful reduction of the allele-specific primers to a point where they amplify alleles but do not go to primer-dimer.

Some primer mixes only detect very rare alleles (such as HLA-A*4301 or B*4802) and are consequently difficult to positively test for unless reference DNA samples are available. If reference samples are not available test the individual primers in different combinations to estimate the optimal concentrations. For example, if the HLA-A*4301 primer mix (PM12) is not positively tested, the sense primer (primer 174) which is specific for A*2901-3 as well as A*4301, could be tested in conjunction with another antisense primer that also detects A*2901-3. Similarly the antisense primer (primer 298) could be tested and the optimal concentration of primers could be extrapolated to the A*4301-specific primer mix. If a primer cannot be tested in this way because it's sequence is unique to a rare allele it is best to use it at the highest possible concentration that does not produce false-positives.

Testing TDMH.

Each batch of TDMH should be tested in comparison with the previous batch before general use. It is best to test several different DNA samples of different phenotypes to ensure that the buffer is efficient for most primer mixes. The most common defect found when testing TDMH is that the control bands appear strong but the allele bands appear weak, or even nonexistent. This is commonly caused by an imbalance in the $MgCl_2$:dNTP ratio: either too high a concentration of $MgCl_2$ or too low a concentration of dNTP's has been used. It is thought that as dNTP's efficiently chelate $MgCl_2$ an excess of dNTP's sequesters free $MgCl_2$ and thus deprives *Taq* of the magnesium that it requires as a cofactor.

Troubleshooting

1. All reactions have failed (no allele, no control-specific amplicons).

This may be because of either poor quality or insufficient DNA: Test another DNA sample previously shown to work to test reagents and PCR machine. If poor quality DNA is suspected using less DNA with 50% more *Taq* may work. If it looks like there is lots of DNA by gel electrophoresis then it could be heparin or protein contamination. If heparin contamination is suspected use the heparinase protocol. If protein contamination is suspected try re-extracting by adding 20% v/v 6M NaCl to the remaining DNA and an equal volume of chloroform, vortex, centrifuge at high speed in a microfuge for 5 min, extract the aqueous DNA phase and ethanol precipitate as usual.

If DNA samples shown to previously work start failing it is possible that one of the PCR ingredients is faulty or that the DNA sample is degrading over time. Always keep a batch of working frozen stock ingredients so that trouble shooting can be made easier. Fluctuations can be due to variation in *Taq* supply.

2. Generally weak reactions.

- Usually due to insufficient or poor quality DNA. Try adding more DNA: if this does not work see the above section on failures.
- Incorrectly made buffer or poor/dilute *Taq*. Remake buffer or try increasing *Taq* concentrations. Some laboratories use twice or three times the *Taq* concentration that we use.
- Inefficient PCR machine: not all PCR machines work well for this PCR-SSP protocol. If reactions are always weak try elongating some of the PCR program sections or try lower annealing temperatures at the start of the program (68°C instead of 70°C).

3. Too many allele-specific amplicons in one locus.

- Possible new allele: Try to confirm by PCR mapping techniques (Krausa *et al*., 1995; Vilches *et al*., 1995) or by using another molecular method such as sequencing or SSOP.
- Sample contaminated with another DNA sample: Most such contamination would yield extra bands at all loci tested but it is possible to get a combination of alleles in two samples so that the contamination was only noticed at one locus. Most accidental contamination involves

small amounts of contaminant being introduced to a larger amount so contaminating bands are typically weak but consistent.

- Sample contaminated with a locus-specific amplicon from another part of the laboratory: try to minimise contamination by maintaining good laboratory procedures and spatial separation of pre and post-amplification areas.
- Incorrectly made up or contaminated primer mix: Retest suspected primer mix and re-synthesise primer mix if faulty.

4. Too many allele-specific amplicons in all loci.

- PCR machine error: If the PCR program is interrupted and restarted (especially at the early stages) multiple bands are seen due to the low stringency PCR induced. Use a PCR machine which gives error messages when programs have been interrupted.
- Sample or PCR buffer contamination. Remake solutions if contaminated.

5. No allele-specific amplicons at one locus.

- Homozygous example of a new allele not detected by the given PCR reactions. This is unlikely.
- Incorrectly made primer mixes: ensure all primer mixes are tested before use.
- Incorrect buffer mixture: If the dNTP to $MgCl_2$ ratio is incorrect it can affect one locus more than another so that it appears as if there are no alleles at one particular locus. For unknown reasons, the HLA-B locus, and especially the primer mixes specific for B*44, B*08, B*51, Bw4 and Bw6 are most susceptible to this phenomenon. Classically false-negative allele amplifications due to incorrect $MgCl_2$ concentrations are associated with much stronger control amplicons and much weaker than normal allele-specific amplicons.

6. Individual reaction failure.

Approximately 0.5-1% of PCR-SSP reactions spontaneously fail for no apparent reason. Possible causes include: incomplete PCR reaction, PCR inhibitory contaminant in an individual well, or failure of individual PCR vessels. If a reaction has failed and no primer or primer-dimer is visible on the gel it is likely that either the agarose well was incomplete or the reaction was not loaded into the gel properly.

7. Allele-specific bands present but no controls.

- Degraded DNA may produce only small amplicons such as the allele-specific amplicons but not larger amplicons such as the control amplicon.
- Insufficient PCR extension time: try increasing the time the PCR program spends at the extension temperature (72°C)
- PCR machine needs re-calibration.
- Concentration of control primers is too low.

8. Control-specific amplicons but no alleles.

- Magnesium concentration too high: re-calibrate TDMH.
- PCR program is inefficient. Try different PCR programs.
- Poor fit of PCR tubes/plate into PCR block: The bottom of the PCR vessel must be in direct contact with the PCR block otherwise the correct temperature will not be applied to the PCR reactions. If the fit is suspect dip the vessels in a little light paraffin oil to coat the exterior of the vessel before placing in the PCR machine.
- Insufficient pressure from above. If pressure is not applied to the PCR plate the plate may lift out of the block slightly or the thermoseal may peel off. Either way you end up with different PCR thermodynamics which can produce allele dropout.

9. Part of the typing has worked well, but the remainder has failed.

- PCR machine failure. This is a common failure if a PCR machine is used intensively. Test block uniformity by amplifying 96 identical reactions in one plate. If a problem does exist contact a PCR service engineer.
- PCR plate not placed in machine properly.
- Uneven pressure applied during PCR.
- Gel artifact caused by insufficient ethidium bromide.

Updating the typing system.

The ever increasing number of HLA alleles makes updating large PCR-SSP typing systems very difficult: each new allele must be cross-referenced with the two (or more) *cis*-located polymorphisms identified in each primer mix and internal mismatches with primer lengths must also be considered. This is a difficult, time consuming task which frequently leads to errors being made. To facilitate updating various primer mixes sets we have developed a computer program known as “PCR-SSP Manager Program” (Bunce *et al.*, 1998). This program allows all new HLA sequences to be aligned. Once a new allele is inserted, the specificities of all the primers and consequently the primer mixes is adjusted and the new updated specificity list for a tray of reactions is produced. Furthermore, the program can assist the investigator developing new primer mixes by suggesting new primer mixes to sort out the inevitable conundrums created by new alleles. Added to this are various interpretation facilities which make the program an invaluable tool for anyone using PCR-SSP for HLA typing. This program is now available on request from the Oxford Transplantation Immunology Laboratory.

Inevitably further primer mixes must be included to accommodate new alleles and higher resolution requirements; indeed we now use 192 reactions for class I, 96 reactions for DR and DQ and 96 reactions for DP. Many of these extra reactions will shortly be published or have already been published (Gilchrist *et al.*, 1998). Most PCR-SSP primer mixes taken from papers using different PCR protocols and parameters can be successfully adapted to the universal method presented here by ensuring that the primer temperatures are 60°C or 62°C and that the working concentration of the primers is properly evaluated prior to general use.

Materials

1. DNA preparation.

1.1. Red cell lysis buffer (RCLB):

- ☑ 0.144M ammonium chloride (NH_4Cl)
- ☑ 1mM sodium bicarbonate ($NaHCO_3$)

- Dissolve 15.4g of NH_4Cl and 1.68g of $NaHCO_3$ in two litres of ddH_20.

1.2. Nuclear lysis buffer (NLB):

- ☑ 10mM Tris-HCl pH8.2
- ☑ 0.4M Sodium chloride (NaCl)
- ☑ 2mM disodium EDTA pH 8.0 (Na_2EDTA)

- Dissolve 23.37g of NaCl in 900ml of distilled water. Add 10ml 1M Tris-HCl pH8.2 and 10ml Na_2EDTA pH8.0 and make up to one litre with distilled water.

1.3. 10% w/v sodium dodecyl sulphate (SDS).

- In a fume hood, dissolve 100g of sodium dodecyl sulphate in one litre of ddH_20. Store at approximately 20°C to prevent precipitate forming.

1.4. NLB+SDS buffer.

- Combine 300ml of NLB with 20ml of 10% w/v SDS. Store at approximately 20°C to prevent precipitate forming (N.B. The precitate redissolves upon warming).

1.5. 95% ethanol

- Combine 950ml of absolute ethanol and 50ml ddH_20.

1.6. 70% ethanol

- Combine 700ml of absolute ethanol and 300ml ddH_20.

1.7. 6M NaCl

- Dissolve with warming 350.64g of sodium chloride in 800mls of ddH_20 and then make up to one litre with ddH_20. (N.B. This is a saturated solution).

2. Ingredients for primer mixes.

2.1. Primers

- Synthesise or purchase primers (from Table 5.1) resuspended in ddH_20 at a concentration of 2000μg/ml and store frozen until required.

2.2. Cresol red 6mg/ml stock.

- Dissolve 3g of cresol red sodium salt (Sigma, C9877) in 500ml ddH_20. Pass through a 0.22 micron filter and store frozen in 1ml volumes.

2.3. Stock solutions of control primers.

- For the 796bp control amplification used in all primer mixes except the Bw4 and Bw6 mixes, autoclave 2 litres of ddH_20.
- When cold, add 1.5µl/ml each of primer 63 and primer 64 along with 10µl/ml of cresol red and filter through a 0.22 micron filter.
- For the 256bp control amplification used in the Bw4 and Bw6 mixes autoclave 20ml of ddH_20. When cold, add 3µl/ml each of primers 210 and 211 along with 10µl/ml of cresol red and filter through a 0.22micron filter. The control stocks must be tested (see methods) prior to freezing in aliquots.

3. PCR ingredients

3.1. 25mM magnesium chloride

- Add 1ml 1M stock solution (Sigma, M1028) to 39ml ddH_20. Note that stock solutions deteriorate over a period of 6 months, so when a new bottle is opened dispense in 1ml volumes and freeze.

3.2. dNTP mix

- Combine 0.4ml of each dNTP (dCTP, dATP, dTTP, dGTP) from 100mM stock (Promega, U1240).

3.3. 10x Base buffer

☑ 670mM Tris-base pH8.9

☑ 166mM Ammonium sulphate

☑ 1%v/v Tween 20 (Polyoxyethylenesorbitan monolaurate) (Sigma, P9416)

- Dissolve 40.568g Tris base in 400ml dH_2O and adjust to pH 8.9 with conc. HCl. Dissolve 10.96g of ammonium sulphate in the Tris solution. Filtered through a 0.22 micron filter into an autoclaved bottle. Add 5ml of Tween and make up to 500ml with ddH_20. Store at -70°C.

3.4. TDMH buffer (200ml recipe). This when combined with all other PCR ingredients gives a final $MgCl_2$ concentration of 1.9mM.

- ☑ 33.3ml x10 base buffer
- ☑ 25.1ml 25mM fresh $MgCl_2$
- ☑ 140.4ml freshly autoclaved water
- ☑ 1.215ml dNTP mix (i.e. all 4 mixed together)

- Test TDMH buffer (see Methods) before freezing in 13.3ml aliquots.

4. Setting up PCR reactions

- The method is described in the Methods section. The extra ingredient required is 5units/ml *Taq* polymerase (Bioline).

5. Gel electrophoresis

5.1. Orange G loading buffer

- Combine 300ml of glycerol, 250ml of 2xTBE, 550ml distilled water and 0.25g orange G (Sigma, O7629). Store at 20°C.

5.2. 2x and 0.5x TBE buffer

- To make 2x TBE dissolve 216g of Tris-base and 110g of boric acid in 9 litres of distilled water. Add 8ml of 0.5M EDTA pH 8.3 and make up to 10 litres with ddH_20.
- To make 0.5x TBE combine 750ml of distilled water with 250ml of 2xTBE.

5.3. 1% agarose (one litre).

- ☑ 10g electrophoresis grade agarose (Helena BioSciences, 8201-03)
- ☑ 1l of 0.5x TBE
- ☑ 10μl of 10mg/ml ethidium bromide (E1510, Sigma)

- Dissolve, by heating in a microwave, 10g of agarose (Helena BioSciences, 8201-03) in 400ml 0.5xTBE. Top up to one litre with 0.5x TBE and add 10ml of 10mg/ml ethidium bromide solution. Agarose solutions can be stored at 50°C for up to one week.

Specialist equipment.

Very little in the way of specialist equipment is required if the laboratory already performs molecular biological assays. Listed below are the main items of equipment required for PCR-SSP.

Specialist plastics

- 96-well PCR plates. Advanced Biotechnologies AB-0600.
- 96-well plate sealers. Costar 6524

Dispensing equipment

- 96-well dispenser. Robbins Scientific Hydra-96
- 8-channel electronic multi dispenser. Anachem EDP-Plus M8

PCR Machines with 96-well or 384-well block (384-well blocks work well for small volume PCR in either 384 or 96-well format PCR plates).

- Hybaid PCR Express. Hybaid HB-PX-02

Horizontal gel rigs with combs suitable for multichannel loading.

- 30x25cm horizontal gel rig. Flowgen. G3-0403
- 1mm 26 well sample combs. Flowgen. G3-0416

Large 312nm transilluminator

- Flowgen. T7-0174

Gel imaging systems.

There are many gel imaging systems available but a Polaroid Land Camera gives excellent results. However the film is relatively expensive compared to non-film based imaging systems.

- Polaroid MP4 land camera system. Sigma MP-4P

- N.B. if using Polaroid camera system you will also need to use Polaroid Type 667 Black and White film in conjunction with Wratten 2A and Wratten 22 filters)

Suppliers Addresses.

Anachem: 20 Charles Street, Luton, Bedfordshire LU2 OEB, England

Advanced Biotechnologies: Units B1-B2, Lonmead Business Centre, Blenheim Road, Epsom, Surrey KT19 9QQ, England

Costar: 10, The Valley Centre, Gordon Road, High Wycombe, Bucks HP13 6EQ, England

Flowgen: Lynn Lane, Shenstone, Lichfield, Staffordshire WS14 OEE, England

Hybaid: Action Court, Ashford Road, Ashford, Middlesex TW15 1XB, England

Robbins Scientific (Europe): Greville Court, 165 High Street, Knowle, Solihull, West Midlands B93 OLL, England

Sigma Chemicals: Fancy Road, Poole, Dorset BH12 4XA, England

References

Aldener, A and Olerup, O (1993). Characterization of a novel DQB1 (DQB1*0609) allele by PCR amplification with sequence-specific primers (PCR-SSP) and nucleotide sequencing. *Tissue Antigens* **42**: 536-538

Anasetti, C, Amos, D, Beatty, PG, Appelbaum, FR, Bensinger, W, *et al.* (1989). Effect of HLA compatibility on engraftment of bone marrow transplants in patients with leukemia or lymphoma. *N Engl J Med* **320**: 197-204

Atkinson, K, Farewell, V, Storb, R, Tsoi, MS, Sullivan, KM, *et al.* (1982). Analysis of late infections after human bone marrow transplantation: role of genotypic nonidentity between marrow donor and recipient and of nonspecific suppressor cells in patients with chronic graft-versus-host disease. *Blood* **60**: 714-720

Baan, CC, Vaessen, LM, ten Kate, F, Schreuder, GM, Claas, FH, *et al.* (1993). Rejection of a kidney graft mismatched only for the HLA-C locus and an HLA-BW22 split. *Transplantation* **55**: 438-439

Barnardo, MC, Davey, NJ, Bunce, M, Brookes, PA, Lechler, RI, *et al.* (1996). A correlation between HLA-C matching and donor antirecipient CTL precursor frequency in bone marrow transplantation. *Transplantation* **61**: 1420-1423

Barnardo, M. C. N. M., Bunce, M., Thursz, M. and Welsh, K. I. (1997). Analysis of the molecular epitopes of anti-HLA antibodies using a computer program, OODAS; Object Oriented Definition of Antibody Specificity. In: *Genetic diversity of HLA: functional and medical implications*, Vol 2. (Ed. Charron, D), pp.132-134. EDK, Sevres, France

Baxter-Lowe, LA, Eckels, DD, Ash, R, Casper, J, Hunter, JB, *et al.* (1992). The predictive value of HLA-DR oligotyping for MLC responses. *Transplantation* **53**: 1352-1357

Beatty, PG. (1992). Results of allogeneic bone marrow transplantation with unrelated or mismatched donors. *Semin Oncol* **19**(3 Suppl 7), 13-19

Bodmer, JG, Marsh, SG, Parham, P, Erlich, HA, Albert, E, *et al.* (1990). Nomenclature for factors of the HLA system, 1989. *Tissue Antigens* **35**: 1-8

Bodmer, JG, Marsh, SGE, Albert, ED, Bodmer, WF, Bontrop, RE, *et al.* (1995). Nomenclature for factors of the HLA system, 1995. *Tissue Antigens* **46**: 1-18

Bodmer, JG, Marsh, SGE, Albert, ED, Bontrop, RE, Charron, D, *et al.* (1997). Nomenclature for factors of the HLA system, 1996. *Tissue Antigens* **49**: 297-321

Browning, MJ, Krausa, P, Rowan, A, Bicknell, DC, Bodmer, JG, *et al.* (1993). Tissue typing the HLA-A locus from genomic DNA by sequence-specific PCR: comparison of HLA genotype and surface expression on colorectal tumor cell lines. *Proc Natl Acad Sci U S A* **90**: 2842-2845.

Bunce, M, Barnardo, MC and Welsh, KI (1994). Improvements in HLA-C typing using sequence-specific primers (PCR-SSP) including definition of HLA-Cw9 and Cw10 and a new allele HLA-"Cw7/8v". *Tissue Antigens* **44**: 200-203.

Bunce, M, Barnardo, MC, Procter, J, Marsh, SGE, Vilches, C, *et al.* (1996). High resolution HLA-C typing by PCR-SSP: identification of allelic frequencies and linkage disequilibria in 604 unrelated random UK Caucasoids and a comparison with serology. *Tissue Antigens* **48**: 680-691

Bunce, M, Barnardo, MC and Welsh, KI. (1998). The PCR-SSP Manager Computer Program: A tool for maintaining sequence alignments and automatically updating the specificities of PCR-SSP primers and primer mixes. *Tissue Antigens* **52**: 159-175

Bunce, M, Fanning, GC and Welsh, KI. (1995a). Comprehensive, serologically equivalent DNA typing for HLA-B by PCR using sequence-specific primers (PCR-SSP). *Tissue Antigens* **45**: 81-90

Bunce, M, O'Neill, CM, Barnardo, MC, Krausa, P, Browning, MJ, *et al.* (1995b). Phototyping: Comprehensive DNA typing for HLA-A, B, C, DRB1, DRB3, DRB4, DRB5 and DQB1 by PCR with 144 primer mixes utilising sequence-specific primers (PCR-SSP). *Tissue Antigens* **46**: 355-367

Bunce, M, Taylor, CJ and Welsh, KI. (1993). Rapid HLA-DQB typing by eight polymerase chain reaction amplifications with sequence-specific primers (PCR-SSP). *Hum Immunol* **37**: 201-206

Bunce, M and Welsh, KI. (1994). Rapid DNA typing for HLA-C using sequence-specific primers (PCR-SSP): identification of serological and non-serologically defined HLA-C alleles including several new alleles. *Tissue Antigens* **43**: 7-17

Chapman, JR, Taylor, C, Ting, A and Morris, PJ. (1986). Hyperacute rejection of a renal allograft in the presence of anti-HLA-Cw5 antibody. *Transplantation* **42**: 91-93

Charron, D, Arnaiz-Villena, A, Bignon, , Busson, M, Christiansen, F, *et al.* (1997). Unrelated donor bone marrow transplantation (UD-BMT): 12th Internataional Histocompatibility Workshop study. In: *Genetic diversity of HLA: functional and medical implications.* Vol 1. (Ed. Charron, D), pp.459-465. EDK, Sevres, France

Chien, A, Edgar, DB and Trela, JM. (1976). Deoxyribonucleic acid polymerase from the extreme thermophile Thermus aquaticus. *J Bacteriol* **127**: 1550-1557

Fanning, GC, Bunce, M and Welsh, KI. (1997). PCR-haplotyping using 3' mismatches in the forward and reverse primers: Application to the biallelic polymorphisms of TNF and LTa. *Tissue Antigens* **50**: 23-31

Fugger, L, Morling, N, Ryder, LP, Odum, N and Svejgaard, A. (1990). Technical aspects of typing for HLA-DP alleles using allele-specific DNA in vitro amplification and sequence-specific oligonucleotide probes. Detection of single base mismatches. *J Immunol Methods* **129**: 175-185

Gilchrist, FC, Bunce, M, Lympany, PA, Welsh, KI and du Bois, RM. (1998). Comprehensive HLA-DP typing using polymerase chain reaction with sequence-specific primers and 95 sequence-specific primer mixes. *Tissue Antigens* **51**: 51-61

Jordan, F, McWhinnie, AJ, Turner, S, Gavira, N, Calvert, AA, *et al.* (1995). Comparison of HLA-DRB1 typing by DNA-RFLP, PCR-SSO and PCR-SSP methods and their application in providing matched unrelated donors for bone marrow transplantation. *Tissue Antigens* **45**: 103-110

Knipper, AJ, Hinney, A, Schuch, B, Enczmann, J, Uhrberg, M, *et al.* (1994). Selection of unrelated bone marrow donors by PCR-SSP typing and subsequent nonradioactive sequence-based typing for HLA DRB1/3/4/5, DQB1, and DPB1 alleles. *Tissue Antigens* **44**: 275-284

Krausa, P, Barouch, D, Bodmer, JG and Browning, MJ. (1995). Rapid characterization of HLA class I alleles by gene mapping using ARMS PCR. *Eur J Immunogenet* **22**: 283-287

Krausa, P, Bodmer, JG and Browning, MJ. (1993). Defining the common subtypes of HLA A9, A10, A28 and A19 by use of ARMS/PCR. *Tissue Antigens* **42**(2), 91-99

Krausa, P and Browning, MJ. (1996). A comprehensive PCR-SSP typing system for identification of HLA-A locus alleles. *Tissue Antigens* **47**: 237-244

Kwok, S, Kellogg, DE, McKinney, N, Spasic, D, Goda, L, *et al.* (1990). Effects of primer-template mismatches on the polymerase chain reaction: human immunodeficiency virus type 1 model studies. *Nucleic Acids Res* **18**: 999-1005

Laforet, M, Froelich, N, Parissiadis, A, Pfeiffer, B, Schell, A, *et al.* (1997). A nucleotide insertion in exon 4 is responsible for the absence of expression of an HLA-A*01 allele. *Tissue Antigens* **50**: 347-350

Lanchbury, JS, Hall, MA, Welsh, KI and Panayi, GS. (1990). Sequence analysis of HLA-DR4B1 subtypes: additional first domain variability is detected by oligonucleotide hybridization and nucleotide sequencing. *Hum Immunol* **27:** 136-144

Lopez-Larrea, C, Sujirachato, K, Mehra, NK, Chiewsilp, P, Isarangkura, D, *et al.* (1995). HLA-B27 subtypes in Asian patients with ankylosing spondylitis. Evidence for new associations. *Tissue Antigens* **45**:169-176

Lorentzen, DF, Iwanaga, KK, Meuer, KJ, Moritz, TL and Watkins, DI. (1997). A 25% error rate in serologic typing of HLA-B homozygotes. *Tissue Antigens* **50**: 359-365

Magor, KE, Taylor, EJ, Shen, SY, Martinez-Naves, E, Valiante, NM, *et al.* (1997). Natural inactivation of a common HLA allele (A*2402) has occurred on at least three separate occasions. *The Journal of Immunology* **158**: 5242-5250

Mallon, E, Bunce, M, Wojnarowska, F and Welsh, KI. (1996). HLA-C locus genotyping in a UK population with psoriasis: confirmation that Cw*0602 is a disease susceptibility factor in type I psoriasis, and evidence for differential frequency of ^{73}Ala in male and female type I psoriatics. *J. Invest. Dermatology* **109**: 183-186

Marsh, SGE. (1998). HLA Class II region sequences, 1998. *Tissue Antigens* **51:** 467-507

Mason, PM and Parham, P. (1998). HLA class I region sequences, 1998. *Tissue Antigens* **51:** 417-466

Mignot, E., Kimura, A, Latterman, A, Grumet, F, Mayer, G, *et al.* (1997). HLA class II studies in non DRB1*1501 patients with narcolepsy-cataplexy. In: *Genetic diversity of HLA: functional and medical implications.* Vol 1. (Ed. Charron, D), pp.437-441. EDK, Sevres, France

Miller, SA, Dykes, DD and Polesky, HF. (1988). A simple salting out procedure for extracting DNA from human nucleated cells. *Nucleic Acids Res* **16**: 1215

Mytilineos, J, Lempert, M, Middleton, D, Williams, F, Cullen, C, *et al.* (1997). HLA class I typing of 215 "HLA-A, B, -DR zero mismatched" kidney transplants. *Tissue Antigens* **50**: 355-358

Mytilineos, J, Scherer, S and Opelz, G. (1990). Comparison of RFLP-DR beta and serological HLA-DR typing in 1500 individuals. *Transplantation* **50**: 870-873

Newton, CR, Graham, A, Heptinstall, LE, Powell, SJ., Summers, C, *et al.* (1989). Analysis of any point mutation in DNA. The amplification refractory mutation system (ARMS). *Nucleic Acids Res* **17:** 2503-2516

Olerup, O, Aldener, A and Fogdell, A. (1993). HLA-DQB1 and -DQA1 typing by PCR amplification with sequence-specific primers (PCR-SSP) in 2 hours. *Tissue Antigens* **41**: 119-134

Olerup, O and Zetterquist, H. (1992). HLA-DR typing by PCR amplification with sequence-specific primers (PCR-SSP) in 2 hours: an alternative to serological DR typing in clinical practice including donor-recipient matching in cadaveric transplantation. *Tissue Antigens* **39**: 225-235

Opelz, G, Mytilineos, J, Scherer, S, Dunckley, H, Trejaut, J, *et al.* (1991). Survival of DNA HLA-DR typed and matched cadaver kidney transplants. The Collaborative Transplant Study. *Lancet* **338**: 461-463

Opelz, G, Scherer, S and Mytilineos, J. (1997). Analysis of HLA-DR split-specificity matching in cadaver kidney transplantation: a report of the Collaborative Transplant Study. *Transplantation* **63**: 57-59

Otten, HG, Tilanus, MG, Barnstijn, M, van Heugten, JG and de Gast, GC. (1995). Serology versus PCR-SSP in typing for HLA-DR and HLA-DQ: a practical evaluation. *Tissue Antigens* **45**: 36-40

Petersdorf, EW, Setoda, T, Smith, AG and Hansen, JA. (1994a). Analysis of HLA-B*44 alleles encoded on extended HLA haplotypes by direct automated sequencing. *Tissue Antigens* **44**: 211-216

Petersdorf, EW, Stanley, JF, Martin, PJ and Hansen, JA. (1994b). Molecular diversity of the HLA-C locus in unrelated marrow transplantation. *Tissue Antigens* **44**: 93-99

Poli, F, Bianchi, P, Crespiatico, L, Terragna, C, van den Berg-Loonen, E, *et al.* (1996). Characterization of a new DRB5 allele (DRB5*0105) by PCR-SSP and direct sequencing. *Tissue Antigens* **47**: 338-340

Procter, J, Crawford, J, Bunce, M and Welsh, KI. (1996). A rapid molecular method (PCR-SSP) to genotype for ABO blood group and secretor status and it's potential for organ transplants. *Tissue Antigens* **50**: 475-483

Sadler, AM, Petronzelli, F, Krausa, P, Marsh, SG, Guttridge, MG, *et al.* (1994). Low-resolution DNA typing for HLA-B using sequence-specific primers in allele- or group-specific ARMS/PCR. *Tissue Antigens* **44**: 148-154

Santamaria, P, Reinsmoen, NL, Lindstrom, AL, Boyce-Jacino, JJ, Fara, AJ, *et al.* (1994). Frequent HLA class I and DP sequence mismatches in serologically (HLA-A, HLA-B, HLA-DR) and molecularly (HLA-DRB1, HLA-DQA1, HLA-DQB1) HLA-identical unrelated bone marrow transplant pairs. *Blood* **83**: 280-287

Satsangi, J, Jewell, DP, Welsh, K, Bunce, M and Bell, JI. (1994). Effect of heparin on polymerase chain reaction. *Lancet* **343**: 1509-1510

Savelkoul, PH, de Bruyn-Geraets, DP and van den Berg-Loonen, EM. (1995). High resolution HLA-DRB1 SSP typing for cadaveric donor transplantation. *Tissue Antigens* **45**: 41-48

Schipper, RF, Oudshoorn, M, D'Amaro, J, van der Zanden, HGM, de Lange, P, *et al.* (1996). Validation of large data sets, an essential prerequisite for data analysis: an analytical survey of the Bone Marrow Donors Worldwide. *Tissue Antigens* **47**: 169-178

Speiser, DE, Tiercy, JM, Rufer, N, Chapuis, B, Morell, A, *et al.* (1994). Relation between the resolution of HLA-typing and the chance of finding an unrelated bone marrow donor. *Bone Marrow Transplant* **13**: 805-809

Speiser, DE, Tiercy, JM, Rufer, N, Grundschober, C, Gratwohl, A, *et al.* (1996). High resolution HLA matching associated with decreased mortality after unrelated bone marrow transplantation. *Blood* **87**: 4455-4462

Tindall, KR and Kunkel, TA. (1988). Fidelity of DNA synthesis by the Thermus aquaticus DNA polymerase. *Biochemistry* **27:** 6008-6013

Ting, A and Morris, PJ. (1978). Matching for B-cell antigens of the HLA-DR series in cadaver renal transplantation. *Lancet* **1**: 575-577

Tonks, S, Marsh, SGE, Bunce, M, Moses, JH, Krausa, P, *et al.* (1997). HLA Class I DNA typing study. In: *Genetic diversity of HLA: functional and medical implications.* Vol 1. (Ed. Charron, D), pp.199-215. EDK, Sevres, France

Vilches, C, Bunce, M, de Pablo, R, Herrero, MJ and Kreisler, M. (1995). Anchored PCR cloning of the novel HLA-Cw*0704 allele detected by PCR-SSP. *Tissue Antigens* **46**: 19-23

Wu, DY, Ugozzoli, L, Pal, BK and Wallace, RB. (1989). Allele-specific enzymatic amplification of beta-globin genomic DNA for diagnosis of sickle cell anemia. *Proc Natl Acad Sci USA* **86**: 2757-2760

Young, NT, Roelen, D, Bunce, M, Dallman, MJ, Morris, PJ, *et al.* (1997). Alloreactive helper T-lymphocyte precursor frequencies correlate with HLA-DRB1 antigen amino acid residue mismatches. In: *Genetic diversity of HLA: functional and medical implications.* Vol 2. (Ed. Charron, D), pp. 501-503. EDK, Sevres, France

Yu, N, Ohashi, M, Alosco, S, Granja, C, Salazar, M, *et al.* (1997). Accurate typing of HLA-A antigens and analysis of serological deficiencies. *Tissue Antigens* **50**: 380-386

CHAPTER 6

PCR-SSOP TYPING

D. Middleton
Northern Ireland Histocompatibility and Immunogenetics Laboratory
Belfast City Hospital and School of Biology and Biochemistry
Queen's University
Belfast BT9 7TS

Introduction

This chapter describes the use of sequence-specific oligonucleotide probes (SSOP) as a method for DNA typing of HLA alleles. The methods employ polymerase chain reaction (PCR) amplification of the HLA alleles for a given HLA locus, followed by probing of the PCR product with labelled SSOP. Polymorphism within the HLA system seems to have resulted from *gene conversion*, during which small nucleotide sections of one allele (usually no more that 100 bases long) are transferred non-reciprocally to another allele, and also from nucleotide substitutions. A corollary of gene conversion is that many sequence motifs are not allele-specific but may be shared by two or more, and often multiple, HLA alleles. Therefore in PCR-SSOP typing, a battery of probes is used which ultimately determine an allele-specific pattern of sequence motifs, with the result that individual HLA alleles may be identified.

The PCR-SSOP method consists of labelling the probes with digoxigenin (DIG) and detecting hybridisation of these probes to a complementary sequence present in the PCR-amplified HLA alleles of individuals. Hybridisation is detected by adding an anti-digoxigenin antibody conjugated with alkaline phosphatase (ALP). The ALP enzyme reacts with CSPD, a chemiluminescent substrate, and emitted photons of light are detected by autoradiography.

The number of HLA alleles reported in the last decade has risen at a rapid rate. Thus, whereas in January 1991 there were 25 HLA-A, 32 HLA-B and 34 HLA-DR alleles registered, the corresponding numbers in March 1999 were 132, 266 and 222 (S. Marsh, personal communication). To define every HLA allele at a given locus would require a large number of probes (in excess of 100 for certain loci) and the typing system would constantly need up-dating to take account of each newly discovered allele. A further complication is that, in certain individuals heterozygous at a given HLA locus, patterns of SSOP hybridisation may appear identical to those present in another heterozygous individual possessing two different alleles.

Here, we describe the use of a two-tier PCR-SSOP system. The first level of resolution is equivalent to very good serology and results in the definition of an allele group, for example, HLA-A*02. Dependent on the results of this initial typing, a second PCR, specific for that group of alleles, is performed and a further set of probes is used to give definition at the allele level. Thus the number of probes required is kept to a minimum and, in all but exceptional circumstances, only the high resolution system needs alteration to take account of newly defined alleles. The PCR primers used for each HLA locus are listed in Table 6.2.

HLA-A, -B and -C primers

The primers used for HLA-A, -B and -C generate a locus-specific product spanning exon 2, intron 2 and exon 3. For HLA-B, a mixture of two 3'-primers is required because HLA-B*7301 differs in intron 3 from all other known alleles at this locus, and an extra primer is required to amplify this allele. In testing for HLA-B*27 alleles only, which many laboratories perform for association with ankylosing spondylitis, this extra primer is not required. Instead, the probe BL12 detects a sequence which is only found in HLA-B*27 alleles and HLA-B*7301. Thus, omitting the primer 3 BIN3-AC (Table 6.2) ensures that HLA-B*7301 is not amplified, and that the BL12 probe is specific for alleles of HLA-B*27.

HLA-DRB primers

The primers for HLA-DRB generate a product from exon 2: this product is not specific for the HLA-DRB1 locus, but amplifies alleles of other HLA-DRB loci (e.g. HLA-DRB3). Thus it is necessary to include a further amplification for alleles of HLA-DRB1*03, -DRB1*11, -DRB1*13 and -DRB1*14. This is referred to as the HLA-DRB3/11/6 group.

Protocols

In the protocols described below, each probe is hybridised to two different membranes in the same hybridisation bottle, and the reagents are prepared accordingly. The PCR-SSOP method is thus very suitable for typing large numbers of samples – for example, we simultaneously test 192 samples including controls (96 each on two membranes). However, the volume of reagents used can be scaled down appropriately if a laboratory is not performing tests on large numbers of samples: for example, only a single membrane per bottle need be hybridised.

Since in these protocols the number of probes is kept to a minimum, not all polymorphic nucleotide positions are tested. This might theoretically lead to a failure in detecting new alleles, but despite this we have previously discovered 13 new alleles recognised by their unique probe-hybridisation patterns. In a medium resolution typing system, many examples are observed where a combination of two HLA alleles gives the same probe-hybridisation pattern as a different combination of two alleles. However in the system described below, few anomalies exist. For example, there are theoretically only eight anomalous combinations at the HLA-A locus involving alleles representing different serological groups (Table 6.1).

HLA-A alleles				
Combination 1		Combination 2		f*
2501	2501	2501	2603/05	1
0101	3401	3601	6601	2
30	6601	30	2603/05	
2501	7401	3201	6601	
2501	3201	3201	2603/05	10
7401	6601	7401	2603/05	
02	6602	0216	3401	
02	34	0203	68	6

Table 6.1. Anomalous combinations of HLA-A alleles in PCR-SSOP. **f* = frequency per 5000 Caucasian individuals (Northern Ireland).

There are more anomalous combinations at the HLA-B locus than at the HLA-A locus. For example in the Northern Ireland population, anomalies with the highest frequency are:

- HLA-B*7 cannot be distinguished from HLA-B*81 in the presence of HLA-B*40 (*f* = 0.9%);
- HLA-B*15 homozygosity cannot be distinguished from HLA-B*15 present with HLA-B*35 (*f* = 0.4%);
- HLA-B*15 cannot be distinguished from HLA-B*35 or HLA-B*53 in the presence of either HLA-B*49 or HLA-B*51 (*f* = 0.4%).

Clinical relevance

Renal transplantation

It has been shown that more accurate HLA-DR typing using DNA techniques leads to a significant increase in graft survival (Opelz *et al.* 1991). Using serological techniques, it has been impossible to reach any conclusion on the effects of matching for HLA-DQ and -DP in kidney transplantation. With the advent of DNA technology, there have been indications that matching for HLA-DQ may have some benefit in graft survival (Sengar *et al.* 1987; Middleton *et al.* 1992a), but the question remains difficult to answer because of the strong linkage disequilibrium between HLA-DR and -DQ. Initially, no effect of matching for HLA-DP alleles was found in transplants from a single centre (Middleton *et al.* 1992a), or in transplants selected from multiple centres with no mismatching at the HLA-A, -B and -DR loci (Middleton *et al.* 1992b). However an effect of HLA-DP matching in transplants with varying degrees of HLA-A, -B and -DR matching has

Locus	Primers	*Location* and sequence 5' - 3'	Band size (bp)
HLA-A GENERIC	A15	*94 (intron 1) → 116* GAGGGTCGGGCG(A)GGTCTCAGCCA	863
	AL#AW	*13 (intron 3) → 274 (exon 3)* TGGCCCCTGGTACCCGT	
HLA-B GENERIC	5 BINI-57M	*36 (Intron 1) → 57* GGGAGGAGC(A)G(A)AGGGGACCGCAG	970
	3 BIN3-37M	*68 (Intron 3) → 37* AGG(C)CCATCCCCGG(C)CGACCTAT	
	3 BIN3-AC	*68 (Intron 3) → 37* AGGCCATCCCGGGCGATCTAT	
HLA-B27	5 BINI-57M	see above	970
	3 BIN3-37M	see above	
HLA-C GENERIC	5 CIN1-61	*42 (Intron 1) → 61* AGCGAGGG(T)GCCCGCCCGGCGA	937
	3 BCIN3-12	*35 (Intron 3) → 12* GGAGATGGGGAAGGCTCCCCACT	
HLA-DRB GENERIC	AMP-A*	*15 (intron1) → 24 (exon2)* CCCCACAGCACGTTTCT(C)TG	274
	AMP-B	*279 (exon2) → 260* CCGCTGCACTGTGAAGCTCT	
HLA-DRB 3/11/16 GROUP	3/11/6 GF	*17 (exon2) → 38* GTTTCTTGGAGTACTCTACGTC	263
	AMP-B	*279 (exon2) → 260* CCGCTGCACTGTGAAGCTCT	

Table 6.2. HLA-A, -B, -C and -DRB primers used for PCR-SSOP typing. Parentheses surrounding individual bases indicate a degenerate base at this location

been reported in second but not first transplants (Middleton *et al.* 1997). Although no allowance has been made for linkage disequilibrium, it is known that linkage between HLA-DP and -DR is limited compared to that between HLA-DQ and HLA-DR.

A recent study using PCR-SSOP examined HLA-A and -B specificities in cadaveric kidney transplants that had zero mismatches for HLA-A and -B (typed by serology) and HLA-DR (typed by restriction fragment length polymorphism (RFLP) (Mytilineos *et al.* 1997)). This study did not take the resolution of typing to the allele level, but still found a difference in graft survival of 15% between those transplants with zero mismatches for HLA-A, and -B after testing with medium resolution PCR-SSOP, compared to transplants which were found to have mismatches at either HLA-A or -B.

Bone marrow transplantation

The adoption of DNA typing methods have meant that most laboratories typing for bone marrow transplantation no longer rely on the mixed lymphocyte culture (MLC) test. In addition, they have enabled HLA testing before birth, in order to ascertain if the cord blood would be suitable to use for a sibling requiring a stem cell transplantation. The application of high resolution DNA typing for HLA alleles in bone marrow transplantation has revealed that nearly 20% of transplants that were initially matched for HLA-DR by serology were not matched at the allele level, and that there was a significant correlation between HLA-DRB1 mismatches and decreased survival (Petersdorf *et al.* 1995). Other groups have observed a significant correlation between HLA class I mismatches and graft-versus-host disease (GVHD) (Spencer *et al.* 1995, Davies *et al.* 1995).

Bone marrow registries

The application of DNA techniques has played a major role in the typing of bone marrow registry donors. However, the fact that many new alleles defined by DNA typing have not been characterised at the serological level will make it difficult to standardise results obtained by the two methods. At present over 3.9 million donors registered by the United States Marrow Donor Program have only serologically defined HLA-A and -B types, and approximately 40% of the one million HLA-DR typed donors are typed only by serology (Hurley *et al.* 1997).

Laboratories which have previously submitted serological data to bone marrow donor registries may, on implementing DNA techniques for HLA class I, regard it as prudent to re-examine those donors previously reported with serological "blanks". This should lead to the identification of those alleles which have previously been difficult or impossible to find by serological methods, and which are absent or present only at a very low frequency on the donor registry (Williams *et al.* 1997). DNA techniques will also be useful in typing non-Caucasian donors for bone marrow registries. Typing of non-Caucasians by serological methods has always proved difficult since the majority of HLA antisera available have been derived from Caucasians.

Cost implications have meant that the degree of resolution in donor typing for bone marrow registries is not at the highest level. However, the ability to conveniently store DNA samples has meant that if a donor is initially selected on the basis of a medium resolution type, he or she can quickly be re-typed at a high resolution without valuable time being wasted.

Methods

1. *Materials*

- ☑ Buffer 1 (4x) (0.4M maleic acid, 0.6M NaCl pH7.5). Add 300ml 4M NaCl and 400ml 2M maleic acid followed by 200ml 4M NaOH to approximately 800ml dH_2O. Add 27g NaOH pellets. (N.B. a white precipitate forms when all reagents are added - this will disappear as the pH approaches 7). Cool to room temperature and adjust pH to 7.5 by adding 4M NaOH dropwise. Adjust volume to 2 litres with dH_2O and sterilize by autoclaving.

- ☑ Buffer 2 (2% blocking reagent (see below) in Buffer 1). Combine 768ml 5% blocking reagent (in Buffer 1), 288ml 4x Buffer 1 and 864ml dH_2O. Leave 5% blocking reagent at room temperature for 10 min before use.

- ☑ Buffer 3 (0.1M Tris-HC1, 0.1M NaCl, 0.05M $MgCl_2$, pH9.5). Add approximately 1400ml dH_2O to 200ml 1M Tris-HCl (pH9.5) and 50ml 4M NaCl. Add 100ml of filter-sterilised 1M $MgCl_2$ and mix. Adjust pH to 9.5 and make up to 2 litre with dH_2O. Do not autoclave as precipitates tend to form. Store at room temperature for up to one week.

- ☑ Hybridisation buffer. Make up by combining the following reagents. 192ml 2% blocking reagent, 144ml 6x SSPE, 48ml 5x Denhardts, 48ml 0.1% N-lauroylsarcosine, 0.96ml 0.02% SDS and make up to 480ml with dH_2O.

- ☑ Washing buffer (0.3% Tween 20 in Buffer 1). Add 14.4ml Tween 20 to 1200ml 4x buffer 1 and make up to 4800ml by adding dH_2O.

- ☑ Blocking Reagent (Boehringer, Lewes, England, 1096176: 5% in Buffer 1). Prepare 2 litres of 1x Buffer 1 by combining 500ml 4x Buffer 1 with 1500ml dH_2O. Add 100g blocking reagent in parts, with vigorous mixing using a magnetic stirrer, to approximately 1600ml 1x Buffer 1. As the blocking reagent is supplied in 50g tubs, there is no need to weigh out. Heat to 65°C until blocking reagent is dissolved. Allow to cool to room temperature and make up to 2 litre with Buffer 1. Sterilize by autoclaving and store at 4°C.

- ☑ Cresol Red (10mg/ml, sodium salt, Sigma, St Louis, Mo, C9877). Add 200mg to some dH_2O taken from a measured 20ml of dH_2O in a sterile universal. Resuspend in the remaining volume. Filter sterilize, dispense into 1ml aliquots and freeze at -20°C.

☑ CSPD (Boehringer 1655884). Vortex and centrifuge CSPD in a microcentrifuge for 1 min before use. Dilute CSPD stock solution (25mM, 11.6mg/ml) 1:100 in Buffer 3.

☑ Denhardts (50x) (1% polyvinyl pyrrolidone (PVP), 1% Ficoll, 1% bovine serum albumin (BSA)). Prepare 200ml of 2% PVP and 2% Ficoll by adding 4g of each to 180ml dH_2O. (Prepare this solution in a fume cupboard. PVP is harmful if inhaled). Dissolve with gentle mixing and make up to 200mls with dH_2O. Sterilize by autoclaving and cool to room temperature. Slowly add 4g of BSA to 200ml of above solution with gentle mixing. When the BSA has dissolved make up to 400ml with dH_2O, mixing well. Filter solution through 0.45μm filter and aliquot. Do not autoclave. Store at -20°C. Leave to thaw at 4°C the evening before it is to be used.

☑ Anti-digoxigenin-alkaline phosphatase (anti-DIG-ALP) conjugate (Boehringer 1093274). Immediately prior to use, remove anti-DIG-ALP stock conjugate (0.75U/μl) from the refrigerator, vortex for 15 sec and centrifuge for 1 min in a microcentrifuge. Make a 1:10,000 dilution of the conjugate in Buffer 2 (i.e. 192μl of anti-DIG-ALP conjugate in 1920ml of Buffer 2).

☑ EDTA (0.5M, pH8.0). Slowly add 186.1g of EDTA (Na_22H_2O salt) to 800ml dH_2O. Adjust the pH to 8.0 using 4M NaOH. Make up to 1 litre with dH_2O and sterilize by autoclaving.

☑ Ethidium bromide (10mg/ml, Sigma, E-1510).

☑ Gel loading buffer (GLB). Slowly add 8g sucrose to 10ml dH_2O and mix by inversion until dissolved. Then add 1ml 1M Tris (pH7.6), 2ml 0.5M EDTA, 1ml 10% SDS, 0.02g cresol red. Make up to 20ml with dH_2O. Do not autoclave.

☑ dH_2O. Double distilled H_2O or equivalent. Note that dH_2O used to set up PCR is of ultra high purity quality.

☑ $MgCl_2$. Supplied with *Taq* enzyme.

☑ dNTP mix (Pharmacia Biotech, St Albans, England, 27-2094).

☑ NH_4 Buffer. Supplied with *Taq* enzyme.

☑ N-Laurolysarcosine (1%). A barrier face mask should be worn when weighing. Dissolve 10g N-laurolysarcosine in approximately 800ml dH_2O. Adjust volume to 1 litre with dH_2O and autoclave.

☑ Nylon membrane (Boehringer, 1417 240).

☑ PCR plates: 96 well (Advanced Biotechnologies, Epsom, England, AB-0366).

☑ Size Marker (ΦX174/*Hae* III (0.1mg/ml, Promega, Southampton, England, G1761)). Add 450μl dH_2O to vial of the size marker. Add 20μl of GLB to 12μl (1.2μg) of the size marker and 8μl of TE buffer. Store at 4°C.

☑ Sodium dodecyl sulphate (10%) (SDS). This reagent is extremely harmful if inhaled. Wear a mask when working with SDS powder. Also wear gloves. Wash skin thoroughly if in contact with SDS. Wipe down work area after use. Preferably add SDS to dH_2O in fume cupboard. SDS sometimes comes out of solution but will go back on heating. Add 100g of SDS in parts to approx 800ml dH_2O. As SDS is supplied in 100g tubs there is no need to measure. Apply heat (up to 68°C) if necessary to assist dissolution. Allow to cool to room temperature and adjust the volume to 1 litre. Do not autoclave.

☑ Saline sodium phosphate EDTA (20x) (SSPE) (3M NaCl, 0.2M NaH_2PO_4, 0.02M EDTA pH7.4). Add 350.6g NaCl followed by 48g NaH_2PO_4 to approx 1600ml dH_2O. Then add 80ml 0.5M EDTA (pH8.0). Adjust the pH to 7.4 using 4M NaOH. Adjust volume to 2 litres and sterlize by autoclaving.

☑ Saran Wrap, (Genetic Research Instrumentation, Felsted, England, SW1).

☑ 2 x SSPE/0.1% SDS. Combine 240ml 20xSSPE and 24ml 10% SDS. Make up to 2400ml with dH_2O.

☑ 5 x SSPE/0.1% SDS. Combine 600ml 20x SSPE and 24ml 10% SDS. Make up to 2400ml with dH_2O.

☑ Sodium saline citrate (2x, pH7.0) (SSC). 0.3 M NaCl + 0.03M tri-sodium citrate.

☑ *Taq* enzyme (Bioline, London, England, M958013).

☑ Thermofast Plate (Advanced Biotechnologies, AB-0600).

☑ 1M Tris pH7.6. Add 242.28g Tris base to 1400 ml dH_2O. Adjust the pH to 7.6 by adding 100ml conc. HCl (take care - wear a mask and goggles and where possible perform this in a fume cupboard). Allow the solution to cool to room temperature before making final adjustments to the pH. Make up to 2 litres with dH_2O and sterilize by autoclaving. If the 1M solution has a yellow colour, discard it and obtain better quality Tris. More than 100 ml conc. HCl may be required.

☑ Tris borate EDTA (10x) (TBE). Add 216g Tris, 110g orthoboric acid and 80ml 0.5M EDTA to 1400ml dH_2O. Adjust volume to 2 litres with dH_2O and sterilize by autoclaving.

☑ Tris-EDTA (TE) Buffer (10mM Tris, 1mM EDTA pH7.6). Combine 10ml 1M Tris pH7.6 with 2ml 0.5M EDTA and make up to 1 litre with dH_2O. Sterilize by autoclaving and store in aliquots.

Component	Stock conc	Master mix (components in µl)					
		HLA-A GENERIC	HLA-B GENERIC	HLA-B27	HLA-C GENERIC	HLA-DRB GENERIC	HLA-DRB 3/11/6
dH_2O		8220	12345	4155	8300	8280	8300
Cresol Red	10mg/ml	100	150	50	100	100	100
NH_4 buffer	10x	1000	1500	500	1000	1000	1000
$MgCl_2$	50mM	300	450	150	300	300	300
dNTPs	20mM each	100	150	50	100	100	100
Each primer (n=2 or 3: see Table 6.2)	25µM	120	120	40	80	100	80
Taq polymerase	5U/µl	40	45	15	40	20	40

Table 6.3. PCR master mixes

2. *PCR*

2.1. Heat DNA samples to be tested to 60°C for 5-10 min, vortex and centrifuge for 5 sec in a microcentrifuge.

2.2. Prepare 10ml of mastermix for the appropriate locus (Table 6.3). Use dH_2O of ultra high purity quality. Dispense 100µl slowly into tubes of the 96 well plate. Take care to avoid splashes and air bubbles at the bottom of the tubes. When all tubes have been filled, cover the 96 well plate with a sterile microtitre tray lid. Cresol red is used to help visualise DNA solutions in the dot blotting process.

2.3. Add 1µl DNA sample to each well from position 1A.1H, 2A.2H etc. Only one row at a time should be uncovered by the lid. Leave two wells with mastermix only to act as negative controls, and leave an appropriate number of wells for control DNA (see Tips, Quality Control and Troubleshooting). When a complete row of DNA samples has been added, place a strip of 8 caps over these samples and press down gently. When DNA samples have been added to all tubes and caps are in place, use a cap sealing tool to ensure that all caps are pushed firmly into place.

2.4. Centrifuge the plate for 1 min at 1000rpm, place in a PCR machine and run the appropriate cycle programme (Table 6.4). After amplification, if the PCR samples are not to be processed immediately, store at -20°C.

3. *Electrophoresis of PCR products*

3.1. Add 4.5g of agarose to 300ml 1xTris-borate EDTA (TBE), boil and allow the solution to cool to 65°C. It is important to stir the agarose while cooling to prevent lumps forming.

	PCR step				
	1	2		3	4
Locus	Hold	Cycles	No of cycles	Hold	Hold
HLA-A GENERIC	96°C/5 min	96°C/1 min 60°C/30 sec 72°C/1 min	35	72°C/5 mins	15°C/forever
HLA-B GENERIC and B27 TESTING	96°C/5 mins	96°C/30 sec 65°C/30 sec 72°C/45 sec	32	72°C/5 mins	15°C/forever
HLA-C GENERIC	96°C/5 mins	96°C/1 min 66°C/30 sec 72°C/1 min	30	72°C/5 mins	15°C/forever
HLA-DRB GENERIC	96°C/5 mins	96°C/1 min 55°C/1 min 72°C/1 min	30	72°C/5 mins	15°C/forever
HLA-DR 3/11/6	96°C/5 mins	96°C/1 min 64°C/1 min 72°C/1 min	10	72°C/5 mins	15°C/forever
		then			
		96°C/1 min 56°C/1 min 72°C/1 min	20		

Table 6.4. PCR amplification conditions.

3.2. While the agarose is cooling prepare 96-well gel template by placing the casting tray in the gel sealer - take care to ensure gel sealer is not over-tightened otherwise the casting tray may separate when agarose is added.

3.3. Place the sealed casting tray on top of a levelling table and adjust the feet of the levelling table until centred each way.

3.4. Once the agarose has cooled to 65°C add 15μl of ethidium bromide (10mg/ml) and mix gently. (N.B. ethidium bromide is mutagenic)

3.5. Pour the molten agarose solution into the level casting tray. Immediately push any air bubbles to edges of the template using a pipette tip.

3.6. Insert four 24-slot combs into the gel, with equal spacing between the combs. Allow gel to set for approximately 1 hour at room temperature.

3.7. Add 1 litre of 1 x TBE to an electrophoresis tank. Carefully remove the combs from the set gel. Remove the gel from the gel sealer. Place the gel in a tank containing 1 x TBE buffer. Ensure the gel is covered by buffer to a depth of 2 to 3mm.

3.8. Add 4μl of each PCR product to a 96 well Thermofast plate. Ensure product is visible in each well. Add 8μl GLB to each well. Spin the plate for 1 min to ensure mixing.

3.9. Load 10μl of size marker into the first well of each of the four rows.

3.10. Using an octapipette carefully load 10μl of sample into each well of the gel. Care must be taken to ensure the octapipette is orientated properly when adding the samples to the gel.

3.11. Place the lid of the electrophoresis system on to the electrophoresis tank, connect the electrodes to the power pack and electrophorese the samples at 250V, 250mAmp for 20min.

3.12. Once electrophoresis is complete, remove the gel from the tank and photograph under UV light. Check size of PCR product against size marker to ensure correct product has been amplified (Table 6.2).

4. *Dot blotting of membranes*

We use a Robbins Hydra dot blotting machine which enables us to make as many replicate membranes as required from the PCR product. Other laboratories use different equipment and some may dot blot by hand.

4.1. After PCR products have been dispensed onto the membranes, allow to air dry for at least 20 min.

4.2. Carefully place membranes (DNA face up) onto 2 sheets of Whatman 3MM paper soaked in 0.4M NaOH. Leave for 10 min. When placing membranes onto Whatman paper, take care to ensure that: the membrane is not dragged over denaturation pad; all of the membrane soaks up the 0.4M NaOH; that there are no air bubbles beneath the membrane.

4.3. Transfer each membrane on to Whatman 3MM paper soaked in 10XSSPE. Leave for 5 min.

4.4.Gently wash in 2xSSPE and allow to air dry for at least 25 min.

4.5.Wrap membranes in Saran Wrap and place (DNA face down) on UV transilluminator for 4 min. Ensure that all the UV lights are fully on during the procedure, do not switch transilluminator off between each step. Place a glass plate on top of membranes to hold them flat during this procedure. Store the membranes wrapped in tin foil at 4°C if not using immediately.

5. *Dehybridisation of membrane*

If the preparation of the required number of membranes proves difficult, an alternative method is to dehybridise used membranes (a maximum of 3 at a time in the same solution) as follows:

5.1. Rinse membranes in dH_2O for 5 min at room temperature.

5.2. Wash membranes in 0.4M NaOH, 0.1% SDS at 45°C for 30 min.

5.3. Wash membranes in 2 x SSC for 30 min at room temperature.

5.4. Check dehybridisation is complete by exposing membranes overnight to X-ray film and developing in the usual manner.

5.5. Store membrane flat at 4°C in a sealed plastic bag if not using immediately.

6. *3' end-labelling of SSOP*

The labelling reagents may be obtained in kit form (Boehringer, Cat No: 1362372).

6.1. Remove all reagents from freezer (except terminal transferase - this should be removed just before use) and allow to thaw. Vortex reagents briefly, and centrifuge in a microcentrifuge for 5 sec.

6.2. Combine the following: 4µl Reaction Buffer (5x), 4µl $CoCl_2$ (25mM), 1µl digoxigenin (DIG)-ddUTP (1mM), 1µl terminal transferase (50 units), 100 pmoles probe. Make up to 20µl with dH_2O. Vortex samples briefly, microcentrifuge for 5 sec and incubate at 37°C for 30 min in a water bath.

6.3. Microcentrifuge for 5 sec and place on ice for 5 min. Add 80µl dH_2O, vortex briefly and microcentrifuge for 5 sec. Aliquot in volumes appropriate to the amount of probe used (Tables 6.5 to 6.9) and store at -20°C.

7. *Prehybridisation, hybridisation and stringent SSPE washes*

Each probe is simultaneously hybridised to two different membranes, each containing 96 DNA samples.

7.1. Hand roll the membranes length-wise to form a cylinder. Place two membranes in a hybridisation bottle. One membrane should have the DNA side of the membrane facing the glass, while the second membrane should have the DNA side facing inwards in the bottle.

7.2. Add 20ml of freshly prepared hybridisation buffer. Screw cap on tightly and clamp to the rotisserie of a Robbins incubator (pre-set at 45°C). Rotate the bottles for 1 h.

Probe	Sequence 5' - 3'	Wash temp °C	Picomoles used	Nucleotide position	
				Exon 2	Exon 3
W (A94)	TTCTTCACATCCGTGTC	50	50	22-38	
A (56R)	GAGAGGCCTGAGTAT	46	40	163-177	
B (62LQ)	TGGGACCTGCAGACA	48	50	178-192	
C (62G)	GACGGGGAGACACGG	52	20	181-195	
O (62RN)	GACCGGAACACACGG	52	20	181-195	
D (62EG)	GAGGAGACAGGGAAA	46	40	184-198	
Y (A276)	GGCCCACTCACAGACT	52	50	204-219	
E (73I)	TCACAGATTGACCGA	45	40	211-225	
X (A290)	CTGACCGAGTGGACCT	51	40	218-233	
R (A26)	TGACCGAGCGAACCTG	54	40	219-234	
F (77S)	GAGAGCCTGCGGATC	50	20	226-240	
Z (A347)	CTCACACCATCCAGA	45	70		5-19
T (95V)	CACACCGTCCAGAGG	48	40		7-21
P (114EH)	TATGAACAGCACGCC	46	30		67-81
G (131R)	CGCTCTTGGACCGCG	52	40		121-136
H (142TK)	ACCACCAAGCACAAG	46	40		154-168
I (149T)	TGGGAGACGGCCCAT	50	40		169-183
J (150V)	GAGGCGGTCCATGCG	60	20		172-186
K (151R)	GCGGCCCGTGTGGCG	60	20		175-189
1 (A525)	TGAGGCGGAGCAGTTG	54	40		183-198
N (156Q)	GAGCAGCAGAGAGCC	52	20		190-204
Q (156W)	GAGCAGTGGAGAGCC	50	10		190-204
L (161D)	CTGGATGGCACGTGC	50	20		208-222
V (A551)	TGGAGGGCACGTGCGT	56	40		209-224
M (163R)	GAGGGCCGGTGCGTG	54	20		211-225
S (A355)	GGCGAGTGCGTGGAGTGGC	68	10		214-232
U (A357)	GGCGAGTGCGTGGACGGGC	68	10		214-232

Table 6.5. Probes used in HLA-A typing by PCR-SSOP

Probe	Sequence 5' - 3'	Wash temp °C	Picomoles used	Nucleotide position	
				Exon 2	Exon 3
31 (B89)	GGTATTTCGACACCGCC	56	40	17-33	
32 (B156)	GGACGGCACCCAGTT	52	40	84-98	
33 (B168)	GTTCGTGCGGTTCGA	50	40	96-110	
09 (BL09)	GAGTCCGAGAGAGGAGCC	57	6	123-140	
01 (BL01)	GAGGAAGGAGCCGCGGGC	64	20	129-146	
02 (BL02)	GAGGACGGAGCCCCGGGC	64	40	129-146	
07 (BL07)	GAGGATGGCGCCCCGGGC	64	60	129-146	
34 (B249)	TTGGGACGGGGAGAC	50	40	177-191	
24 (BL24)	GGGAGACACAGATCTCCA	55	40	185-202	
05 (BL05)	ACACAGATCTTCAAGACC	55	14	190-207	
10 (BL10)	GATCTACAAGGCCCAGGC	58	10	195-212	
12 (BL12)	ATCTGCAAGGCCAAGGCA	56	20	196-213	
18 (BL18)	ACTGACCGAGTGAGCCTG	58	20	217-234	
35 (B73)	ACTGACCGAGTGGGCCTG	63	40	217-234	
20 (BL20)*	AGCGGAGCGCGGTGCGCA	64	40	233-250	
21 (BL21)	CGGAACCTGCGCGGCTAC	62	40	235-252	
22 (BL22)	CGGACCCTGCTCCGCTAC	61	30	235-252	
23 (BL23)	CGGATCGCGCTCCGCTAC	62	40	235-252	
27 (BL27)	CTCACACTTGGCAGAGGA	56	20		5-22
36 (B348)	TCACACCATCCAGAGG	49	50		6-21
37 (B354)	CATCCAGGTGATGTAT	46	40		12-27
28 (BL28)	CCAGTGGATGTATGGCTG	56	40		15-32
38 (B361)	AGGATGTTTGGCTGC	48	40		19-33
26 (BL26)	CTGCGACCTGGGGCCCGA	65	40		30-47
30 (BL30)	GGCATAACCAGTTAGCCT	54	50		65-82
39 (B409)	TATGACCAGGACGCCT	55	40		67-82
40 (B427)	GACGGCAAAGATTACA	46	40		85-100
41 (B499)	ACCCAGCTCAAGTGG	47	40		157-171
42 (B505)	CGCAAGTTGGAGGC	46	40		163-176
43 (B532)	GAGCAGCTGAGAGCCT	52	40		190-205
44 (B539)	GAGAACCTACCTGGA	46	40		197-211
45 (B553a)	GAGGGCCTGTGCGT	48	40		211-224
46 (B553b)	GAGGGCACGTGCGT	48	40		211-224
47 (B566)	TGGAGTCGCTCCGC	48	40		224-237
48 (B597)	GAAGGACACGCTGGA	52	40		255-269
49 (B599)	AGGACAAGCTGGAGCG	52	40		257-272

Table 6.6. Probes used in HLA-B typing by PCR-SSOP

Probe	Sequence 5' - 3'	Wash temp °C	Picomoles used	Nucleotide position	
				Exon 2	Exon 3
15 (C2D6)	AGCCCCGGGCGCCGT	56	35	137-151	
1 (C2EALL)	GGGTGGAGCAGGAGGG	56	20	152-167	
3 (C2G2)	AGTGAACCTGCGGAAACTG	59	25	225-243	
2 (C2G1)	TGAGCCTGCGGAACCTG	56	30	227-243	
17 (C2H303)	CCAGAGCGAGGCCAGT	54	25	258-2 (intron 2)	
21 (C3A14)	CTCCAGTGGATGTTTGGC	56	25		13-30
4 (C3A1)	TCCAGTGGATGTGTGGC	54	25		14-30
19 (C3A4)	CAGAGGATGTTTGGCTGC	56	20		16-33
12 (C3A7023)	AGGATGTCTGGCTGCGA	54	25		19-35
7 (C3A212)	TGTACGGCTGCGACCTG	56	20		23-39
22 (C3C15)	GGCATGACCAGTTAGCC	54	25		65-81
18 (C3CA)	GTATGACCAGTCCGCCT	54	25		66-82
20 (C3D58)	GCCCTGAATGAGGACCT	55	30		103-119
6 (C3E1203)	TCCTGGACTGCCGCGG	56	25		124-139
5 (C3E12)	GGACCGCTGCGGACAC	56	25		128-143
11 (C3G17712)	CGCAAGTTGGAGGCGG	54	25		163-178
13 (C3G716)	GGCCCGTGCGGCGGA	56	25		177-191
23 (C3G8013)	GCCCGTACGGCGGAG	54	25		178-192
8 (C3G2612)	TGAGGCGGAGCAGTGGA	57	25		183-199
14 (C3G16)	GCGGCGGAGCAGCAGA	57	25		184-199
9 (C3H2)	GGAGGGCGAGTGCGTG	57	25		210-225
16 (C3H3)	GGAGGGCCTGTGCGTG	56	25		210-225
10 (C3J17)	GCTCCGCGGATACCTG	54	25		231-246

Table 6.7. Probes used in HLA-C typing by PCR-SSOP

Probe	Sequence 5' - 3'	Wash temp °C	Picomoles used	Nucleotide position Exon 2
09 (1007)	GAAGCAGGATAAGTTTGA	50	10	24-41
03 (1008N)	GAGGAGGTTAAGTTTGAG	54	2	25-42
07 (1004)	GAGCAGGTTAAACATGAG	56	4	25-42
08 (1006)	TGGCAGGGTAAGTATAAG	50	10	25-42
06 (1003)	GTACTCTACGTCTGAGTG	56	4	27-44
02 (1002)	AGCCTAAGAGGGAGTGTC	56	30	29-46
18 (DR18)	CTACGGGTGAGTGTTAT	48	40	32-48
10 (2810)	GCGAGTGTGGAACCTGAT	56	10	66-83
01 (2801)	CGGTTGCTGGAAAGATGC	60	6	73-90
25 (DR25)	CGGTTCCTGGACAGATA	52	40	73-89
11 (DRB12)	CAGGAGGAGCTCCTGCGC	58	4	100-117
13 (DRB6)	CAGGAGGAGAACGTGCGC	62	7	100-117
22 (DR22)	CGGCCTAGCGCCGAGTA	58	50	163-179
05 (5703)	GCCTGATGAGGAGTACTG	54	20	165-182
15 (DRB14/1)	GGCCTGCTGCGGAGCACT	64	4	164-181
26 (DRB ALL)	TGGAACAGCCAGAAGGAC	56	40	181-198
14 (7031)	CTGGAAGACAAGCGGGCCG	60	30	202-220
16 (DRB13)	TGGAAGACGAGCGGGCCG	64	3	203-220
24 (DR24)	AGCGGAGGCGGGCCGAG	62	40	206-222
17 (7012) *	ACCGCGGCCCGCCTCTGC	66	30	207-224
23 (7005) *	ACCGCGGCCCGCTTCTGC	66	40	207-224
12 (DRB8)	GCGGGCCCTGGTGGACAC	64	20	213-230
04 (7004)	GGCCGGGTGGACAACTAC	62	1	217-234

Table 6.8. Probes used in HLA-DRB typing by PCR-SSOP

Probe	Sequence 5' - 3'	Wash temp °C	Picomoles used	Nucleotide position Exon 2
1 (DR19)	CGGTACCTGGACAGAT	50	40	73-88
2 (5703)	GCCTGATGAGGAGTACTG	54	20	165-182
3 (DRB14/1)	GGCCTGCTGCGGAGCACT	64	4	164-181
4 (7031)	CTGGAAGACAAGCGGGCCG	60	30	202-220
5 (DRB13)	TGGAAGACGAGCGGGCCG	64	3	203-220
6 (DR24)	AGCGGAGGCGGGCCGAG	62	40	206-222
7 (7012)	ACCGCGGCCCGCCTCTGC	66	30	207-224
8 (7005)	ACCGCGGCCCGCTTCTGC	65	40	207-224
9 (DRB8)	GCGGGCCCTGGTGGACAC	64	20	213-230
10 (7004)	GGCCGGGTGGACAACTAC	62	1	217-234
11 (5701)	GCCTGATGCCGAGTACTG	58	40	165-182

Table 6.9. Probes used in HLA-DR3/11/6 group typing by PCR-SSOP

7.3. Immediately before the incubation is complete, thaw appropriate aliquots of DIG-labelled oligonucleotide probe, vortex briefly and centrifuge for 5 sec in a microcentrifuge

7.4. Add an appropriate number of picomoles of probe (Tables 6.5 to 6.9) to 20ml of pre-warmed (45°C) hybridisation buffer and mix by inversion.

7.5. Remove the hybridisation bottle from the incubator and pour off the hybridisation buffer into a disposable collection container. Add 20ml of hybridisation buffer containing the DIG-labelled probe, and incubate the bottle for 1 h at 45°C.

7.6. Remove the bottle from the incubator and pour off the fluid into a disposable collection container.

7.7. Add 100ml of 2xSSPE, 0.1% SDS. Re-cap the bottle, place inside a Robbins incubator (pre-set to 25°C) and incubate for 10 min. Make sure the temperature does not rise above 25°C.

7.8. Discard the fluid and repeat Step 7.7.

7.9. Remove the bottle from the incubator. Uncap the bottle and using forceps carefully remove the membranes from the bottle, prior to discarding fluid, directly into a small plastic tray containing 200ml 5xSSPE, 0.1% SDS, which has been heated to the appropriate temperature (Tables 6.5 to 6.9). Place one membrane DNA face down and the other membrane DNA face up into the washing solution. Incubate with shaking for 40 min. Check temperature reading and record any variation on the hybridization record sheet. If the temperature varies more than 2°C above or below the required temperature, abandon the hybridization.

7.10. Remove the membranes from the tray, blot dry, but do not allow the membrane to dry out. Wrap the membrane in Saran Wrap, and store in tin-foil at 4°C, until ready to perform chemiluminescent detection.

8. *Chemiluminescence detection*

All steps are performed at room temperature with shaking using a platform shaker. Use separate enzyme storage boxes for different buffer solutions and keep light-tight. Use one enzyme box for a maximum of three membranes at the same time.

8.1. Add 240ml anti-DIG-ALP conjugate in buffer 2 to the enzyme box. Place membranes into the boxes DNA side down. Incubate for 15 min on shaker.

8.2. Transfer membranes to 300ml of washing buffer and incubate for 15 min on shaker. Discard washing buffer and replace with fresh washing buffer and incubate for a further 15 min.

8.3. Transfer membrane to 300ml of buffer 3 and incubate for 5 min on shaker.

8.4. Remove from buffer 3, place 2 membranes back to back in a plastic bag. Add 20ml of CSPD (1:100 dilution) and reseal the bag. Place the bag on a platform shaker, cover with tinfoil and shake for 5 min at room temperature.

8.5. Pour off CSPD fluid into 20ml plastic tube for re-use (up to 5 times). Carefully remove the membrane from the bag, blot off excess liquid and wrap in Saran Wrap. Store at -20°C if using on more than 1 day, but note that CSPD should only be frozen once.

8.6. Tape two membranes to one X-ray film and place a second film on top. Expose the top film for 5 min and check the intensity of the dots. Depending on these results process the second film accordingly. It may be necessary to re-expose the membrane to a third or fourth film for a further period of time, depending on dot intensity.

8.7. Record the probe reaction for each sample and analyse according to the known patterns (Tables 6.10 to 6.14) using a computer programme.

Tips, Quality Control And Troubleshooting

1. We do not routinely determine the concentration of DNA in each isolation. When isolating DNA the amount of TE buffer added to the pellet of DNA is judged by eye. However, we regularly assess approximately 10% of samples to ensure that the DNA is at an appropriate concentration. For our methods we normally store the DNA at a concentration of approximately 0.1μg/μl.

	Probes																										
HLA-A* alleles	A	B	C	D	E	F	G	H	I	J	K	L	M	N	O	P	Q	R	S	T	U	V	W	X	Y	Z	1
0101							+			+			+					+					+		+	+	
0102							+			+			+					+							+	+	
2.1			+				+	+												+		+	+		+		
0202			+				+	+									+					+	+		+		
0203			+				+	+	+								+			+		+	+		+		
0204/17			+				+	+														+	+		+		
0205/08			+				+	+									+					+			+		
0206/10/21			+				+	+												+		+			+		
0211			+		+		+	+												+		+	+	(+)			
0212/13			+				+	+						+						+		+	+		+		
0214			+				+	+														+			+		
0216			+				+	+											+	+			+		+		
0219			+				+							+						+		+	+		+		
0222			+				+	+									+			+		+	+		+		
0301/03N							+					+											+	+		+	+
0302							+					+		+									+	+		+	
1101/02/03							+						+	+										+		+	
1104							+							+								+		+		+	
2301				+			+				+											+			+		
2402/03/05				+			+							+								+			+		
2404				+			+							+				+				+			+		
2406				+			+										+					+			+		
2407				+			+							+								+					
2408			+				+							+								+			+		
2409N				+			+							+								+			+		
2410				+			+						+	+											+		
2413				+			+															+			+		
2414				+			+							+						+		+			+		
2501						+	+		+				+		+		+								+	+	
2502						+	+		+				+		+		+									+	
2601/02							+		+				+		+		+	+							+	+	
2603/05/06							+		+				+		+		+								+	+	
2604							+		+						+		+	+							+	+	
2607			+				+		+				+				+	+							+	+	
2608							+		+				+	+	+			+							+	+	
68011/012/02							+	+							+		+					+		+		+	
6803							+	+							+		+					+		+	+	+	
6804					+		+	+							+		+					+		(+)		+	
6805							+	+							+		+					+			+	+	
6901							+	+							+					+		+		+			
2901/02/03		+					+				+							+				+				+	
3001	+						+									+						+		+		+	
3002	+						+									+						+			+	+	
3003							+									+						+			+	+	
3004	+						+									+	+					+			+	+	
31012	+				+		+				+											+		(+)		+	
3201						+	+				+											+	+		+	+	
3202						+	+							+								+	+		+	+	
3301/03					+		+				+				+							+		(+)		+	
3401							+		+						+		+					+		+		+	
3402							+		+						+							+		+		+	+
3601							+			+								+				+	+		+	+	
4301		+					+		+				+				+	+							+	+	
6601							+		+				+		+		+							+		+	
6602							+		+						+		+		+					+		+	
6603							+		+						+		+		+					+	+	+	
7401/02/03							+				+											+	+	+	+	+	
8001							+											(+)			+		+		+	+	

Table 6.10. HLA-A PCR-SSOP probe-hybridisation patterns. "2.1" represents the alleles 0201, 0207, 0215N, 0218 and 0220. (+) indicates that a probe is positive in practice where not predicted from its sequence. The alleles listed in all Tables for this Chapter are from ASHI, April 1997.

Probe	HLA-B allele																																													
	7.2	0703	0708	0801	0802	0803	0804	1301/02	1303	14	18	2701	2702	27.2	2708	35.3	3508/18	35.4	3515	3519	3520	3701	3702	3801	3802	39.2	39.3	4001	40.2	4005	4007	4008	4101	4102	4201	4402	44.1	4404	4405	4406	4408	4410	4501	4601	4701	4702
01																				+								+	+	+	+	+	+	+		+	+	+	+			+	+		+	+
02											+					+	+	+	+		+	+	+																	+						
05			+	+	+	+										+	+	+	+	+											+	+								+						
07								+	+																																+			+		
09	+	+	+	+	+	+	+			+		+	+	+	+									+	+	+	+								+											
10	+																																		+											
12												+	+	+	+																															
18																																												+		
20					+			+	+			+													+											+	+	+	+		+	+				
21	+	+	+	+			+			+	+				+	+	+	+	+	+	+					+	+	+	+	+	+	+	+	+	+								+	+		+
22														+								+	+																						+	
23						+							+											+																+						
24								+	+													+	+				+	+	+	+			+	+		+	+	+	+		+	+	+		+	+
26																+	+		+	+	+																					+	+			
27																																	+										+			
28										+																																				
30								+	+																																	+				
31				+	+	+	+																																							
32											+																																			
33																																														
34																																														
35																																														
36																						+																								
37																																														
38																																										+			+	+
39																																				+	+	+		+	+					
40																																														
41								+																																						
42																												+			+															
43								+	+	+	+	+	+	+	+	+		+	+	+	+		+					+	+	+	+	+					+					+			+	+
44																								+	+	+	+																			
45									+							+	+	+		+	+									+						+	+		+	+	+	+	+	+		
46				+	+	+	+			+	+											+		+	+	+	+						+	+	+			+								
47																																				+	+	+	+	+	+	+	+			
48				+	+	+	+																										+	+	+											
49	+	+	+																										+			+														

Table 6.11a HLA-B PCR-SSOP probe-hybridisation patterns (see also Table 6.11b & c).

Probe	HLA-B allele																																												
	4801/03	4802	4901	5001	51.1	5105/08	5107	52	53	5401	55.1	5503	5504	5506	56.1	5603	5701/03	5702	5704	5801	5802	5901	67	7301	78	8101	8201	15.3	1502/21	1503	1505/25	1506	1508	1509	15.5	15.4	1513/17	1514	1516	1520	1522	1523	1524	1527	1529
01			+	+																																									
02					+	+	+	+	+											+	+				+																+				
05					+	+			+													+			+								+								+				+
07																	+	+	+									+	+		+	+	+			+	+	+	+	+			+	+	
09	+	+									+	+	+	+	+	+						+	+	+		+	+			+				+	+							+			+
10										+	+	+	+		+	+							+			+	+																		
12																								+																					
18												+																																	
20																																													
21	+	+		+						+	+	+	+	+	+	+							+	+	+	+	+	+	+	+	+	+	+	+	+	+		+		+	+			+	+
22																																													
23			+		+	+	+	+	+								+	+	+	+	+	+															+		+			+	+		
24	+	+	+	+				+																				+		+	+	+						+		+			+	+	
26		+	+	+					+											+	+						+													+					
27			+	+																																			+						
28																					+																								
30										+	+	+			+							+					+																		
31																																													
32																																													
33										+																																			
34																	+	+	+	+	+																								
35																								+																					
36																																													
37																	+	+	+																										
38																											+					+												+	
39																			+																										
40					+	+	+	+																	+									+											
41																																													
42	+																									+																			
43	+	+	+	+	+		+	+	+	+	+	+	+	+	+		+			+	+	+		+	+	+			+	+	+	+		+	+		+		+	+		+			+
44																							+																						
45		+	+	+	+	+	+	+	+						+	+	+	+	+	+	+				+			+	+	+	+	+	+	+	+	+	+	+	+	+	+	+	+	+	+
46										+	+	+	+	+								+	+																						
47																											+											+							
48																																													
49	+																									+																			

Table 6.11b HLA-B PCR-SSOP probe-hybridisation patterns (see also Table 6.11a & c).

HLA-B: Designation of groups	
7.2	0702 0704 0705 0706 0707
14	1401 1402
18	1801 1802 1803
4001	40011 40012
40.2	4002 4003 4004 4006 4009
44.1	44031 44032 4407
51.1	51011 51012 51021 51022 5103 5104 5106
39.2	39011 39013 3903 3904 3905 39061 39062 3907 3909 3910 3911 3912
39.3	39021 39022 3908
35.3	3501 3502 3503 3504 3505 3506 3507 35091 35092 3510 3511 3513 3521
35.4	3512 3516 3517
27.2	2703 2704 27052 27053 2706 2707 2709 2710 2711
15.3	1501 1504 1507 1512 1519 1526N 1530 1532 1533 1534 1535
15.4	1511 1515 1528 1531*
15.5	1510 1518 1537
55.1	5501 5502 5505
56.1	5601 5602
67	67011 67012
78	7801 78021 78022
52	52011 52012

Table 6.11c. HLA-B: Designation of groups. *N.B. 1531 full sequence data not available for probes B532 and B553A.

	Probes																						
HLA-Cw*	1	2	3	4	5	6	7	8	9	10	11	12	13	14	15	16	17	18	19	20	21	22	23
01	+	+		+																			
02021	+						+	+	+									+					
02022/024	+		+				+	+	+									+					
02023	+		+					+	+									+					
0302	+	+														+		+					
0303	+	+														+	+						
0304	+	+														+							
04	+		+																+				
0501	+		+																	+			
0602	+		+					+							+			+					
7.1*	+	+									+		+					+					
0702	+	+									+	+	+					+					
0703	+	+										+	+					+					
0704	+	+									+		+		+								
0707	+		+								+		+					+					
0801/03	+	+																		+			+
0802	+	+																		+			
1202	+	+			+		+	+										+					
1203	+	+				+		+										+					
1204	+		+					+										+					
1301	+	+			+		+	+							+			+					
14	+	+																+			+		
1502/03	+		+																			+	
1504	+		+															+					
1505	+		+																				
1601	+	+											+	+				+					
1602	+		+										+	+				+					
17	+		+						+	+	+												
18	+		+												+				+				

Table 6.12. HLA-C PCR-SSOP probe-hybridisation patterns.
*7.1 represents 0701, 0705, 0706.

HLA-DR allele		1	2	3	4	5	6	7	8	9	10	11	12	13	14	15	16	17	18	22	23	24	25	26
		Probes																						
1	1.1	+																+						+
	01022	+																						+
	0103	+															+							+
2	15.2		+																				+	+
	1503/1607		+																					+
	16.1		+																				+	+
	1604		+										+										+	+
	1608		+											+									+	+
3	3.1				+		+							+										+
	3.2						+							+										+
	0304				+		+																	+
	0308				+	+	+							+										+
4	4.2							+			+						+					+	+	+
	4.3							+			+										+	+	+	+
	4.5							+			+											+	+	+
	4.6							+			+									+		+	+	+
	4.7							+			+							+				+	+	+
	4.8							+			+							+		+		+	+	+
	0409							+			+									+	+	+	+	+
	0412							+			+		+							+		+	+	+
	0415					+		+			+											+	+	+
	0418							+			+		+									+	+	+
	0422				+			+			+											+	+	+
11	11.2					+	+										+						+	+
	11.4					+	+																+	+
	11.16					+	+							+			+						+	+
	1105/30					+																	+	+
	1107				+	+	+																+	+
	1109					+	+							+									+	+
	1117					+	+															+	+	+
	1122					+		+															+	+
	1123/25					+	+						+										+	+
	1126					+	+											+					+	+
12	12.1											+							+					+
	1204					+						+							+					+
	1205																		+					+

HLA-DR allele		1	2	3	4	5	6	7	8	9	10	11	12	13	14	15	16	17	18	22	23	24	25	26
		Probes																						
13	13.2						+							+			+						+	+
	13.3						+																+	+
	13.5						+							+									+	+
	13.6						+													+			+	+
	13.8						+										+						+	+
	13031/32						+								+					+			+	+
	1304						+										+			+			+	+
	1310						+							+	+								+	+
	1313						+						+							+			+	+
	1315/27						+							+			+							+
	1317																+		+				+	+
	1318						+						+	+									+	+
	1319						+										+							+
	1326						+							+										+
14	14.1						+									+						+	+	+
	14.3						+						+	+										+
	14.4						+							+				+						+
	14.5						+															+	+	+
	14.7						+							+				+					+	+
	1404/28															+			+			+	+	+
	1410							+								+						+	+	+
	1411					+													+			+	+	+
	1413						+							+				+		+				+
	1415												+						+				+	+
	1416						+									+	+						+	+
	1418						+							+								+		+
	1419						+							+							+			+
	1420						+											+						+
	1421						+							+							+		+	+
	1422/25						+									+							+	+
	1423						+															+	+	+
	1424						+							+										+
	1426						+									+						+		+
7	0701								+		+											+		+
8	8.2												+						+	+			+	+
	8.3												+						+				+	+
	0808												+			+			+				+	+
9	09012									+	+											+		+
10	1001			+																				+

Table 6.13a. HLA-DRB PCR-SSOP probe-hybridisation patterns

HLA-DRB: Designation of groups	
1.1	0101 01021 0104
15.2	15011 15012 15021 15022 1504 1505 1506
16.1	16011 16012 16021 16022 1603 1605
3.1	03011 03021 0303 0305 0306 0307
3.2	03012 03022 0311
4.2	0402 0414
4.3	04011 04012 0413 0416 0421
4.5	0403 0406 0407 0420
4.6	0411 0417 0424
4.7	0404 0408 0419 0423
4.8	04051 04052 0410
11.2	1102 1103 1111 1114 1121
11.4	11011 11012 11013 11041 11042 1106 11081 11082 1110 1112 1113 1115 1118 1119 1124 1127 1129
11.16	1116 1120
12.1	1201 12021 12022 12031 12032
13.2	1301 1302 1316 1320 1328 1329
13.3	1307 1311 1314 1325
13.5	1305 1306 1309
13.6	1312 1321 1330
13.8	1308 1322 1323 1324
14.1	1401 1407
14.3	1403 1412 1427
14.4	1402 1406 1429
14.5	1405 1408 1414
14.7	1409 1417
8.2	0801 08031 08032 0805 0806 0810 0812 0814 0816
8.3	08021 08022 08041 08042 0807 0809 0811 0813 0815

Table 6.13b. HLA-DRB: Designation of groups

HLA-DRB alleles		Probes 1	2	3	4	5	6	7	8	9	10	11
DR3	3.1	+									+	+
	3.2	+										+
	3.3										+	+
	0308	+	+								+	
DR11	11.1		+									
	11.2		+			+						
	11.3		+							+		
	1107		+								+	
	1117		+				+					
	1126		+					+				
DR13	13.1					+						+
	13.2/1424											+
	1303				+							
	1304					+						
	1310				+							+
	1313									+		
	1318/14.3									+		+
	1327	+				+						+
	13.4											
DR14	14.1			+			+					
	14.2							+				+
	14.4						+					
	14.5						+					+
	14.6								+			+
	14.7			+								
	1413							+				
	1416			+		+						

Table 6.14a. HLA-DR3/11/6 subgroup PCR-SSOP probe-hybridisation patterns

HLA-DR3/11/6: Designation of groups	
3.1	03011 0304 0305 0306
3.2	03012 0311
3.3	03021 03022 0303 0307
11.1	11011 11012 11013 11041 11042 1106 11081 11082 1109 1110 1112 1113 1115 1118 1119 1124 1127 1129
11.2	1102 1103 1111 1114 1116 1120 1121
11.3	1123 1125
13.1	1301 1302 1308 1315 1316 1319 1320 1322 1323 1324 1328 1329
13.2	1305 1306 1307 1309 1311 1314 1325
1303	13031 13032
13.4	1312 1321 1326 1330
14.1	1401 1407
14.2	1402 1406 1409 1417 1420 1429
14.3	1403 1412 1427
14.4	1405 1408 1418
14.5	1414 1423
14.6	1419 1421
14.7	1422 1425 1426

Alleles not amplified by this system:
1105 1122 1130
1317
1404 1410 1411 1415 1428

Table 6.14b. HLA-DR3/11/6: Designation of groups

2. When setting up a PCR wear a separate lab coat, wear gloves and change them frequently, and perform all work in pre-PCR room using dedicated equipment. Pipettes should not be removed from pre-PCR room. Pipettes are labelled according to reagents and must only be used for these reagents. The use of tips with filters is advisable. When preparing the mastermix thaw out following reagents: $MgCl_2$, dNTPs, PCR buffer and appropriate primers. Vortex each reagent briefly, centrifuge in a microcentrifuge for 5 sec and place in an ice bucket (PCR buffer and $MgCl_2$ should be centrifuged for 2 min). *Taq* polymerase should always be added last, after vortexing and centrifuging, and just prior to dispensing the master mix. The aliquoted master mixes should not be left on the bench too long (a maximum of 15 min - *Taq* loses activity once diluted in buffer). Switch on the PCR machine for at least 10 min prior to use to allow the machine to heat up. The PCR machine should be situated in the post-PCR room.

3. After setting up a PCR, wash work areas with 16% sodium hypochlorite. Soak all racks used to hold samples in 16% sodium hypochlorite for approx 30 min, and rinse thoroughly in water. Pipettes should be wiped with 16% sodium hypochlorite, followed by dH_2O. Wipe the microcentrifuge, vortex, freezer handle etc with 16% sodium hypochlorite. Expose the working area including pipettes etc to UV light for 60 min.

4. When performing a PCR on 96 samples there may be one or two samples which are not amplified. Therefore we always run a gel to ensure that we have sufficient product. This enables the PCR-SSOP method to be well controlled. On some occasions the product is deemed weak and this sample will always be repeated. Good amplification always gives a clean and clear cut SSOP hybridisation while almost all the problematic typing results we have encountered have been due to poor amplification. Interpretation of weak hybridisation signals can give an incorrect result.

5. When determining the conditions necessary for this technique one important aspect is to ensure that the amplification is equally effective for both alleles. On some occasions when determining amplification conditions we have found that a PCR product was obtained where only one of two known alleles could be detected. Therefore, if a laboratory is setting up a technique for the first time, ensure that there is no differential amplification by testing various combinations of alleles.

6. When implementing new probes to the system we initially use a wash temperature which is equivalent to the melting temperature of the probes. This is equal in °C to 2x (number of A + T bases) + 4x (number of G + C bases). Thereafter we adjust the wash temperature by 1°C either up or down according to the probe reaction at the melting temperature. We also start with 20 pmoles of probe and adjust accordingly.

Note on the use of tetramethylammonium chloride (TMAC)

We do not recommend the use of TMAC for washing hybridisation membranes because of its toxic properties: also, in our experience it does not necessarily, as claimed, permit the use of a single wash temperature. Thus a significant number of water-baths may be required. In our own laboratory, one individual normally performs 16 simultaneous hybridisations. Thus if a laboratory is defining alleles at three loci (HLA-A, -B, and -DRB), probes can be selected for simultaneous use according to a common wash temperature, thus eliminating the requirement for a large number of water-baths.

7. When the probe conditions (i.e. number of picomoles and wash temperature) have been determined it is worthwhile to keep a record on the performance of the probes, i.e. whether the probe is not giving an adequate signal with its positive control or whether it is cross-reacting with controls with which it should be negative. On occasions the conditions for the probes may need to be altered. This in a way is similar to the use of HLA sera, where after long term storage, some specificities can change. If a probe appears to be giving strong false-positive reactions, we will initially increase the wash temperature by 1°C; or if giving weak false-positive reactions, we will decrease the probe concentration by approximately 20%. If a probe appears to be giving false-negative results we will decrease the wash temperature by 1°C. If a probe is giving weak reactions, we will initially increase the probe concentration by approximately 20%. One way to monitor the performance of the probes is to record the length of time needed for autoradiography exposure. If this varies to such an extent that it takes more than 30 minutes to achieve a good signal, the conditions of the probe should be altered.

8. Many of the probes used in this laboratory are DIG-labelled during their manufacture, adding the digoxigenin moiety to 5'-amino-linked oligonucleotides by incubating with a digoxigenin ester under mild alkaline conditions.

9. Enough controls should be included so that each probe will have two positive reactions. In addition, control DNA should be included as negative controls, which contain alleles with sequences which are closely related to the sequence which the probe detects and with which the probe might cross-hybridize. This is especially important when initially determining the optimum conditions for the probe to work. To maintain consistency between membranes we try to use the same controls. If a laboratory finds it difficult to have a large enough supply of the same control DNA it may consider cloning control DNA by long range amplification (Curran *et al.*, 1996). This gives material to use in as many tests as needed. This is especially important when the control DNA has been obtained from an external source.

10. It is normal practice in this laboratory for chemiluminescence detection to be performed on 24 membranes at the same time. All membranes are processed up to the end of step 8.2. Thereafter, membranes are processed in groups of six simultaneously, leaving the remaining membranes in the washing buffer.

11. In this laboratory we always ensure two independent readings of the hybridisation patterns. We do not believe in recording a result according to the strength of the reaction (e.g. 1, 2, 4, 6, 8 as in serology). The result should be recorded as positive or negative. If in doubt it should be repeated. In the future it will be beneficial for laboratories if a scanning mechanism is made available for reading the membranes as mistakes are possible in the transmissions of results. We

believe it is important that probe patterns are analysed objectively. To overcome subjectivity, laboratories should consider using an appropriate computer programme.

12. A commercially available method similar to that described in this chapter is now available (Lifecodes Corporation, Stampford, CT) whereby probes are supplied already labelled with alkaline phosphatase. This removes the requirement for digoxigenin labelling of probes and the use of anti-digoxigenin antibody.

Equipment

☑ Enzyme Boxes (Boehringer, 800058).

☑ Gel Sealer and Casting Tray (Merck Ltd, Poole, England, 306/7252/12).

☑ Robbins Hybridisation Incubator (Robbins Scientific, Sunnyvale, CA, 1040-60-2).

☑ Robbins Hydra (Robbins Scientific, 1029-60-1).

References

Curran, MD, Williams, F, Earle, JAP, Rima, BK, Van Dam, MG, *et al.* (1996). Long range PCR amplification as an alternative strategy for characterizing novel HLA-B alleles. *Eur. J. Immunogenetics* **23**: 297

Davies, SM, Shu, XO, Blazra, BR, *et al.* (1995). Unrelated donor bone marrow transplantation: influence of HLA-A and B incompatibility on outcome. *Blood* **86**: 1636

Hurley, CK, Noreen, H, Hunter, J, *et al.* (1997). The search for HLA-matched donors: a summary of HLA-A*, -B*, -DRB1/3/4/5/* alleles and their association with serologically defined HLA-A, -B, -DR antigens. *Tissue Antigens* **50:** 401

Middleton, D, Savage, D, Trainor, F and Taylor, A. (1992a). Matching for various HLA class II loci in cadaveric renal transplantation using DNA techniques. Transplantation using DNA techniques. *Transplantation* **53**: 1138

Middleton, D, Mytilineos, J, Savage, D, *et al.* (1992b). Matching for HLA-DPB1 alleles in zero mismatched HLA-A, -B, -DR renal transplants. *Transplant Proc* **24:** 2439

Middleton, D, Mytilineos, J, Deufel, A, Williams, F and Opelz, G. (1997). Impact of HLA-DPB eptiope matching in kidney graft survival. *Eur J Immunogenet* **24:** 54

Mytilineos, J, Lempert, M, Middleton, D, Williams, F, Scherer S, *et al.* (1997). HLA class I DNA typing of 215 HLA-A, -B, -DR zero mismatched kidney transplants. *Tissue Antigens* **50**: 355

Opelz, G, Mytilneos, J, Scherer S, *et al.* (1991). Survival of DNA HLA-DR typed and matched cadaver kidney transplants. *Lancet* **338**: 461

Petersdorf, EW, Longton, GM, Anasetti, C, *et al.* (1995). The significance of HLA-DRB1 matching on clinical outcome after HLA-A, B, DR identical unrelated donor marrow transplantation. *Blood* **86**: 1606

Segnar, DPS, Couture, RA, Raman, S, Jindal, SL and Lazarovits, AI. (1987). Role of class I and class II HLA antigens in cadaveric renal transplantation. *Transplant Proc* **19**: 3422

Spencer, A, Szydio, RM, Brookes, PA, *et al.* (1995). Bone marrow transplantation for chronic myeloid leukaemia with volunteer unrelated donors using ex vivo or in vivo T-cell depletion: major prognostic impact of HLA class I identity between donor and recipient. *Blood* **86**: 3590

Williams, F, Mallon, E and Middleton, D. (1997). Development of PCR-SSOP for HLA-A typing of bone marrow registry donors. *Tissue Antigens* **49**: 61

CHAPTER 7

SEQUENCING-BASED TYPING

J. Ross
United Kingdom Transplant Support Service Authority
Fox Den Road
Bristol BS34 8RR, England

Introduction

DNA sequencing techniques, developed originally in the 1970s, had by the end of the 1980s become sufficiently rapid, cheap and simple to be considered as a means of tissue typing. Since then sequencing-based typing (SBT) methods have been developed and refined, taking advantage of new enzymology, improved DNA labelling approaches and advances in automated sequencer instrumentation such that there are now well established SBT methods for all of the classical class I and class II HLA genes.

This chapter summarises the main methods currently available for dideoxy-mediated chain termination sequencing, which is now by far the most popular approach used for DNA sequencing, and includes a review of the SBT literature. Where appropriate, examples have been chosen to highlight the options currently available in terms of sequencing chemistry, automated sequencer platform and SBT analysis software. However, no attempt has been made to describe in detail any of the methods used and the reader is referred to the references cited for detailed methodological information. A discussion focusing upon the potential role of SBT in tissue typing laboratories and some of the likely future developments concludes the chapter.

Dideoxy-mediated chain termination DNA sequencing

The dideoxy-mediated chain termination method evolved from the +/- sequencing technique originally described in 1975 (Sanger and Coulson, 1975). The +/- method proved too inaccurate to become widely accepted and it was not until the introduction of chain-terminating dideoxynucleotide triphosphates (ddNTPs) (Sanger *et al.*, 1977) that enzymatic methods of DNA sequencing were used extensively.

Figure 7.1 provides a summary of the steps involved in dideoxy-mediated chain termination sequencing and these steps are listed below:

1. The region of DNA to be sequenced is amplified in some way and then denatured to produce single stranded DNA.

2. A sequencing primer is annealed to the single stranded DNA.

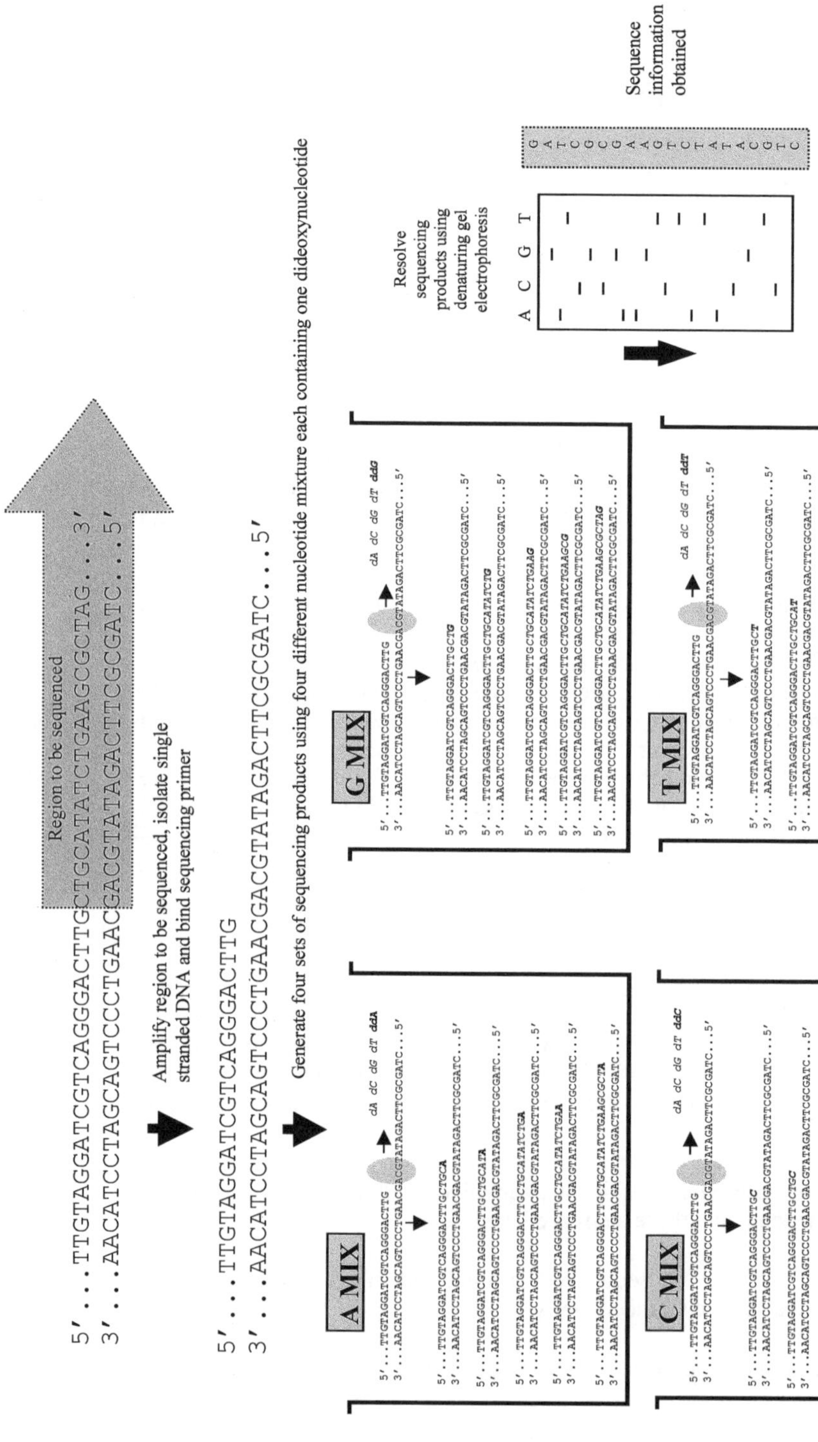

Figure 7.1. Steps involved in dideoxy-mediated chain termination DNA sequencing

3. Dideoxynucleotide chain termination DNA sequencing then takes advantage of the fact that a growing chain of nucleotides, extending in the 5' to 3' direction, will terminate if, instead of a conventional deoxynucleotide, a 2'3'dideoxynucleotide becomes incorporated. By performing four separate reactions, each containing a DNA polymerase and a small amount of one of the four dideoxynucleotides in addition to all four deoxynucleotides, four separate sets of chain-terminated fragments can be produced.

4. Following the replication/termination step, these chain terminated fragments will remain bound to the single stranded DNA molecule which has acted as a template. By heating these partially double stranded molecules and/or adding a denaturing agent such as formamide, the single stranded chain termination molecules can be released from their template and separated using high resolution denaturing gel electrophoresis.

5. The sequence of the original region of DNA is then finally deduced by examining the relative positions of the dideoxynucleotide chain termination products in the four lanes of the denaturing gel.

This is the basic procedure which all modern gel-based enzymatic DNA sequencing utilises and has not changed over the two decades since its discovery.

In contrast to the continuity of this basic procedure, the various reagents, equipment and methodological strategies for carrying out DNA sequencing have undergone constant evolution to improve the simplicity, speed and reliability of the process. The following list presents some of the major technical developments which have occurred and subsequently become incorporated into the SBT methods discussed later in this chapter.

1. *Use of PCR fragments as initial template material (Figure 7.2.1).*

If the DNA sequences flanking the region to be analysed are known, PCR provides a rapid means of obtaining large amounts of template material and cuts out any recombinant DNA steps which were needed, prior to the use of PCR, at the start of the sequencing strategy to obtain sufficient material for sequencing.

2. *Streptavidin/biotin linkage to isolate single stranded DNA (Figure 7.2.2).*

The inclusion of a biotin labelled PCR primer allows single stranded DNA to be isolated rapidly as the resulting biotin labelled strand of the PCR product can be immobilised to a streptavidin solid support followed by alkali denaturation to remove the non-biotinylated strand.

3. *DNA sequencing enzymology improvements*

Developments in the DNA polymerase used for sequencing have led to a continuing improvement in the characteristics of the enzymes used for DNA sequencing. For example T7 DNA polymerase is now used in preference to

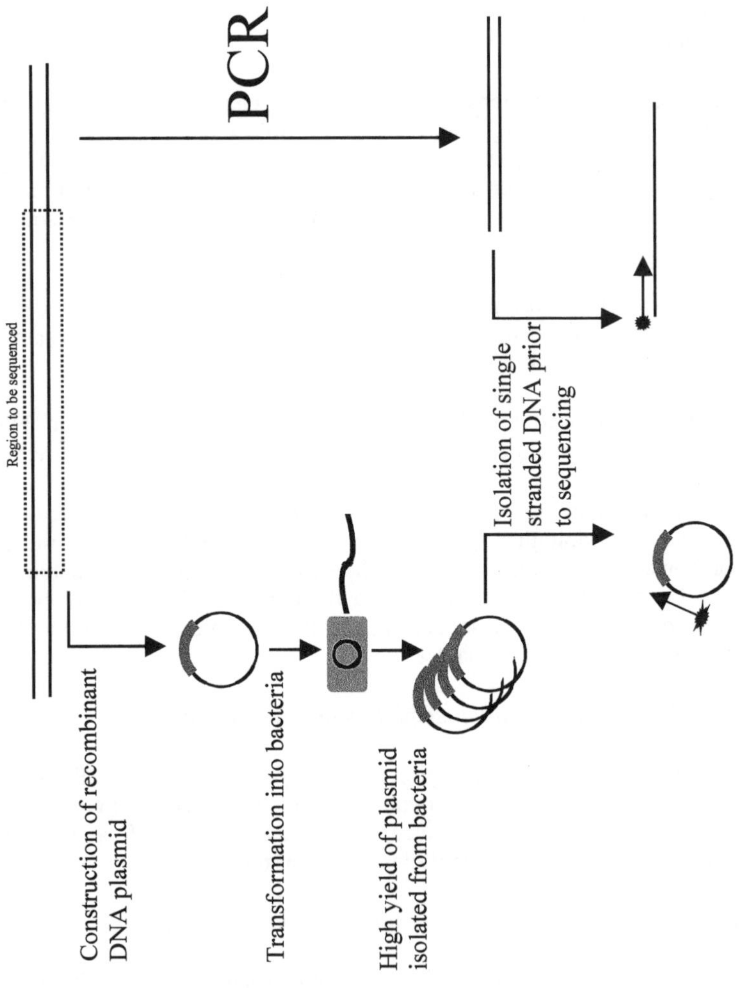

Figure 7.2.1. Comparison of PCR and recombinant DNA-based amplification of DNA for sequencing purposes.

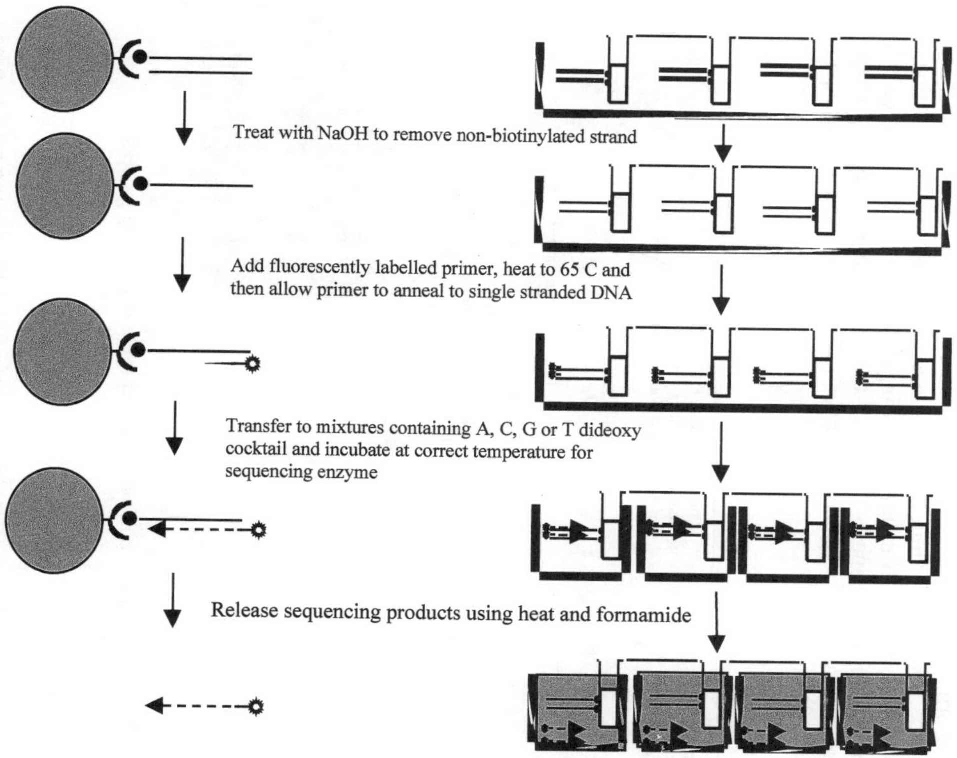

Figure 7.2.2. Use of streptavidin-coated magnetic beads or combs to isolate single stranded DNA and facilitate subsequent sequencing steps

Klenow polymerase as it incorporates dNTPs and ddNTPs at a more even rate and with a higher processivity.

Another area of sequencing enzyme development has occurred in the use of thermostable DNA polymerases. Polymerases derived from *Thermus aquaticus* have been engineered to produce enzymes such as Thermosequenase which can be used in a process referred to as cycle sequencing. Starting with a PCR product, an initial denaturation step is used to produce single stranded DNA templates. Following primer annealing, Thermosequenase is used to perform the sequencing reaction at a temperature high enough to avoid PCR product reformation. This approach has the added advantage of allowing the template to be 'recycled' - hence the name 'cycle sequencing' - following the sequencing reaction, for repeated rounds of denaturation, sequencing primer hybridisation and DNA sequencing (Figure 7.2.3).

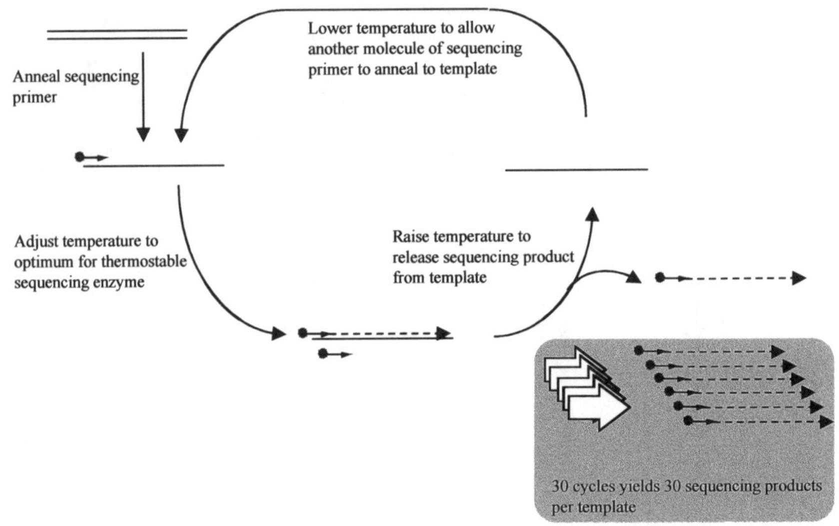

Figure 7.2.3. *Taq* polymerase-based cycle sequencing process.

4. *Fluorescent dye labelling*

The use of radiolabelled nucleotides as a means of detecting sequencing products has been increasing replaced with fluorescent labelling methods with benefits in terms of ease of use, label stability and safety. Labelling can be of the sequencing primer, the deoxynucleotides or the dideoxynucleotides. The development of four colour dyes also brought advantages to sequencing strategies as all four sets of sequencing products could be run on a single lane resulting in a four fold increase in the number of samples which could be loaded on to a gel. Linking one of these four dyes to each of the four dideoxynucleotides also had the advantage of removing the need to perform the four dideoxynucleotide sequencing reactions separately thus further simplifying the sequencing procedure.

5. *Automated sequencing machine development*

A widening range of automated sequencing machines are now available, all of which detect fluorescently labelled sequencing products following either vertical slab gel or capillary electrophoresis. The list of instruments currently available and the details of the manufacturers with their addresses are given in Table 7.1.

Manufacturer	Product	Contact details	
PE Biosystems	377, 310 and 3700	Tel. Fax. Web site	01925 825650 01925 282502 www.perkin-elmer.com/ab
Amersham Pharmacia Biotech	ALFexpress II and Megabase	Tel. Fax. Web site	0870 6061921 01494 542179 www.biotech.pharmacia.se/autodna
Licor	4000 and 4200 systems	Tel. Fax. Web site	01908 247700 01908 247724 www.licor.com
Visible Genetics Inc.	MicroGene Clipper and Long-Read Tower	Tel. Fax. Web site	33 0 160 871300 (France) 33 0 160 871301 (France) www.visgen.com
Beckman Coulter	CEQ 2000	Tel. Fax. Web site	01494 441181 01494 447558 www.beckmancoulter.com

Table 7.1. Automated sequencing machines and the contact details of the instrument manufacturers.

6. *Sequence analysis software*

All of the automated sequencing machines transfer the data they generate directly to a collection computer preventing the need for manual analysis of 'raw' sequence data. This computer holds all the software for general sequence capture, processing and analysis and is specific to the sequencer of each company. It is the automatic detection of sequence products and conversion of the collected data into sequence information which led to the term 'automated DNA sequencing machine'. The term is something of a misnomer as the physical steps involved in generating the dideoxy-chain termination products are still performed manually.

Specific software packages for the analysis of particular genes have also been developed and, in the case of SBT, were essential to make the method viable as a means of tissue typing.

Establishment of the SBT concept

DNA sequencing has been used to analyse HLA genes since shortly after the emergence of the chemical degradation (Maxim and Gilbert, 1977) and enzymatic methods (Sanger *et al.*, 1977), the latter of which is described above. The 1984 HLA Workshop consequently included several reports of class I and class II HLA sequence data (Albert *et al.*, 1984) and throughout the remainder of that decade the DNA sequence of all of the classical class I and class II loci were established. At the same time the scale of HLA polymorphism was becoming apparent. The laborious cloning strategies, which were originally used to uncover the extent of HLA polymorphism, were not realistically considered at this stage as a viable means of tissue typing.

The use of direct sequencing of PCR-amplified DQA and DRB alleles first led to speculation that DNA sequencing might represent a means to rapidly determine tissue types at the allelic level (Gyllensten and Erlich, 1988; Kaneoka *et al.*, 1991). The first attempt to develop a comprehensive approach to SBT, for both HLA class I and class II, involved the use of RNA as the starting material (Santamaria *et al.*, 1992; 1993). The approach used is summarised in Figure 7.3.

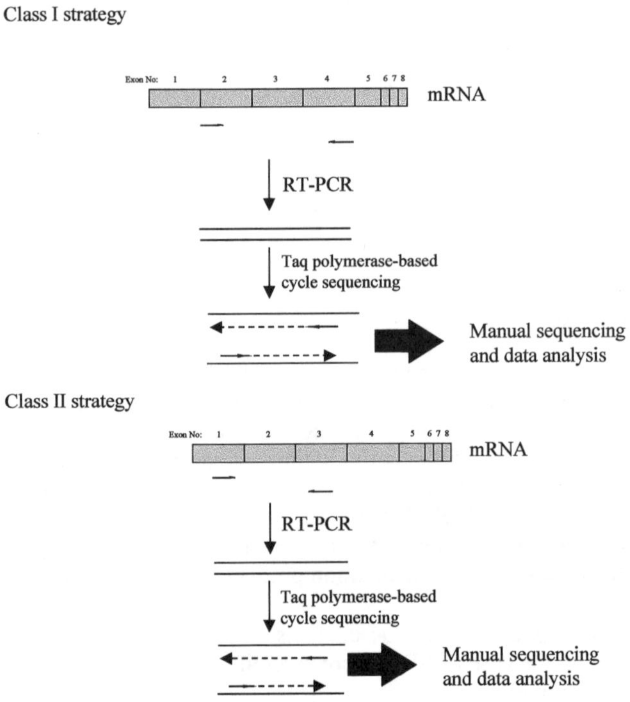

Figure 7.3. Simplified version of the strategies described by Santamaria *et al* (1992; 1993) for HLA Class I and Class II RNA-based SBT.

RNA, isolated from either lymphoblastoid cell lines or peripheral blood, was reverse transcribed using reverse transcriptase and a locus-specific antisense primer to initially produce complementary DNA (cDNA). This cDNA product was then used as the template for a PCR step resulting in amplification of the template as a DNA PCR product. A range of sequencing primers was then used to perform *Taq* polymerase, ^{32}P labelled ATP, direct sequencing of purified PCR products. The products were separated using a 'non-automated' vertical electrophoresis sequencing platform. Finally, sequencing ladders were read manually to interpret the sequence-based type.

This approach was used successfully to perform SBT for the known alleles of DQA, DQB, DRB1, DRB3/4/5, and for HLA-A, -B and -C and demonstrated for the first time the feasibility of SBT as a means of high resolution typing.

The use of RNA provided a simple means of amplifying the relatively short exonic regions of each HLA gene needed for SBT to be applied. The use of simple and rapid RNA isolation procedures was a further strength of this initial SBT approach. However, one of the major disadvantages of using RNA is the need for either previously archived RNA material or the availability of viable material for RNA isolation. As many of the potential uses for SBT involved the use of archived material, for which DNA might well be the only material available, the use of RNA as a starting material was less than ideal. Also, despite its simplicity, the introduction of successful RNA isolation methods into the routine laboratory, given the instability of RNA, seemed an unnecessary hurdle if equivalent DNA-based SBT approaches could be established.

Development of DNA-based sequencing-based typing

Class II

At the same time as the RNA-based approach was being developed, class II DNA-based direct sequencing strategies were being extended to allow all known DRB1, DQB1 and DPB1 alleles to be amplified and sequenced. (Spurkland *et al.,* 1993; Versluis *et al.,* 1993). The methods differed from that described for RNA-based SBT in several key aspects and, particularly in the case of DPB SBT, reflected the way in which sequencing methodologies generally were evolving at the time. The steps involved for DPB SBT are summarised in Figure 7.4.

Using genomic DNA as the starting material, PCR primers, designed to hybridise specifically to the intronic regions flanking exon 2 of the DPB1 locus, were used to amplify a 584 bp fragment. In each PCR one primer was biotinylated at the 3' end producing a biotinylated PCR product which was then bound to streptavidin coated Dynabeads. By placing the resulting PCR product/Dynabead complex in a magnetic rack and treating with NaOH, the non-biotinylated strand of the PCR product was denatured and washed off leaving the biotinylated strand to act as the sequencing template. A four dye, dye-primer T7 polymerase sequencing strategy was then used to sequence the biotinylated PCR strand and the sequencing products analysed on an Applied Biosystems 373A automated sequencer. If necessary the sequencing was performed in both orientations. Sequence analysis

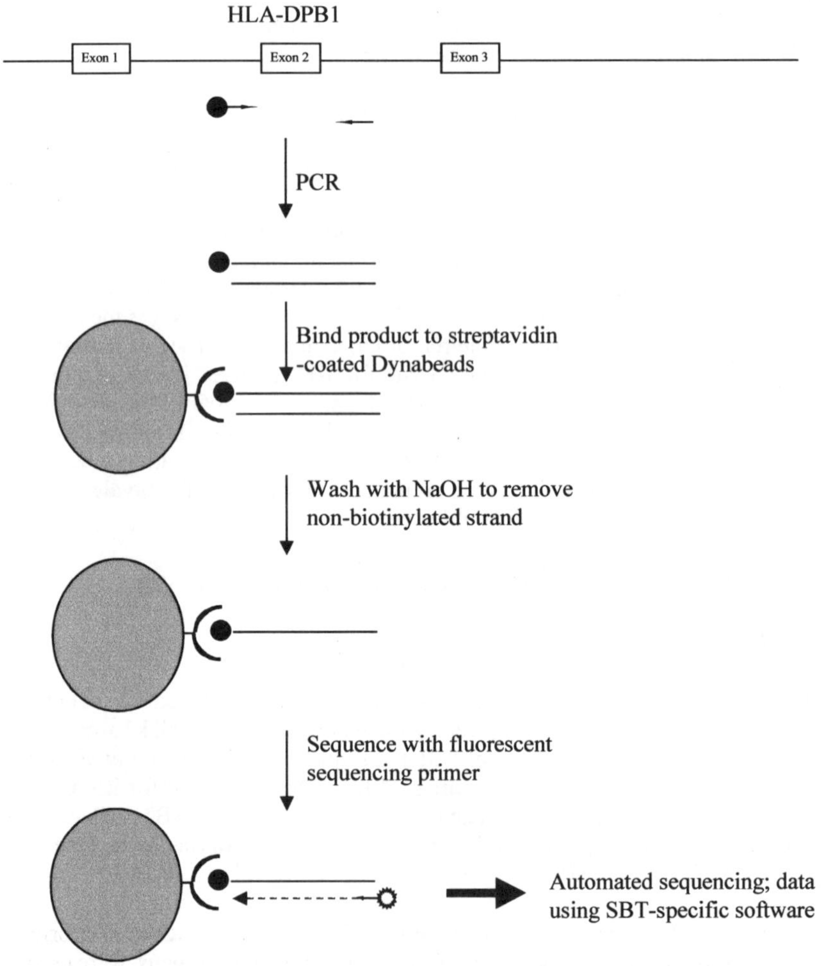

Figure 7.4. HLA-DPB1 SBT strategy to obtain sequence data in the "reverse" orientation. The strategy was also performed using a biotinylated antisense primer and a non-biotinylated sense primer to obtain sequence data in the forward orientation.

was then performed using software specifically designed to compare the newly generated sequence data with a database of all known HLA-DPB sequences (Rozemuller *et al.,* 1993). In this way the DPB type of the sample sequenced could be very rapidly established from either homozygous or heterozygous DPB sequence data.

The SBT strategy developed for HLA-DPB provided the blueprint for the majority of class I and class II SBT methods which have been published since and involved the following key steps.

- Use of genomic DNA as the starting material
- PCR amplification using primers specific to a particular locus or group of alleles
- Fluorescent labelling and the use of dideoxy-mediated chain termination sequencing
- Electrophoresis and sequence data collection using an automated sequencing machine
- Sequence data analysis which included the use of SBT-specific software

Despite the fact that the DRB and DQB SBT strategy, developed at about the same time, shared many of the features described above for DPB, there were also important differences in the approaches used (Spurkland *et al.*, 1993). Firstly, the greater level of polymorphism of DRB1 relative to DPB1, led to a PCR strategy which involved the use of several group specific primers designed to hybridise to regions within exon 2 of DRB1 or DRB3/4/5 (Figure 7.5). A similar PCR strategy was adopted for DQB1 (Figure 7.5). The DRB and DQB1 primer designs originated from the 11th IHWS. The second difference involved the use of a DNA sequencing approach using radioisotopic labelling followed radiographic detection of electrophoresed sequencing products. This approach is often now referred to as 'manual sequencing' to distinguish it from sequencing using fluorescent labelling methods coupled to the use of an automated sequencer. Finally, no SBT-specific software was used for analysis of the manually interpreted sequence data. Despite these differences these initial DRB and DQB SBT methods once again demonstrated the feasibility and utility of SBT, in this case for HLA matching of unrelated bone marrow transplant pairs. The PCR strategies used for DRB and DQB1 have remained largely unchanged in the methods in use today (see below).

Class I

As with other DNA-based tissue typing techniques, class I SBT methodology development lagged slightly behind that of class II. Following the RNA-based class I approach described earlier (Santamaria *et al.,* 1993), the first DNA-based approach to SBT focused upon HLA-C (Petersdorf *et al.,* 1994). Amplification of exon 2 was performed in this instance producing overlapping amplicons (Figure 7.6). 'Tailing' of the PCR primers with M13 sequences allowed PCR products to be sequenced using M13 sequencing primers. Four colour dye-primer *Taq* cycle

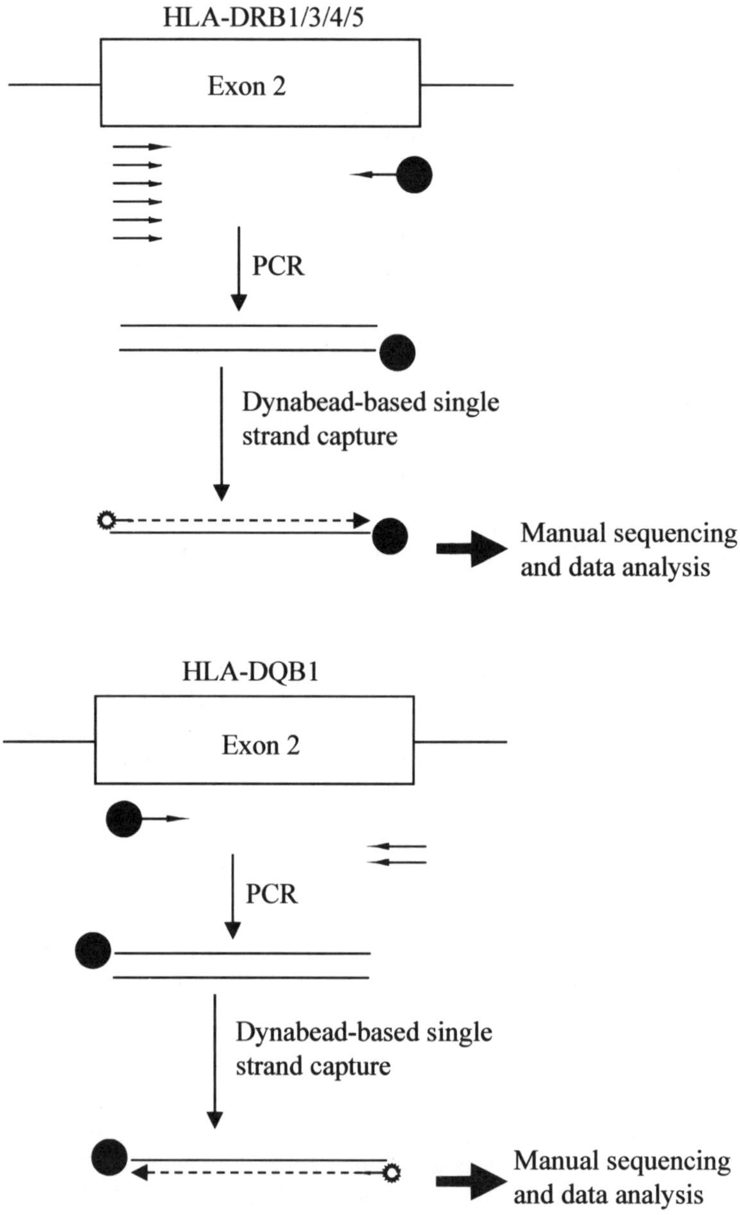

Figure 7.5. HLA-DRB1/3/4/5 and HLA-DQB1 SBT strategies.

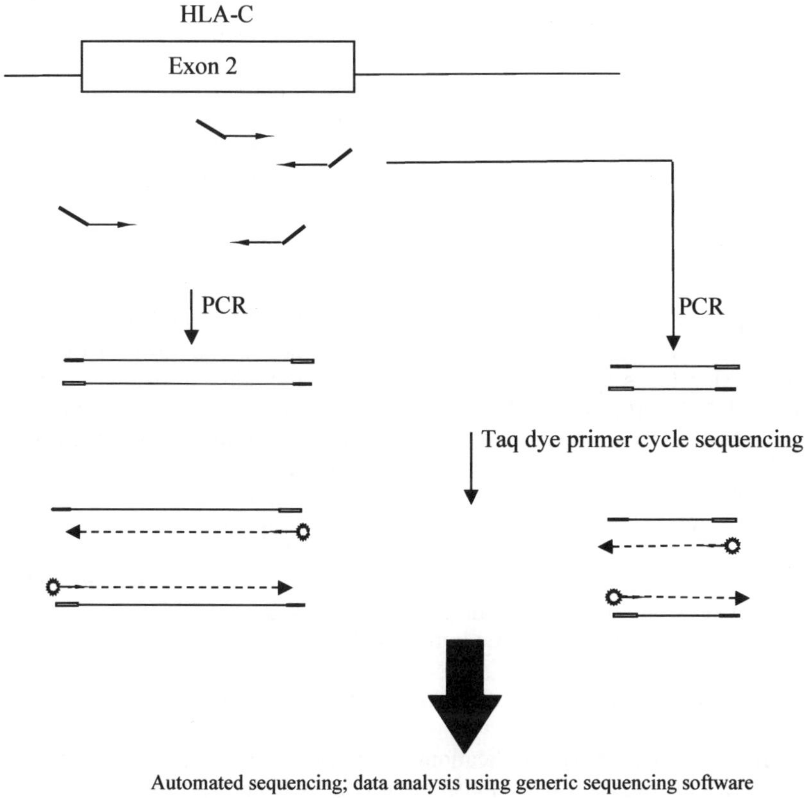

Figure 7.6. HLA-C SBT strategy based upon the use of M13-tailed PCR primers to amplify and facilitate the sequencing of exon 2.

sequencing was then performed and the products electrophoresed on a Applied Biosystems 373A automated sequencer. The analysis of exon 2 alone discriminated all known HLA-C alleles at that time with the exception of the Cw*01 and Cw*08 families and the Cw*0302-0304 and Cw*1501, 1502, Cw*1504 alleles. Exon 3 sequencing was required to resolve these alleles but was not included as part of this approach.

It soon became apparent, based upon the rapidly growing number of identified alleles for each of the class I loci, that any class I SBT strategy would require the sequencing of exons 2 and 3 to allow unambiguous allele assignment. Hence, the next approaches described, in this case for HLA-B, involved the amplification of exon 2, intron 2 and exon 3 as a single PCR product using a panel of PCR primers (Petersdorf *et al.,* 1994; 1995). This was then followed by four colour dye-terminator *Taq* cycle sequencing prior to electrophoresis on a 373A automated sequencer (Figure 7.7). At the time the HLA-B SBT method was published the sequence analysis was performed using the general sequencer analysis software SeqEd.

A simplification of the PCR stage of class I SBT was then proposed, first appearing as an abstract at the 1995 EFI/BSHI meeting (Johnston-Dow *et al.,* 1995). Using locus specific primers designed to hybridise to exons 1 and 5 of either HLA-A, HLA-B or HLA-C, a 2kb PCR product was amplified. The sequences of exons 2 and 3 were then determined using four colour dye-primers which bound to the intronic sequences flanking these exons (Figure 7.8). Electrophoresis was then performed on an Applied Biosystems automated sequencer and the data analysed using Sequence Navigator and Factura software, the latter of which was the first commercially produced SBT analysis software. This method had the additional advantage of allowing exon 4 to be sequenced from the original PCR product, if deemed necessary, using an additional pair of dye-labelled primers which bound to regions flanking exon 4.

Refinement of SBT strategies leading to the current methods

The first wave of SBT publications discussed above allowed many other laboratories to successfully establish rapid HLA sequencing protocols as part of their tissue typing repertoire. The sequencing-based typing component for the Twelfth International Histocompatability Workshop and Conference (IHWC), which was held in June 1996, allowed these SBT methods to be discussed and evaluated in detail for the first time. Organised by Marcel Tilanus and John Francois Eliaou, the SBT component involved the exchange of available methods and the use of DNA reference panels designed to allow the evaluation of different SBT methods. Most of the methods described above were included in this workshop SBT component and some of the approaches outlined below were presented for the first time (Tilanus and Eliaou, 1997). Following the 1996 IHWC, it was clear that SBT had become established as a means of high resolution typing. However, there remained a number of problems associated with the technique. These problems, described below, represented the weaknesses of many of the first SBT strategies.

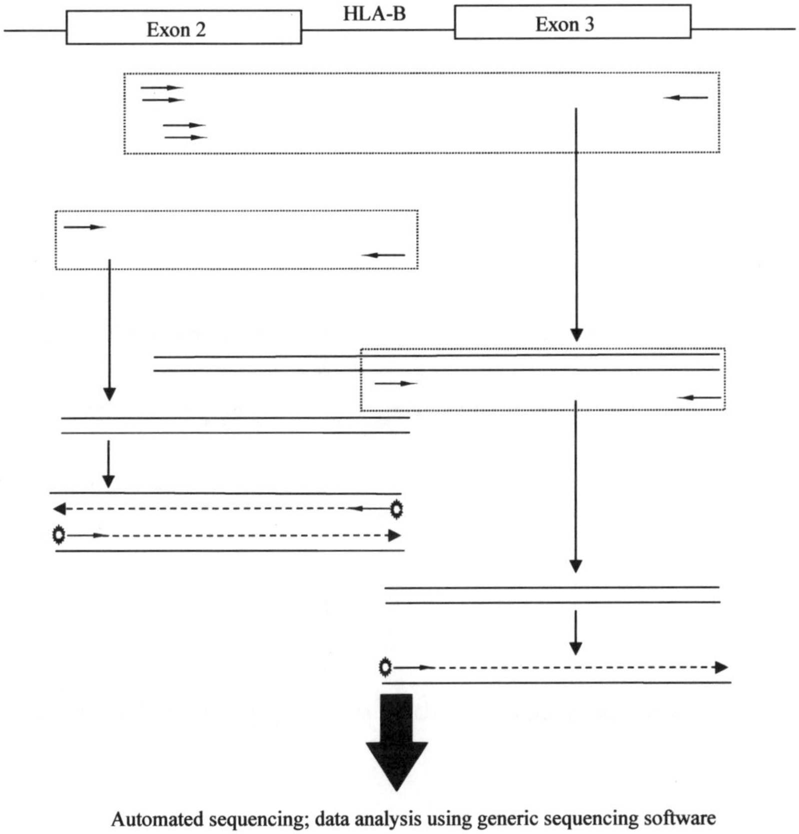

Figure 7.7. HLA-B SBT strategy to amplify and sequence exons 2 and 3.

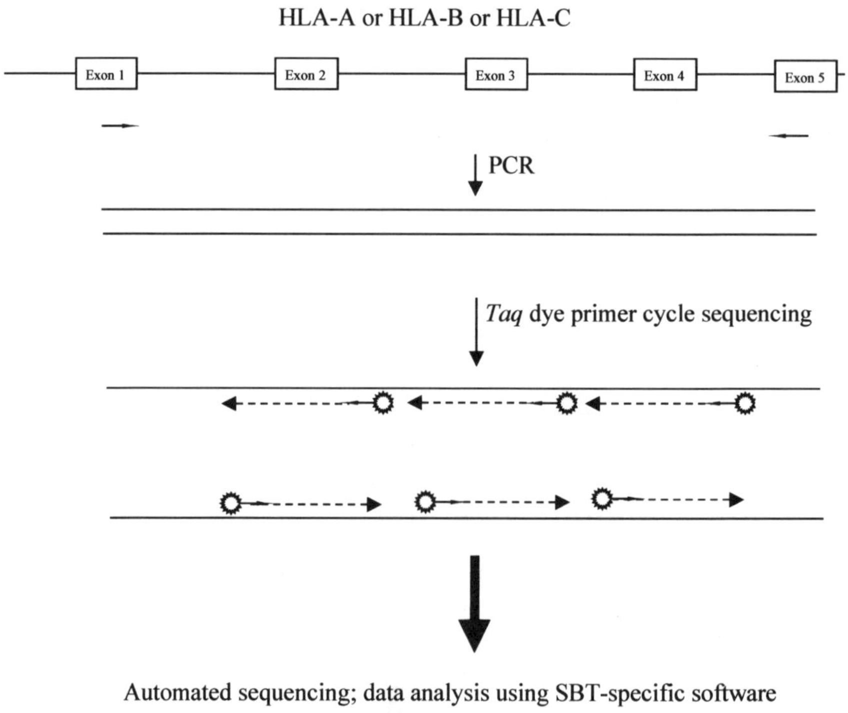

Figure 7.8. General strategy for HLA Class I SBT first proposed by Johnston-Dow *et al.* (1995)

1. *Ambiguous allele combinations*

The phenomenon of ambiguous allele combinations represents perhaps the greatest weakness of the SBT approach. This ambiguity, observed in SBT results for all loci, occurs if two alleles result in a heterozygous sequence which is identical to the heterozygous sequence of a different pair of alleles. Figure 7.9 shows a simplified example to illustrate how the ambiguity arises.

Various analyses have been made of the level of ambiguity for each locus which differ in their outcome depending upon the size of the region analysed and the number of known alleles when the calculations were made (Rozemuller *et al.*, 1996). Clearly as the number of known alleles continues to rise the level of potential ambiguity will also rise.

2. *PCR and sequencing primer design problems*

Sentences along the lines of the following statement appeared in many of the first SBT publications: 'one of the strengths of SBT over other DNA-based typing methods is the ability to detect previously unidentified alleles'. Up to a point statements like this are true but they make at least two assumptions:

- Any new allele will not contain a novel polymorphism at a position corresponding to the 3' end of either the PCR primers or the sequencing primers being used for SBT.
- The SBT method involves sequencing all of the gene being studied or at least all of the highly polymorphic regions.

The first assumption might initially seem a reasonable one to make. However, many of the SBT PCR primers, particularly for class II, were chosen to specifically amplify groups of alleles by using polymorphic positions in the hypervariable regions of the gene to be sequenced. This was done in an attempt to reduce the problem of ambiguous allele combinations mentioned above. By choosing PCR primers which amplified subsets of alleles for a given locus instead of the complete set, the number of potential ambiguities could be reduced.

In the case of the second assumption above, the less of the gene that is sequenced, the greater the chance of a novel polymorphism being missed. Hence, many of the initially described methods had the potential to miss novel alleles by virtue of the regions they did not sequence.

Apart from the attempt to reduce ambiguity, the reason for using SBT PCR primers which lay within the polymorphic exonic sequence regions was the lack of available intronic sequence data for most of the known HLA alleles. The WHO Nomenclature Committee for Factors of the HLA System requires the sequencing of all of exon 2 for class II and all of exon 2 and 3 for class I prior to the designation of an official name to a new allele (Bodmer *et al.*, 1997). As a consequence the majority of submitted HLA allele sequence information is limited to exonic

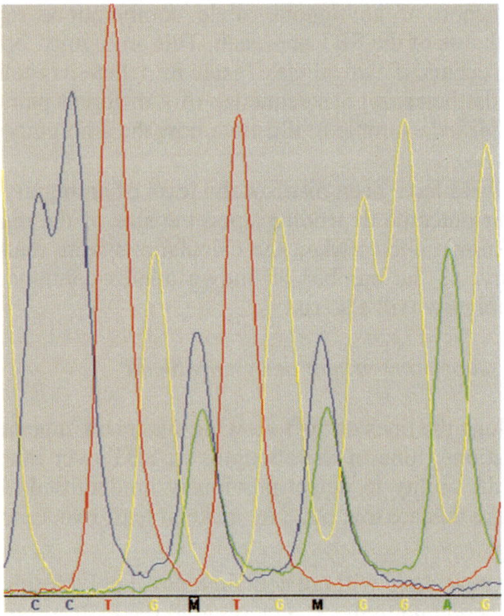

Allele 1	CCTGCTGCGGAG
Allele 2	CCTGATGAGGAG
	↓
Heterozygous sequence for Allele 1 plus Allele 2	CCTGMTGMGGAG

Allele 3	CCTGCTGAGGAG
Allele 4	CCTGATGCGGAG
	↓
Heterozygous sequence for Allele 3 plus Allele 4	CCTGMTGMGGAG

Figure 7.9. An example of ambiguous SBT data generated from an electropherogram showing heterozygous sequence data.

regions. At the time the SBT methods were being developed this made it difficult to use intronic regions to design primers which amplified and sequenced all of the more polymorphic exonic regions.

3. *Allele drop out*

The use of several PCR and/or sequencing primers, as outlined in a number of the SBT approaches discussed above, introduces the risk of preferential amplification and/or sequencing of one allele relative to the other. There are several reports of this in the SBT literature which resulted in the incorrect homozygous designation of a sample.

4. *Methods still too slow, complicated and expensive*

Despite the significant improvements from the original HLA sequencing approaches which involved cloning and the use of manual sequencing, SBT methods remained relatively labour intensive and required the use of expensive reagents and equipment when compared to other techniques.

Clearly, there therefore remained much room for improvement upon many of the first SBT approaches. Most of the more recent SBT publications have, as a consequence, described methods which have sought to overcome one or more of the problems listed above.

A summary of these more recent publications, focusing on each HLA locus separately, is given below. The range of methods described illustrates the many different options in terms of PCR strategy, sequencing chemistry, automated sequencer platform and analysis software which are now available.

HLA-DPB

The DPB SBT strategy, discussed above, which was originally described in 1993 has remained largely unchanged . A method based upon the selective amplification of alleles prior to sequencing was developed to resolve the many ambiguous allele combinations which exist for this locus (Versluis *et al.,* 1995). Using 4 pairs of group-specific amplification primers the vast majority of ambiguous sequences can be resolved.

The only other alterations to the original DPB1 SBT strategy have come about with developments in sequencing chemistry and the adaptation of the method for use on sequencing platforms other than the ABI 373. HLA-DPB1 approaches have therefore now been developed for use with, for example, *Taq* cycle-sequencing chemistry (Rozemuller *et al.,* 1995). Commercial kits for DPB1 SBT are also available from PE Biosystems and Amersham Pharmacia Biotech based upon the original DPB1 strategy.

HLA-DPA

Based upon earlier DPA1 sequence data (Harada *et al.,* 1992; Guethlein *et al.,* 1993) a study of the DNA sequences of exons 2 and 4 of DPA1 was performed using a novel DPA1 SBT strategy (Rozemuller *et al.,* 1995). The approach used was similar to that developed for DPB1 SBT, using DPA1 specific primers to amplify exons 2 and 4 separately prior to 4 colour *Taq* cycle-sequencing and analysis using an Applied Biosystems 373A automated sequencer and the computer based comparison of the sequence data with databases of DPA1 exons 2 and 4 (Figure 7.10). The study identified errors in the earlier DPA1 sequence data and established that exon 2 sequencing of DPA1 was sufficient to identify the known DPA1 alleles.

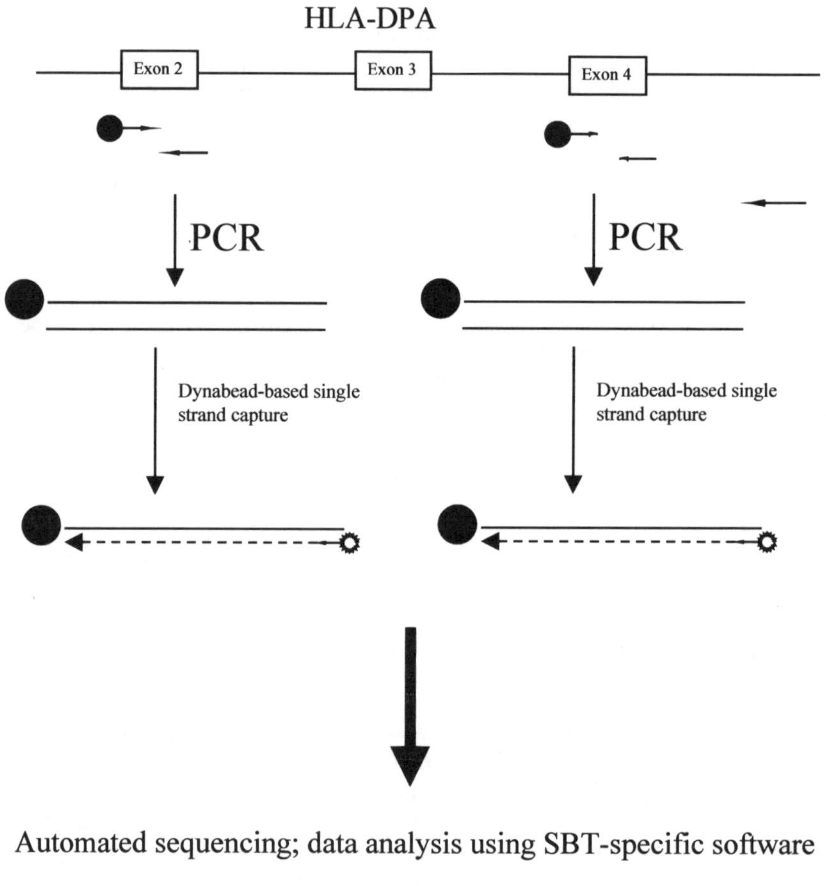

Figure 7.10. HLA-DPA1 SBT strategy involving the PCR and sequencing of exons 2 and 4 of the DPA1 gene. Sequence data from exon 4 SBT established that the analysis of exon 2 alone was sufficient to resolve all known HLA-DPA1 alleles (Rozemuller *et al.* 1995).

HLA-DRB

The adaptation of the DRB strategy, described by Spurkland in 1993, to include automated sequencing and SBT software analysis, followed as the logical development for these methods, using the DPB1 SBT as the model. The use of streptavidin-coated combs in place of magnetic beads was also later introduced to further simplify the technique described for use with the Pharmacia Biotech ALF*express* automated sequencer (Savelkoul *et al.,* 1995). A DRB SBT approach was also developed for use with the range of PE Biosystems sequencing platforms (McGinnis *et al.,* 1995). Originally designed using T7 sequencing chemistry and four colour dye-labelled primers, the recommended method was subsequently improved and simplified to allow four colour dye-terminator cycle sequencing to be used with AmpliTaqFS. The PE Biosystems MatchMaker software was used for DRB analysis of SBT data generated using this approach. This software evolved from the original programmes designed for DPB1 SBT.

A comparison of the DRB SBT methods was performed to evaluate the relative merits of the two published approaches (Voorter *et al.,* 1997). The study concluded that neither the sequencing chemistry nor the automated sequencing machine influences the typing result. However, the use of several primers to amplify the different families of DRB alleles highlighted a problem with false negative reactions in heterozygous samples where one allele was amplified weakly relative to the other allele. The authors concluded that their findings 'implicates that extensive quality control is needed to assure correct typing results'. Both Amersham Pharmacia Biotech and PE Biosystems now sell DRB SBT kits based upon the published methods.

The strategy to sequence only exon 2 for DRB SBT has recently been revised for the DRB3/4/5 genes (Voorter *et al.,* 1997). An extended SBT approach involving the separate amplification of exons 2, 3 and 4 has been developed and allows all DRB3/4/5 alleles to be resolved.

HLA-DQB

The further development of the DQB1 SBT method has followed a similar evolution to DRB SBT. The DQB1 PCR-SSP and sequencing strategy, described by Spurkland in 1993, was adapted for use with solid phase T7 polymerase sequencing using fluorescently labelled sequencing primers and an ALF*express* automated sequencer. The associated SBTyper software was used for the analysis of the sequence data. The primer design of the DQB1-SBT has recently been re-examined to increase the region sequenced and provide a PCR strategy which avoided allele drop out (Voorter *et al.,* 1998). The strategy which has emerged from these changes is shown in Figure 7.11.

HLA-DQA

The DQA1 locus presents a unique problem when designing a class II SBT method. The majority of the polymorphism for this gene is located in exon 2 as with other class II genes, so this is the region which must be sequenced in any SBT

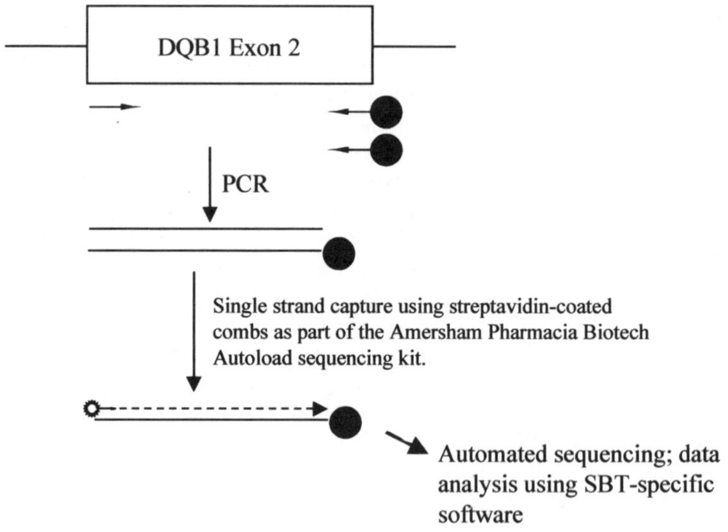

Figure 7.11. HLA-DQB1 SBT strategy using Autoload sequencing reagents.

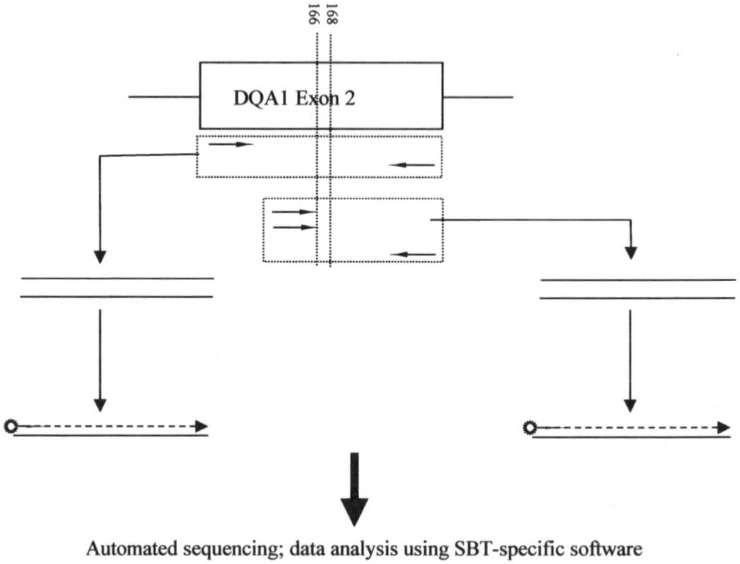

Figure 7.12. HLA-DQA1 SBT strategy (Schaeffer and Charron 1997)

strategy. However, a three base pair deletion from position 166 to 168 representing codon 56 is found in alleles DQA1*0201, DQA1*0401, DQA1*0501-0505, DQA1*06011 and DQA1*06012. Direct PCR and sequencing of exon 2 would therefore result in sequence data which becomes out of phase after this deletion, if alleles heterozygous for this deletion were sequenced together. To overcome this problem a series of specific amplification primers were designed, in addition to a generic DQA1 approach, which allowed specific groups of alleles to be sequenced following a low resolution PCR-SSP test (Figure 7.12) (Schaeffer and Charron, 1997).

HLA-C

At least three different HLA-C DNA-based SBT methods have now been published (Turner *et al.,* 1998; Dunn *et al.,* 1998; van der Viles *et al.,* 1998). Figure 7.13 provides an overview of the strategy used for each approach. All three methods include the sequencing of at least exons 2 and 3, automated sequencing and data analysis using dedicated SBT software.

HLA-C SBT was used, in one of these reports, to type 1823 samples from the National Marrow Donor Program repository in North America. A total of 19 new alleles, or a frequency of approximately 1 new allele per 100 samples typed by HLA-C SBT was observed. This clearly has implications for the true level of polymorphism for HLA-C which may prove to be at least as high as that observed for HLA-A and HLA-B. It also raises questions regarding the ability of other DNA-based techniques to accurately type for HLA-C.

HLA-B

Several strategies for sequencing HLA-B have been published since the initial DNA-based approach described in 1994, not all of which were intended to represent rapid comprehensive methods for performing HLA-B SBT. A novel RNA-based sequencing method has been described which allows the determination of the sequence of all 8 HLA-B exons using 7 sequencing primers (Ellexson *et al.,* 1996). The use of RNA as the starting material places limitations upon this approach as a generally applicable SBT method but the strategy is particularly useful for the rapid characterisation of cDNA clones and provides a rapid means of complete exon sequencing when the characterisation of a newly identified allele is required. An alternative DNA-based approach involving the amplification of a 3.2kb region using primers which hybridise to the 5' and 3' untranslated regions of the HLA-B gene has also been described (Curran *et al.,* 1996). DNA sequencing was then performed using primers specific to either exon 2 or exon 3. The authors mention that sequence data for the promoter region of HLA-B suggests that the PCR strategy used in this approach may lead to amplification difficulties with B*14, B*55 and B*56 alleles. Despite this drawback the approach represents another means of rapidly characterising novel HLA-B alleles. Both of these approaches are outlined in Figure 7.14. Another RNA-based HLA-B sequencing approach has now been described which includes an initial allele separation step performed by the use of denaturing gradient gel electrophoresis (Eberle *et al.,* 1997). Separation of the alleles prior to sequencing

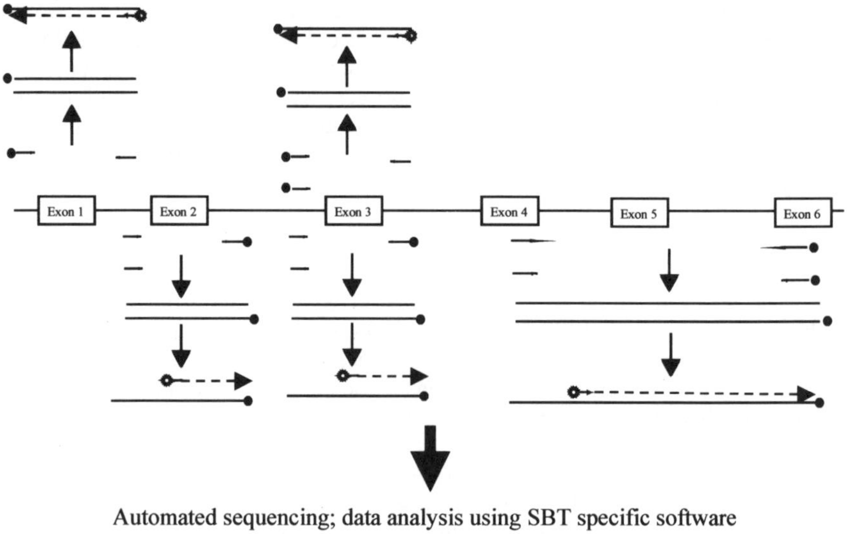

Figure 7.13.1. HLA-C SBT strategy (Van der Viles *et al.,* 1998)

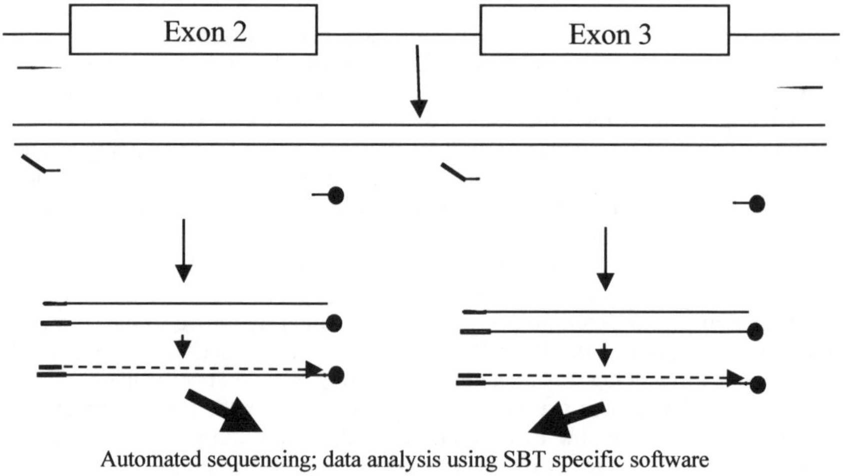

Figure 7.13.2. HLA-C SBT strategy (Turner *et al.,* 1998)

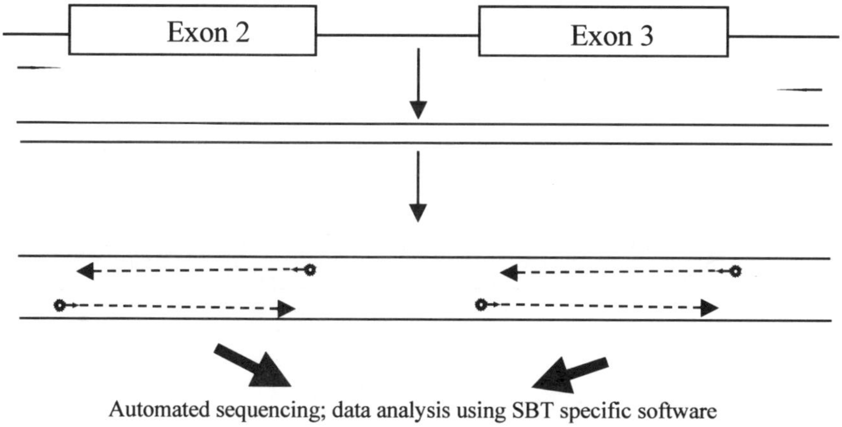

Figure 7.13.3. HLA-C SBT strategy (Dunn *et al.,* 1998)

avoids the ambiguity, discussed earlier, which is inherent in HLA SBT. By supplementing the method with a second amplification and SBT strategy this approach was able to resolve 111 of the 118 known HLA-B alleles.

The DNA-based SBT method for class I employed in our laboratory uses a locus-specific PCR (Cereb *et al.,* 1995). Sequencing of exons 2 and 3 in both directions is achieved using nested sequencing primers, The method has been used with both the ABI 373A and the ALF*express* automated sequencing machines (Figure 7.15) (Hemmatpour *et al.,* 1998; P. Dunn personal communication).

HLA-A

HLA-A SBT has received perhaps the most attention amongst class I sequencing-based methods. The methods outlined below are summarised in Figure 7.16. Once again an RNA-based approach, in this case involving the amplification of exons 1-3 and most of exon 4, has been described (Norgaard *et al.,* 1996). By amplifying this product, performing four colour cycle sequencing with the use of an automated sequencer, all possible combinations of two alleles could be identified (Figure 7.16).

The approach first described by Johnston-Dow *et al.* in 1996 was developed to provide a generic SBT approach for HLA-A which has been extensively tested and is now available as a commercial kit from PE Biosystems (Scheltinga *et al.,* 1997).

Three papers from the same group also focus on HLA-A SBT (Blasczyk *et al.,* 1995; Blasczyk *et al.,* 1996; Kotsch *et al.,* 1997). The most recent strategy the group describe is based upon the use of group specific HLA-A PCR primers which are located in the untranslated regions upstream of exon 1 and the intronic regions

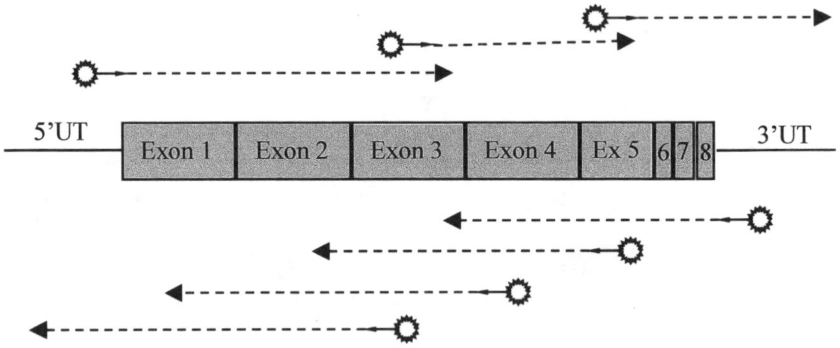

Figure 7.14.1. RNA-based method for sequencing HLA-B.

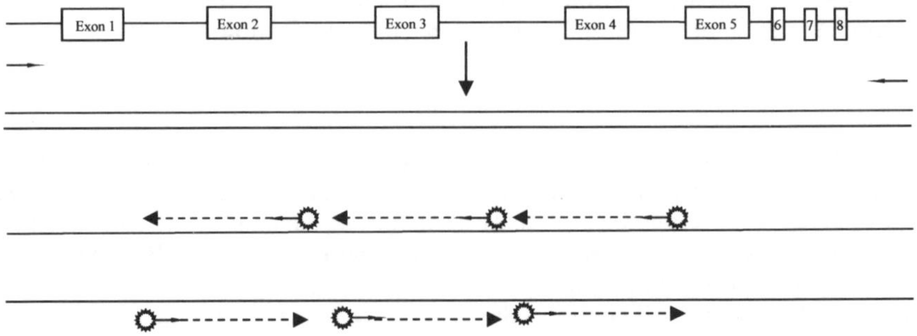

Figure 7.14.2. DNA-based method for sequencing HLA-B.

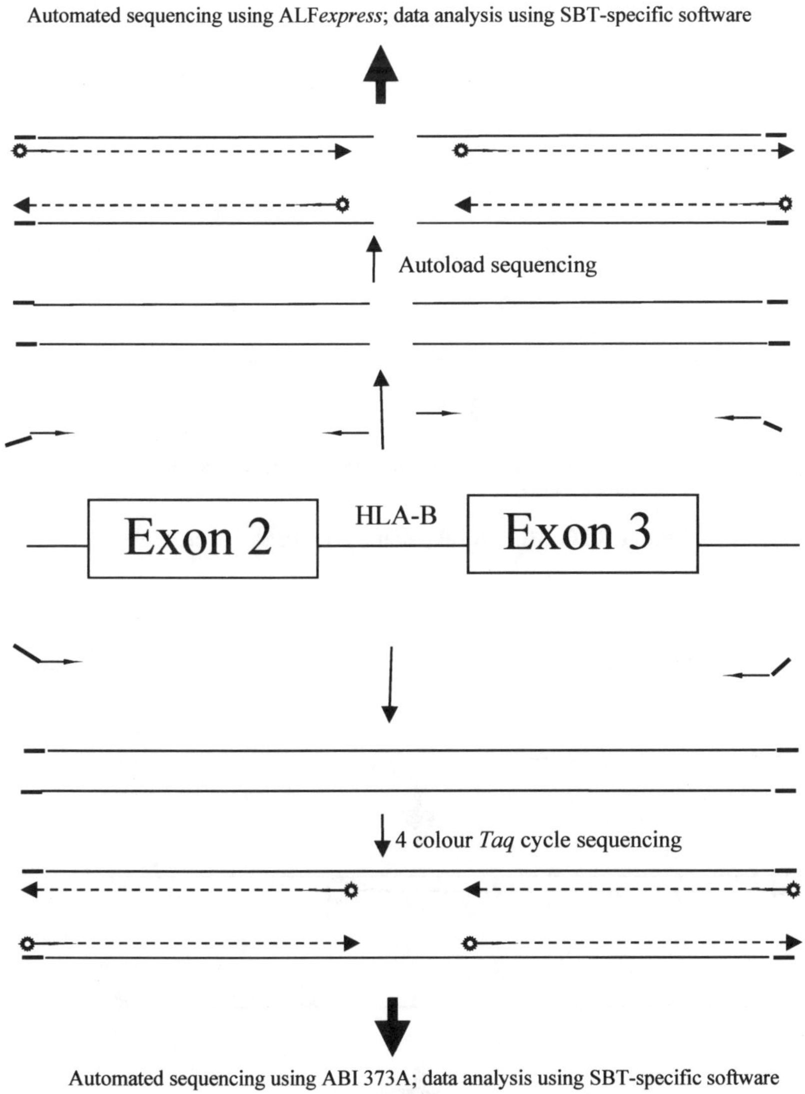

Figure 7.15. HLA-B SBT strategy using intronic primers to amplify and sequence exons 2 and 3 independently.

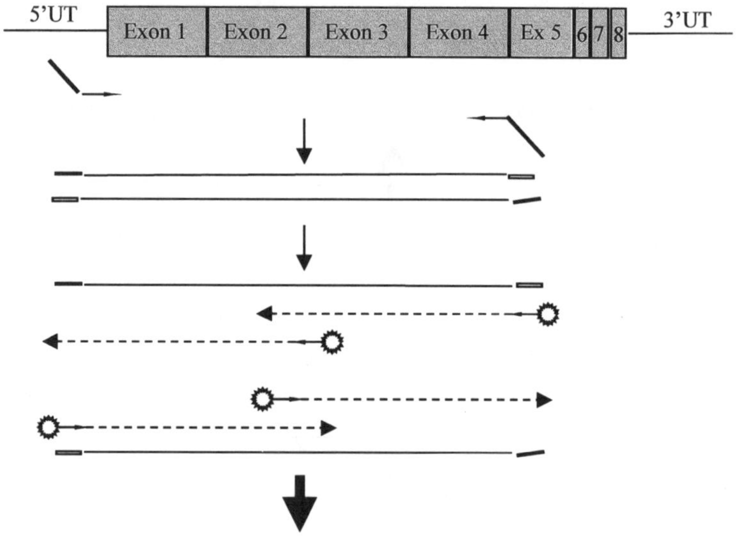

Automated sequencing; data analysis using SBT-specific software

Figure 7.16. HLA-A SBT strategy (Norgaard *et al.,* 1996).

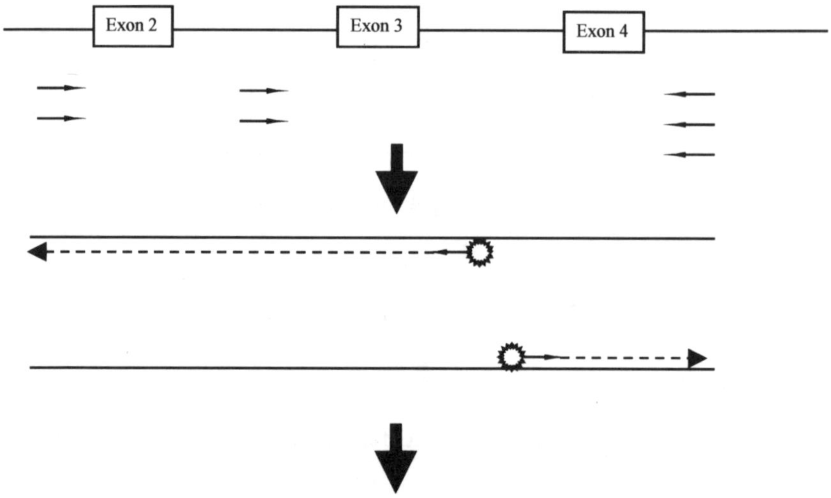

Automated sequencing; data analysis using SBT-specific software

Figure 7.17. HLA-A SBT strategy (Kotsch *et al.,* 1997).

flanking exons 2 and 3. Universal sequencing primers are then used to sequence exons 2 and three unidirectionally. The strategy used is outlined in Figure 7.17. This approach has the advantage of sequencing the majority of alleles as homozygotes, following allele separation by the initial group-specific PCR. The sequencing of homozygotes in turn permitted the use of dye-terminator chemistry in preference to dye-primer chemistry which, at the time of publication, was still considered the method of choice for heterozygote sequencing.

The above review of the literature provides examples of SBT methods for all of the polymorphic classical HLA class I and class II loci. In addition to these published methods, commercial kits for SBT are now available from PE Biosystems, Amersham Pharmacia Biotech and Visible Genetics, the majority of which utilise published methods. Details of these kits can be obtained from the individual suppliers who can be contacted using the addresses provided in Table 7.1.

Future role and direction of SBT

The role of SBT in tissue typing laboratories continues to be debated. Clearly, SBT offers very high resolution tissue typing which, using the most recent developments in sequencing chemistry, automated sequencer platforms and analysis software, can be performed far faster and more reliably than has been possible in the past. However, high resolution PCR-SSP and PCR-SSOP-based methods and kits are now available and RSCA technology is emerging as another high resolution method.

The key feature, unique to SBT, is the ability to detect and type novel alleles. This makes the method ideal for reference laboratories who have a role in identifying novel alleles and resolving ambiguous results obtained by other methods.

As yet there is no strong evidence supporting the importance of high resolution matching in solid organ transplantation, leading to the view that high resolution typing is probably not necessary for solid organ transplantation. This is something of a circular argument, though, as no large scale evaluation of the importance of high resolution matching in solid organ transplantation can be performed until high resolution typing is used on a sufficiently large scale to properly address the question.

For bone marrow transplantation there is a greater consensus that high resolution HLA matching matters in terms of graft outcome. Once again, the large studies using allele level typing to establish what level of matching is required, remain to be carried out (Little and Madrigal, 1999). Despite this, SBT seems most likely to become part of the repertoire of laboratories involved in typing for bone marrow transplantation and there are already many examples of this occurring.

For laboratories with a clear need for high resolution typing, sequencing-based typing can now be considered alongside PCR-SSP, PCR-SSOP and RSCA as a potential method for selection. The SBT methodologies are quite well established, ommercial kits are available and the sequencing equipment required is no longer prohibitively expensive. Perhaps the most significant factor which needs to be considered when evaluating SBT against other methods is the time required to sequence and analyse samples for the loci which will need to be typed. The availability of commercial kits and easily mastered analysis software should allow laboratories to evaluate SBT fully before committing to a particular SBT approach or indeed to SBT at all.

The short term future of SBT will no doubt see the establishment of a greater range of commercial kits for all of the HLA loci including the recently identified MIC genes and other non-classical HLA genes. The extension of the method to other relevant loci such as cytokine genes and minor histocompatabiltiy loci would also seem reasonable to anticipate. A continued refinement of the methods discussed above will also occur as the number of identified alleles continues to rise and the level of knowledge of HLA intron sequence information improves.

The capillary electrophoresis sequencing machines which are now available should offer the possibility to further automate the SBT process and consequently minimise the hands-on time of the method. There remains a need for a rapid and easily automatable allele separation method if the continued increase in identified HLA alleles is not to render the method unable to define unambiguous types. At present the published gel based allele separation methods appear too cumbersome to achieve this task as part of any future automated SBT set up. The longer term future of SBT will undoubtedly involve chip-based sequencing technology. The repeated sequencing of the same locus, which is what SBT represents, is ideally suited to the range of bespoke sequencing biochip methods which are now emerging. Such methods promise rapid, technically simple and ultimately very cheap typing methods. It will then cease to be a question of whether or not one should adopt an approach which obtains all of the DNA-based information which is available. Instead the focus will move to how that information is best used.

References

Albert, ED, Baur, MP and Mayr, WR (1984). *Histocompatibility Testing 1984.* Springer-Verlag, Berlin.

Blasczyk, R, Hahn, U, Wehling, J, Huhn, D and Salama, A (1995). Complete subtyping of the HLA-A locus by sequence-specific amplification followed by direct sequencing or single-strand conformational polymorphism analysis. *Tissue Antigens* **46:** 86-95

Blasczyk, R, Wehling, J, Weber, M and Salama, A. (1996). Sequence analysis of the 2nd intron revealed common sequence motifs providing the means for a unique sequencing based typing protocol of the HLA-A locus. *Tissue Antigens* **47**: 102-110

Bodmer JG, Marsh, SGE, Albert, ED, Bodmer, WF, Bontrop, RE, *et al.*(1997). Nomenclature for factors of the HLA system, 1996. *Tissue Antigens* **46:** 297-321

Curran, MD, Williams, F, Earle, JAP, Rima, BK, van Dam, MG, *et al.* (1996) Long-range PCR amplification as an alternative strategy for characterizing novel HLA-B alleles. *Eur J Immunogenet* **23**: 297-309

Delfino, L, Morabito, A., Longo, A and Ferrara, GB (1998) HLA-C high resolution typing: analysis of exons 2 and 3 by sequence based typing and detection of polymorphisms in exons 1-5 by sequence specific primers. *Tissue Antigens* **52**: 251-259

Dunn, PPJ, Day, S, Harvey, J, Fuggle, SV and Ross, J (1998) Identification of an HLA-C variant allele, Cw*0805, by sequencing based typing. *Tissue Antigens* **52**: 587-589

Eberle, M, Knapp, LA, Iwanga, KK, Domanico, MJ, Aiyer, K, *et al.* (1997) HLA-B typing by allele separation followed by direct sequencing. *Tissue Antigens* **49**: 365-375

Ellexson, M, Stewart, D, Chretien, L, Zhang, W and Hilderbrand, W (1996) Description of a modified sequencing strategy and the molecular characterization of HLA-B*8201. *Tissue Antigens* **47**: 438-441

Guethlein, LA, Bias, WB and Schmeckpeper, BJ (1993) New DP sequences: Three DPA1 and one DPB1. *Tissue Antigens* **41**: 269-272

Gyllensten, UB and Erlich, HA (1988) Generation of single-stranded DNA by the polymerase chain reaction and its application to direct sequencing of the *HLA-DQA* locus. *Proc Natl Acad Sci USA* **85**: 7652-7656

Harada, H, Kimura, A, Dong, RP, Xu, CP, Bhatia, K, *et al.* (1992) Sequencing and population analysis of four novel HLA-DPA1 alleles. *Hum Immunol* **35:** 173-178

Hemmatpour, SK, Dunn, PPJ, Evans, PR, Green, A and Howell, WM (1998) Functional characterization and exon 2-intron 2-exon 3 gene sequence of HLA-B*2712 as found in a British family. *Eur J Immunogenet* **25**: 395-402

Johnston-Dow, L, Chadwick, R, McGinnis, MD, Conrad, MP and Kronick, MN (1995) A strategy for direct sequence analysis of HLA class I genes. *BSHI/EFI 1995,* abstract 297

Kaneoka, H, Lee, DR, Hsu, KC, Sharp, GC and Hoffman, RW (1991) Solid-phase direct DNA sequencing of allele-specific polymerase chain reaction-amplified HLA-DR genes. *Biotechniques* **10:** 30-34

Kotsch, K, Wehling, J, Kohler, S and Blasczyk, R (1997) Sequencing of HLA class I genes based on the conserved diversity of the noncoding regions: sequencing-based typing of the HLA-A gene. *Tissue Antigens* **50**: 178-191

Maxam, AM and Gilbert, W (1977) A new method for DNA sequencing. *Proc Natl Acad Sci USA* **74**: 560-564

McGinnis, MD, Conrad, MP, Bouwens, AGM, Tilanus, MGJ and Kronick, MN (1995) Automated solid-phase sequencing of DRB region genes using T7 sequencing chemistry and dye-labeled primers. *Tissue Antigens* **46:** 173-179

Norgaard, L, Fugger, L, Jakobsen, BK and Svejgaard, A (1997) Sequencing-based typing of HLA-A locus using mRNA and a single locus-specific PCR followed by cycle-sequencing with AmpliTaqFS DNA polymerase, FS. *Tissue Antigens* **49**: 455-465

Petersdorf, EW and Hansen, JA (1995) A comprehensive approach for typing the alleles of the HLA-B locus by automated sequencing. *Tissue Antigens* **46:** 73-85

Petersdorf, EW, Stanley, JF, Martin, PJ and Hansen, JA (1994) Molecular diversity of the HLA-C locus in unrelated marrow transplantation. *Tissue Antigens* **44:** 93-99

Rozemuller, EH and Tilanus, MG (1996) A computerised method to predict the discriminatory properties for class II sequencing-based typing. *Hum Immunol* **46**: 27-34

Rozemuller, EH, Bouwens, AGM, Blast, B and Tilanus, MGJ (1993) Assigment of HLA-DPB alleles by computerised matching based upon sequence data. *Hum Immunol* **37:** 207-212

Rozemuller, EH, Bouwens, AGM, Van Oort, E, Versuis, LF, Marsh, SGE *et al.* (1995) Sequencing-based typing reveals new insight in HLA-DPA1 polymorphism. *Tissue Antigens* **45:** 57-62

Rozemuller, EH, Eliaou, JF, Baxter-Lowe, LA, Charron, D, Kronick, M *et al.* (1995) An evaluation of a multicentre study on HLA-DPB1 typing using solid-phase Taq-cycle sequencing chemistry. *Tissue Antigens* **46:** 96-103

Sanger, F and Coulson, AR (1975) A rapid method for determining sequences in DNA by primed synthesis with DNA polymerase. *J Mol Biol* **94**: 441-445

Sanger, F, Nicklen, S and Coulson, AR (1977) DNA sequencing with chain-terminating inhibitors. *Proc Natl Acad Sci USA* **74**: 5463-5467

Santamaria, P, Lindstrom, AL, Boyce Jacino, MT, Myster, SH, Barbosa, JJ *et al.* (1992) HLA class II 'typing': Direct sequencing of DRB, DQB, and DQA genes. *Human Immunology* **33:** 69-81

Santamaria, P, Lindstrom, AL, Boyce Jacino, MT, Myster, SH, Barbosa, JJ *et al.* (1993) HLA class I sequence-based typing. *Hum Immunol* **37:** 39-50

Savelkoul, PHM, de Bruyn-Geraets, DP and van den Berg-Loonen, EM (1995) High resolution HLA-DRB1 SSP typing for cadaveric donor transplantation. *Tissue Antigens* **45**: 41-48

Schaeffer, V and Charron, D (1997) Sequencing based typing for HLA DQA: a simple method for routine DQA typing. In: *HLA. Genetic diversity of HLA. Functional and Medical Implication.* Vol 2. (Ed. Charron, D), pp.367-369. EDK, Sevres, France

Scheltinga, SA, Johnston Dow LA, White CB, van der Zwan AW, Bakema JE *et al.* (1997) A generic sequencing based typing approach for the identification of HLA-A diversity. *Hum Immunol* **57**: 120-128

Spurkland, A, Knutsen, I, Markussen, G, Vartdal, F, Egeland, T *et al.* (1993) HLA matching of unrelated bone marrow transplant pairs: Direct sequencing of in vitro amplified HLA-DRB1 and -DQB1 genes using magnetic beads as solid support. *Tissue Antigens* **41:** 155-164

Tilanus, MGJ and Eliaou, JF (1997) HLA sequencing based typing. In: *HLA. Genetic diversity of HLA. Functional and Medical Implication.* Vol 1. (Ed. Charron, D), pp237-266. EDK, Sevres, France

Turner, S, Ellexson, ME, Hickman, HD, Sidebottom, DA, FernandezVina, A *et al.* (1998) Sequence-based typing provides a new look at HLA-C diversity. *J Immunol* **161**: 1406-1413

van der Viles, SA, Voorter CEM and van den Berg Loonen EM (1997) A reliable and efficient high resolution typing method for HLA-C using sequence-based typing. *Tissue Antigens* **52**: 558-568

Versluis, LF, Rozemuller, EH, Duran, K and Tilanus, MGJ (1995) Ambiguous DPB1 allele combinations resolved by direct sequencing of selectively amplified alleles. Novel HLA-DPB1 alleles detected in the Ethiopian population. *Tissue Antigens* **46:** 345-349

Versluis, LF, Rozemuller, EH, Tonks, S, Marsh, SGE, Bouwens, AGM *et al.* (1993) High-resolution HLA-DPB typing based upon computerized analysis of data obtained by fluorescent sequencing of the amplified polymorphic exon 2. *Hum Immunol* **38:** 277-283

Voorter, CEM, Rozemuller EH, de Bruyn Geraets, D, van der Zwan AW, Tilanus MGJ *et al.* (1997) Comparison of DRB sequence-based typing using different strategies. *Tissue Antigens* **49**: 471-476

Voorter, CEM, de Bruyn Geraets, D and van den Berg Loonen, EM (1997) High-resolution HLA typing for the DRB3/4/5 genes by sequence-based typing. *Tissue Antigens* **50**: 283-290

Voorter, CEM, Kik, MC and van den Berg Loonen, EM (1997) High-resolution HLA typing for the DQB1 gene by sequence-based typing. *Tissue Antigens* **51**: 80-87

CHAPTER 8

DNA CONFORMATIONAL ANALYSIS

J. R. Argüello and J. A. Madrigal
Anthony Nolan Research Institute
The Royal Free Hospital
Pond Street
London NW3 2QG, England

Introduction

A unique feature of MHC genes is their extensive polymorphism which is mainly encoded by hypervariable regions in exon 2 for HLA class II, and exon 2 and 3 for HLA class I alleles.

Comparison of HLA allelic sequences reveals a patchwork pattern where an individual allele comprises a unique combination of sequence motifs, each of which is shared with other alleles, and only a few alleles have a specific sequence that is not present in other alleles (Parham *et al.*, 1995). This feature of the HLA polymorphism has complicated the application of DNA-based methods that rely on sequence identification to type the HLA genes. An alternative approach, to overcome this problem, is the use of DNA conformational analysis methods which rely on the study of DNA behaviour in nondenaturing polyacrylamide gel electrophoresis (PAGE).

In this chapter, we give a brief description of conventional conformational techniques which have been used for HLA testing. We also describe, in more detail, a method that we have developed recently (Argüello *et al.*, 1998a).

Single strand conformation polymorphism (SSCP)

The SSCP method relies on the fact that single-stranded DNA, in solution, under certain conditions, has a defined secondary structure. This secondary structure is highly sequence-specific and is reflected by differences in the mobility of DNA in nondenaturing PAGE (Orita *et al.*, 1989). Mobility differences can be identified by using radiolabelled or fluorescently labelled primers in the PCR amplification, or by silver staining or ethidium bromide staining of the gel after electrophoresis.

The method typically involves group specific PCR amplification of a discreet segment of genomic DNA, melting of the PCR products, and analysis of the single strands on nondenaturing PAGE.

Polymorphic differences in strand mobility result from the effects of primary sequence changes on the folded structure of a single DNA strand. Because these conformational variations may be subtle, the success of any particular SSCP experiment depends heavily on: the particular nucleotide sequence of the DNA fragments being evaluated, their length and the optimisation of electrophoretic conditions to maximise differential migration among single-stranded DNA fragments. Investigators have used a variety of methods to improve the resolving power of SSCP, such as adding glycerol to polyacrylamide gels, reducing temperatures, increasing the length of the gel and using new polyacrylamide-derived matrix (Dean and Gerrard 1991).

The main application of SSCP in HLA testing has been as a matching technique for bone marrow donor selection (Pursall *et al.,* 1996, Clay *et al.,* 1995). However, it has also been used in combination with SSP for HLA genotyping (Lo *et al.*, 1992).. This involves selection of specific polymorphisms by group specific amplification followed by analysis of allelic variation within each group by SSCP (Hoshino *et al.*, 1992). New HLA alleles have also been identified by this method (Blasczyk *et al.*, 1995a).

The major advantages of SSCP are that it is relatively simple to use, no great technical skills are required, it is inexpensive, no complex enzymatic or chemical reactions are required after PCR amplification, it does not necessarily require expensive instrumentation and can offer high sample throughput.

Although SSCP is the most widely used technique for mutation detection, its application for HLA testing has been restricted by:

- limitations in the length of the DNA fragment to be analysed; the optimal size fragment for sensitive base substitution detection by SSCP is approximately 150 bp, although larger DNA fragments can be used when detection of all potential single nucleotide substitutions is not crucial for the analysis (Sheffield *et al.*, 1993).
- the potential generation of multiple conformations per DNA fragment under identical conditions, as single stranded-DNA fragments with identical nucleotide sequences can adopt several stable conformations resulting in complex banding patterns after electrophoresis.
- poor reproducibility of results due to inter and intra gel variability; which may be the result of small changes in the electrophoresis conditions such as temperature, running time, gel composition, etc.
- the subjective interpretation of electrophoretic banding patterns due to differences in band intensities.
- inability to detect all possible variants.

Methods for SSCP

The method has been described for some HLA loci by Carrington *et al.*, (1992), Lo *et al.*, (1992) and Blasczyk *et al.*, (1995b). For detailed suggestions about how to optimise SSCP reactions, refer to articles such as Sheffield *et al.*, (1993) and Spinardi *et al.*, (1991). To find optimal conditions for SSCP analysis, we suggest adjusting the concentration of polyacrylamide and percentage of glycerol in the gel (from 0% up to 20%) and running the gel at different temperatures (from 4°C to 30°C).

- It is critical to use PCR conditions which minimise unwanted side products, as these can result in artefact bands which interfere with the identification of SSCP bands
- Use only highly purified, salt free template DNA. Salt concentration affect DNA mobility in nondenaturing PAGE
- Do not use degenerate primers to generate PCR templates for SSCP analysis.
- Use the minimum number of PCR cycles to obtain a sufficient quantity of PCR product, usually 30 cycles (or fewer) on 100 ng of genomic DNA.
- The products of amplification reactions must be evaluated for purity by electrophoresis in highly resolving agarose gels.
- Mix equal amounts of PCR product (50-100 ng/µl of DNA) and 95% formamide loading dye (95% formamide, 20 nM EDTA, 0.05% bromophenol blue and 0.05% xylene cyanol, for fluorescently labelled SSCP use dextran blue instead).
- Denature by heating at 95°C for 5 minutes.
- Quickly cool on ice and load 1-20µl of sample, depending on the detection system used.
- Electrophorese DNA under conditions previously determined.
- DNA bands can be identified by ethidium bromide, silver staining, autoradiography or laser, depending on the detection system used.

Heteroduplex analysis

The heteroduplex analysis technique exploits the formation of mismatched DNA duplexes (heteroduplexes), which are formed mainly during the final cycles of the PCR reaction, between coamplified alleles from a particular locus or loci due to primer cross-reaction at sites with similar sequences. During PCR amplification, at the annealing stage of each cycle, a proportion of sense strands of each allele may anneal to anti-sense strands of different allele(s). The resulting molecules contain double-stranded regions in which the nucleotide sequence is complementary but regions of nucleotide sequence mismatch lead to the formation of loops and bulges along the length of the DNA molecule. These cause it to kink, producing a 'drag effect' of the DNA bands during electrophoresis in non-denaturing polyacrylamide gel. Because the molecular conformation of heteroduplexes vary, they may be separated from each other and from the corresponding homoduplexes, thus the banding pattern obtained in PAGE analysis can be useful to compare HLA alleles of a particular donor and recipient in a crossmatch test. Here, genomic DNAs from patient and potential donor are mixed and coamplified in the PCR and the resulting PCR fingerprint is compared with those obtained by separate PCRs for each individual. Matching PCR fingerprints from all three products indicates HLA identity, whereas mismatch is indicated by different patterns and/or the appearance of new heteroduplexes formed by one strand of an allele of donor origin and a second strand from a different allele of recipient origin. The sensitivity of this method can be enhanced by adding PCR product from an HLA allele that is not present in the donor or recipient after the amplification of the samples but before the final annealing stage, this third party PCR product generates new heteroduplexes between otherwise similar PCR fingerprints (Bidwell 1992). However, by doing that the banding pattern may become very complex and difficult to interpret. The presence of multiple duplexes can be overcome by incorporating a label e.g. radioisotope or biotin into one of the strands of the known reference PCR product (Zimmerman *et al.*, 1993) or by isolating single strands from both the tested sample and the known reference PCR product (Argüello *et al.*, 1997).

DNA heteroduplex analysis has been successfully employed in the analysis of HLA class I genes (Martinelli *et al.*, 1996), HLA-DRB (Sorrentino *et al.*, 1991, Bidwell and Hui 1990), DQA1 and DQB1 (Zimmerman *et al.*, 1993 and Carrington *et al.*, 1992) and DPB1 (Clay *et al.*, 1994). In the case of HLA class I genes, heteroduplexes are formed due to coamplification of HLA-A, B, C, E, F, G, H and J. In HLA-DRB, heteroduplexes are formed due to the hybridisation of divergent DRB genes on all DR haplotypes except DR8 (Wood *et al.*, 1991). In HLA-DQA1 and DQB1, heteroduplexes may be formed between PCR products from these loci and, respectively, the DQA2 and DQB2 pseudogene loci. For HLA-DPB1, PCR products may form DNA heteroduplexes if cross-matched with a synthetic molecule referred to as a universal heteroduplex generator (Clay *et al.*, 1994). Simultaneous SSCP and heteroduplex analysis has been described for HLA-A, B and C allotype matching with excellent results (Pursall *et al.*, 1996).

The major application of heteroduplex analysis in HLA testing has been as a rapid screening method for the selection of potential unrelated donor for patients awaiting bone marrow transplantation (Clay *et al.*, 1991), though it can be applied retrospectively to all types of allogeneic transplantation. It has also been used as a mean of separating HLA alleles before typing by conventional techniques (Argüello *et al.*, 1996)

The main advantages of heteroduplex analysis are that is fast, safe, cost-effective, can be easily performed by a routine laboratory, and requires no post-PCR manipulations other than polyacrylamide minigel electrophoresis. Another important advantage of heteroduplex analysis when compared with SSCP is that double stranded DNA appears to adopt a unique conformation under defined conditions, therefore only one band is detected for each duplex. In addition, longer DNA fragments can be analysed. The limitations of heteroduplex analysis are largely those of SSCP, with some additional constraints, for example, when a heteroduplex differs by only one or two mismatches from the homoduplex, the heteroduplex signal is difficult to distinguish due to the increased intensity of the homoduplex signal compared with the heteroduplex as detected by conventional electrophoresis analysis.

Methods for Heteroduplex analysis

PCR amplification

- A set of PCR primers for HLA-A, B and C and PCR conditions are as described by Pursall *et al.* (1996)
- Another set of primers for exon 2 analysis of HLA-A, B, C, E, F, G, H and J, and PCR conditions are as described by Martinelli *et al.* (1996)
- Primers and PCR conditions for HLA class II are as described in the Technical Handbook of the Twelfth International Histocompatibility Workshop

Polyacrylamide gel electrophoresis:

Conditions described are for the Mini-Protean II gel electrophoresis system (Bio-Rad):

- Pour a 12% nondenaturing polyacrylamide (29:1) minigel, using 1x TBE running buffer.
- Add 1µl of 30% ficoll loading buffer (30% Ficoll, 100mM EDTA, 0.05% bromophenol blue and 0.05% xylene cyanol) per 5µl of sample.
- Load 5-10µl of the mixture per well when staining with ethidium bromide.
- Electrophorese at 200 V for 90 to 95 min. The exact time will need to be determined experimentally; the homoduplex band should be allowed to migrate to within 0.5 cm of the end of the gel.
- Stain gels for 10-20 min in 1X TBE containing 0.5 µg/ml ethidium bromide, (destaining is not necessary) and examine using a UV transilluminator.

Reference strand mediated conformation analysis (RSCA)

The majority of the limitations of conventional SSCP and Heteroduplex analysis are derived from one shared factor, that is, the technology used to identify and analyse the results. We have developed a conformational method for high resolution HLA typing called Reference Strand mediated Conformation Analysis (RSCA) (Argüello *et al.*, 1998), which utilises simple DNA manipulations together with laser based instrumentation and computer software, to reproducibly detect differences in DNA conformation. This allows the discrimination of HLA alleles which differ by as little as one nucleotide substitution. RSCA resolves all described limitations of SSCP and Heteroduplex analysis. In addition, RSCA introduces new elements that provide qualitatively improved results and

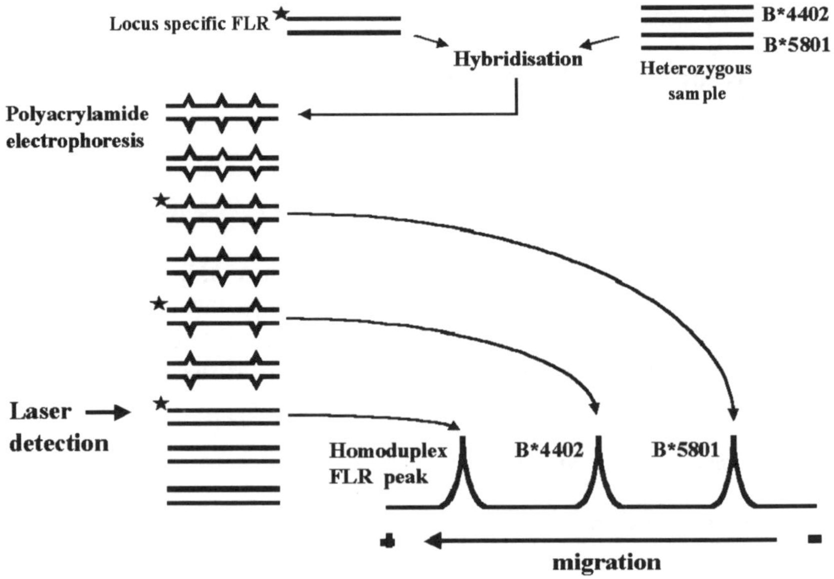

Figure 8.1. DNA from the locus of interest is amplified by PCR. The amplified product is hybridised with a locus specific "reference" DNA molecule. This reference molecule has been prepared such that the sense strand has a fluorescent label attached. Because of similarity between the reference DNA and the sample tested, duplexes will form between the sense and antisense strands of all the DNA molecules. However as the reference sense strand is labelled, only duplexes formed with this strand will be detected after electrophoresis in an automated DNA sequencer instrument with a laser detection system. For example as illustrated, for a heterozygous locus, three duplex "peaks" will be detected.

simplified data analysis, ensuring accuracy and reproducibility in the data generated in addition to HLA typing at the allelic level. A description of the RSCA technique is given in Figure 8.1.

Limitations of DNA conformational techniques and how these are resolved by RSCA

1. *Complex banding patterns*

RSCA utilises a locus specific fluorescent labelled reference (FLR) DNA molecule which is hybridised with the PCR products of the HLA locus to be tested. Because of similarity between the reference DNA and the sample tested, duplexes will form between the sense and antisense strands of all the DNA molecules present in the mixture. However, as only the reference sense strand is labelled, only duplexes formed with this strand will be identified by a laser detection system after electrophoresis in an automated DNA sequencer instrument. As the detected

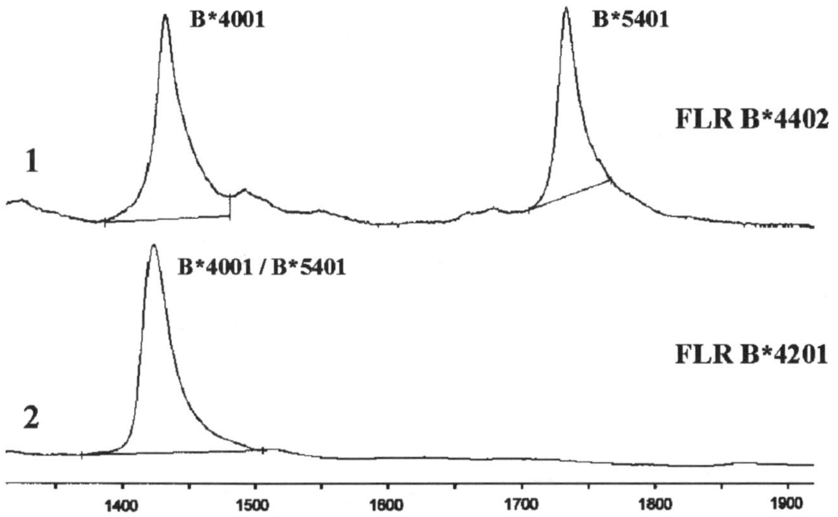

Figure 8.2. The use of two FLRs per sample improves the resolution of duplexes that, despite having different conformations, migrate at a similar rate when duplexed with one of the two FLRs. In lane 2, the HLA alleles B*4001 and B*5401 have overlapping mobilities when hybridised with the FLR B*4201, whereas in lane 1, using a different FLR, B*4402, their mobilities are significantly different.

duplexes have the FLR sense strand in common, the molecular conformation of each duplex generated is in principle unique, as each anti sense strand is different, therefore it is expected that the mobility of each duplex in most cases is also unique, allowing the separation of each HLA allele by electrophoresis. The number of heteroduplexes identified will always equal the number of HLA alleles present in the sample to be tested, in addition to the reference homoduplex band, thus simplifying the banding patterns to be interpreted (Figure 8.1).

2. *Inability to identify all variants*

Unlike other conformational techniques where the conformation of the DNA molecules cannot be manipulated, the use of a reference DNA molecule in RSCA allows control of duplex conformation as several reference strands can be tested in order to achieve optimal separation of difficult samples (Figure 8.2).

3. *Subjectivity of data analysis*

Variation in DNA duplex signal intensity within a sample or between samples may affect their detection and therefore analysis of the results. RSCA makes use of computer software which allows the sensitive analysis of duplexes covering a

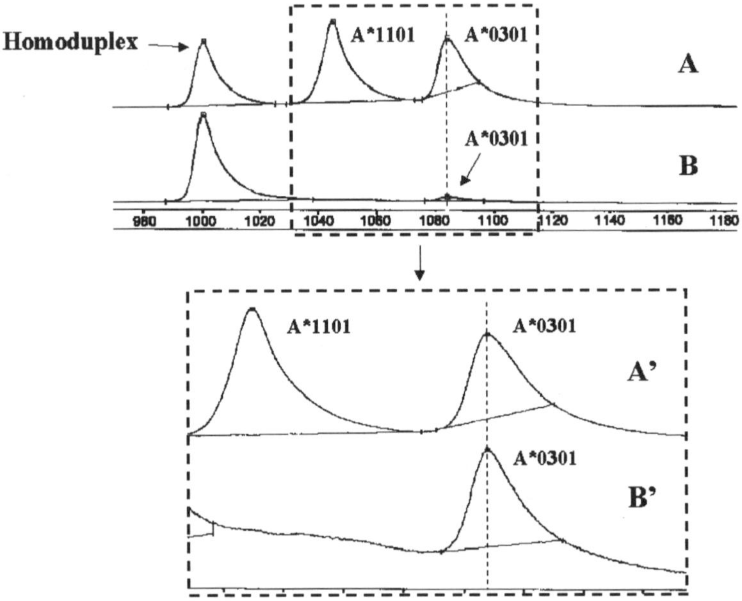

Figure 8.3. Variation in band intensity can be compensated for using computer software. In this example, Lane B, the HLA-A*0301 peak is much smaller than the homoduplex peak in the same lane, and the heteroduplex peaks in the adjacent lane A. Using the Pharmacia ALFexpress Fragment Manager software, the signal from the smaller peak can be amplified (lane B') to allow a direct comparison with duplexes from a different sample (lane A').

wide-spectrum of signal intensities. The same software can compensate for lane to lane variation in duplex band intensities, allowing direct comparisons of two bands with different intensities which otherwise would not be possible (Figure 8.3).

4. *Intra and intergel variability*

Variations in gel composition, buffer, temperature, etc., can affect the mobility of DNA molecules and this makes lane to lane and gel to gel comparisons difficult for conventional conformational analysis. For RSCA, internal control markers in each lane are used to generate a "mobility" scale. Using computer software, data from each lane and multiple gels can be normalised using the internal controls thus allowing direct comparisons (Figure 8.4). Intra and inter gel variability is also improved as described in Section 5.

5. *Limitations relating to distance travelled by DNA in polyacrylamide gels*

The resolution of DNA fragments depends on the effective distance that is migrated during electrophoresis. After conventional electrophoresis of DNA strands generated by Heteroduplex analysis and SSCP (duplexes and single-strands respectively), each DNA species will have migrated a different distance

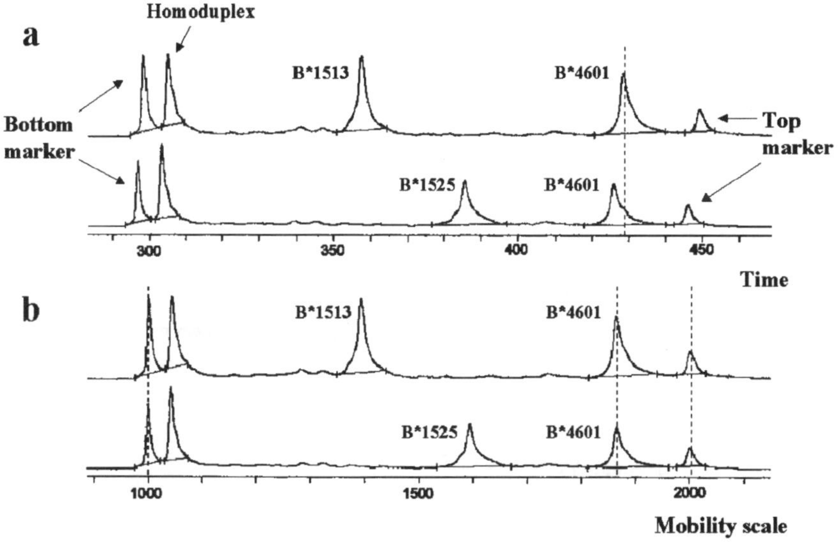

Figure 8.4. (a) Lane-to lane variation can create problems for comparison between lanes. The two lanes contain three constant fluorescent markers: the bottom marker, homoduplex and top marker. Each of these markers travels an identical distance before detection by the laser, but the time taken to travel this distance can vary, making a direct comparison between lanes for accurately defining the type of a DNA duplex (e.g. the B*4601 allele which is present in both lanes) difficult. Both samples depicted are heterozygous for HLA-B, and both share the A*4601 allele in addition to a different second allele, B*1513 and B*1525 respectively. (b) Using Fragment Manager or Allele Links software, arbitrary values can be assigned to the constant markers within each lane. The value of 1000 is assigned to the bottom marker, which in this example is the Cw*0701 homoduplex and the value of 2000 to the top marker B*4201/B*4501 heteroduplex peak. This allows the alignment of all markers with values of 1000 and 2000 in multiple lanes and results in the corresponding alignment of sample heteroduplex peaks as seen for allele B*4601.

whereas the time taken for migration will be constant for all DNA species. This reduces the resolution of DNA strands with slowest mobility, because they have migrated a reduced distance compared with those with faster mobility. In RSCA this problem is overcome by having the detection system at a particular point in the gel at which all measurements are performed (Figure 8.5). In this way each duplex is detected after having run an equal distance. Intra and inter gel variability is also significantly reduced by maintaining the ratio of mobility of each duplex constant in relation to control markers within each lane, as small variations in gel composition across a lane will affect all duplexes equally.

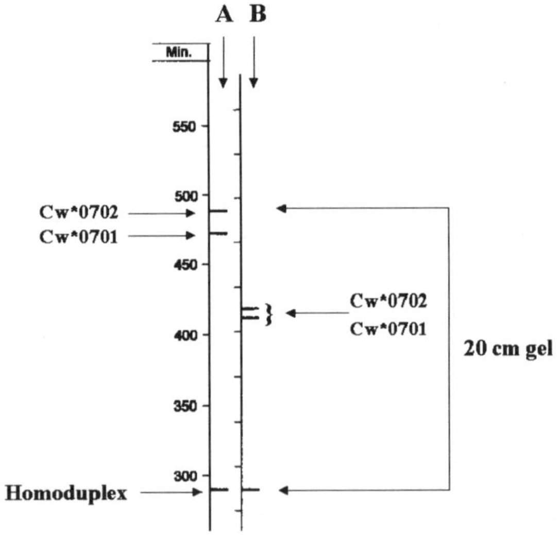

Figure 8.5. Comparison of the separation of duplexes by distance and time. The right hand scale (B) indicates the "banding" position of duplexes separated within 298 minutes, i.e. each duplex indicated as a band has travelled a different distance within 298 minutes. The scale on the left hand side (A) indicates the banding pattern obtained for the same sample in B except that each duplex has migrated an equal distance, 20cm, and the time taken to migrate this distance is indicated on the scale. The two heteroduplex "bands", representing HLA-Cw*0701 and Cw*0702 alleles, which differ by two coding nucleotides in a 909 base pair PCR product are clearly resolved better on scale A than scale B. The data in scale B has been generated by first calculating the rate of migration of duplexes separated by RSCA from scale A, and this represents the position of the heteroduplexes if the gel had been terminated at 298 minutes.

6. *Limitations related to quantity of loaded DNA*

The resolution of duplexes is inversely proportional to the quantity of loaded DNA. The detection systems used currently by SSCP and Heteroduplex analysis (ethidium bromide and silver staining) require a defined minimum amount of DNA for band identification. RSCA requires much less DNA because the detection system is laser based. Analysing low quantities of DNA improves not only the resolution of the duplex bands but also allows very accurate discrimination of duplexes which traverse the laser with time differences of less than one second. By using a sensitive DNA detection system, not only is sample volume reduced, thinner gels can be run thus allowing faster electrophoresis and higher resolution.

7. Discrimination of homoduplexes from heteroduplexes with only one or two mismatches

In conventional Heteroduplex analysis, when homoduplexes and heteroduplexes have similar mobilities, the homoduplex band which is generated from all the alleles present in the sample is always more intense than the heteroduplex bands created by the combination of strands from different alleles. Under these conditions resolution of duplexes is extremely difficult. This problem is overcome with RSCA by the introduction of a FLR DNA duplex such that the ratio between sample and FLR is controlled to allow specific increase in the heteroduplex signal with a concomitant reduction in the homoduplex signal. As only homoduplexes formed from the FLR are visualised, the intensity of this signal is reduced compared with the visualisation of multiple homoduplexes together. Thus heteroduplexes with similar mobility to the homoduplexes can be distinguished using RSCA (Figure 8.6).

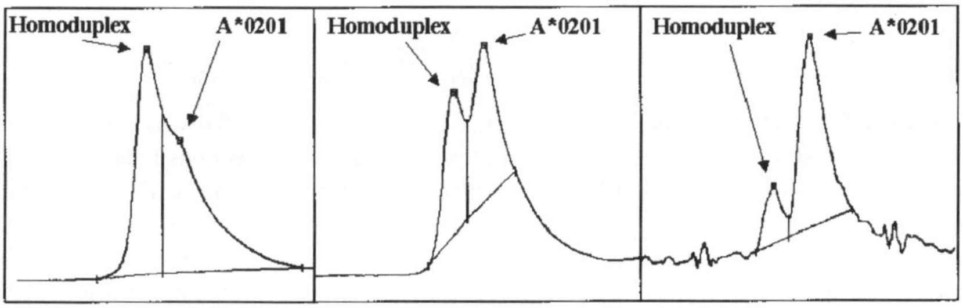

Ratio 1 : 1
FLR : sample

Ratio 1 : 2
FLR : sample

Ratio 1 : 3
FLR : sample

Figure 8.6. The ratio of labelled reference strand to sample, included in the hybridisation step affects the resolution of the heteroduplexes which have a similar mobility to the reference homoduplex. In the first figure, with a ratio of 1:1, the heteroduplex peak can barely be discriminated from the homoduplex peak. Resolution of the heteroduplex peak is improved with a ratio of 1:2 and even greater resolution is achieved with a ratio of 1:3 (reference to sample). This control over the sensitivity of the detection is particularly important when screening for variants which differ by a single nucleotide from the FLR.

RSCA has been developed as a 'one protocol' technique for HLA typing, which allows the assignment of allelic level type, including the identification of alleles differing by silent substitutions (Figure 8.7). At present RSCA has been applied as a typing method for HLA-A, B, C and DPB1 (Argüello *et al.*, 1998; Ramon *et al.*, 1998), and for high resolution HLA matching for DRB, DQA, DQB and DPA (Argüello *et al.*, 1998c). RSCA requires only one pair of PCR primers and two FLR DNAs per locus for the resolution of potentially all HLA alleles, with polymorphisms within exons 2 and 3 for HLA class I and exon 2 for HLA class II, including new alleles, without updating of reagents. One complete RSCA test

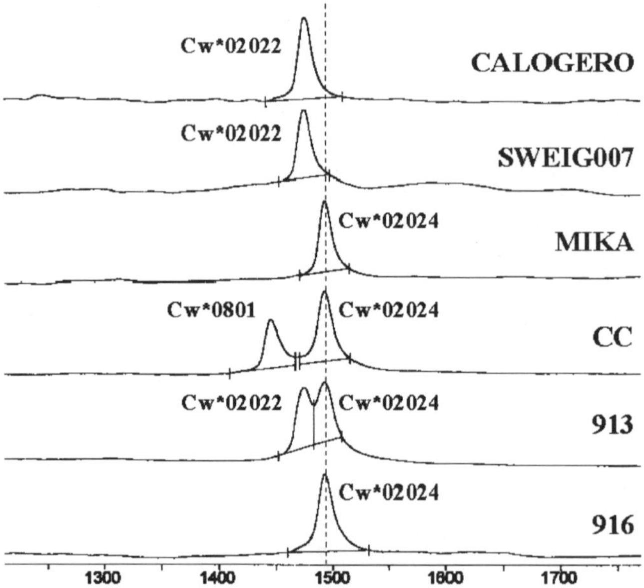

Figure 8.7. Six DNA samples sharing a HLA-C allele, typed originally as Cw*02, were analysed by RSCA and showed that this allele had two different positions in the gel when hybridised with the FLR Cw*0701. Sequencing of sample 913 demonstrated two subtypes of Cw*02, Cw*02022 and Cw*02024, which differ by a synonymous substitution at position 486 in exon 3. Cw*02022 has an adenine and Cw*02024 has a guanine. Sequence analysis of sample 916 demonstrated the presence of the Cw*02024 confirming the heteroduplex mobility for this allele. Samples sharing the Cw*02024 subtype (MIKA, CC, 913 and 916) share also an HLA-B allele (B*1503) suggesting strong linkage desequilibrium between these two alleles, whereas samples sharing Cw*02022 (CALOGERO, SWEIG007 and 913) do not share an HLA-B allele at all.

takes 12 hours, including PCR amplification, agarose gel electrophoresis to confirm presence of PCR product; FLR hybridisation and PAGE (in an ALFexpress, Pharmacia Biotech). Each gel can be re-used up to 5 times. Sample throughput can be increased by purification of the FLR PCR product to remove unincorporated labelled primer thus allowing re-loading of gel every two hours. With the exception of the initial cost of instrumentation, the cost of consumables required for RSCA is comparable with those utilised in other conformational techniques such as SSCP and heteroduplex analysis.

Methods for RSCA

Conditions described are for the ALFexpress electrophoresis instrument (Pharmacia Biotech).

1. PCR amplification

Reagents:

1.1. Master buffer:

☑ 10X NH_4 PCR buffer (Bioline UK).	169μl
☑ dNTPs (12.5mM each, Bioline UK)	12μl
☑ $MgCl_2$ (50mM)	34μl
☑ Distilled H_2O	435μl
Total volume	650μl

1.2. Amplification mixture (per 25μl mixture):

☑ 25 pmol/μl 5' primer	0.5μl
☑ 25 pmol/μl 3' primer	0.5μl
☑ Master buffer	8μl
☑ Taq polymerase (Bioline UK)	0.25μl
☑ Distilled H_2O	13.25μl
☑ DNA (200ng/μl)	2.5μl

1.3. Primers:

The primers used for amplification of HLA class I and II are as described (Cereb *et al.*, 1995 and Charron *et al.*, 1996).

1.4. Thermocycle conditions:

The same program is applied for HLA class I and II loci:

- Step 1: 95°C for 4 min.
- Step 2: 95°C for 30 sec.
- Step 3: 65°C for 50 sec.

- Step 4: 72°C for 30 sec.
- Step 5: Repeat steps 2-4, 32 times.
- Step 6: 72°C for 8 min.

After PCR reaction, run 5µl of the mixture on a 1.5% agarose gel to check for amplification product.

2. Preparation of FLRs:

Locus specific FLRs are prepared from homozygous B-LCLs by PCR as above except the 5' primer for each is labelled with the fluorochrome Cy5 at the 5' end at the time of primer synthesis (Pharmacia Biotech).

HLA-A:	A*0101	(STEINLIN)
	A*0217	(AMALA)
HLA-B:	B*4201	(RSH)
	B*4402	(SP0010)
HLA-C:	Cw*0303	(AMALA)
	Cw*0701	(STEILIN)
HLA-DRB:	DRB1*08021	(SPL)
	DRB1*0101	(plasmid pBActinNeo DRB1*0101 construct)
HLA-DQA1:	DQA1*0101	(KAS 116)
	DQA1*05011	(VAVY)
HLA-DQB1:	DQB1*0402	(BTB)
	DQB2 allele	(BTB)
HLA-DPA1:	DPA1*0103	(T5-1)
	DPA1*02011	(SAVC)
HLA-DPB1:	DPB1*0202	(QBL)
	DPB1*1501	(PLH)

The names in parenthesis are the International Histocompatibility cell lines from which the DNA is used as a template for FLR preparation. Two FLRs are utilised for each locus. For DQB1 analysis, one FLR is the DQB1 allele (DQB1*0402) and the second is the DQB2 allele from the same sample (Argüello *et al.*, 1998c).

3. Hybridisation reaction:

- In a new PCR tube, mix 1µl of each FLR with 3µl of the respective sample PCR product.
- Place PCR tubes in the thermal cycle and perform the following program:

  95°C for 4 min
  55°C for 5 min (to allow reannealing)
  15°C for at least 3 min

- After hybridisation, 0.8µl of 6X Ficoll loading buffer (15% Ficoll, 0.25% bromophenol blue) is added to each tube for HLA-Cw and HLA class II loci. 2µl of this mixture can then loaded in PAGE.
- For HLA-A and B analysis, duplexes are mixed with 2µl of special loading buffer which contain two internal DNA markers and is prepared as described in (4) and (5) below.

4. Preparation of top and bottom marker duplexes for HLA-A typing

- A-locus internal markers used with samples generated with both A*0101 and A*0217 FLRs are prepared as follows.
- The B*5701 allele is amplified by PCR from DNA from the cell line DEM, using unlabelled primers.
- The PCR product is hybridised to the fluorescent labelled B*4201 reference DNA as described above in 'hybridisation reaction' at the ratio of 1:3 (B*4201:B*5701), and mixed with an equal volume of 6X Ficoll loading buffer as described above.
- 2µl of this special loading buffer is added to the appropriate A locus specific sample prior to electrophoresis.
- 2µl of the final mixture can be loaded in the polyacrylamide gel.

5. Preparation of top and bottom marker duplexes for HLA-B typing

- B locus markers for use with samples generated with the B*4201 FLR are prepared by amplifying the B*4601 allele from the cell line TAB089 and hybridising with the fluorescent labelled B*4402 reference DNA at ratio of 1:3 (B*4402:B*4601).
- B locus markers to be used with samples generated with the fluorescent labelled B*4402 reference DNA are prepared by amplifying the B*4501 allele from the cell line OMW and hybridising with the B*4201 reference DNA at a ratio 1:3 (B*4201:B*4501).

6. Post-hybridisation treatment

- After these independent hybridisations, which are performed in a total volume of 160µl, 10µl of fluorescent labelled Cw*0701 PCR product from the cell line STEINLIN, and 170µl 6X Ficoll loading buffer are added.
- 2µl of this special loading buffer is added to the appropriate B locus specific sample prior electrophoresis.
- 2µl of the final mixture can be loaded in the polyacrylamide gel.

7. Preparation of non-denaturing polyacrylamide gel

- Before preparing the gel, clean the plates with 10% Synperonic N detergent (BDH, UK), scrubbing with a brush to ensure that any residual polyacrylamide is removed from the plates.
- Dry the plates with lint-free tissue.
- Wipe the plates (standard size), spacers (0.5mm) and comb (0.5mm) with 96% ethanol .
- Apply bind Silane solution to the top half of both plates.
- The plates can now be clipped together, the comb inserted and fixed with bulldog clips.

7. 1. Bind Silane:

☑ 200ml ethanol (96%)

☑ 300µl acetic acid

☑ 40µl bind Silane (Pharmacia)

7.2. Gel for HLA class I analysis (6% final concentration):

☑ 9.6ml Long Ranger™ Gel solution (FMC BioProducts USA)

☑ 8ml 10X TBE buffer (BioWhittaker, MD, USA)

☑ 61.84ml H_2O

☑ 48µl TEMED (Pharmacia Biotech)

☑ 480µl 10% ammonium persulphate* (Pharmacia Biotech)

7.3. Gel for HLA class II analysis (0.5X MDE solution final concentration):

☑ 20 ml MDE solution (FMC BioProducts USA)

☑ 8ml 10X TBE buffer (BioWhittaker, MD, USA)

☑ 51.5 ml H_2O

☑ 48μl TEMED (Pharmacia Biotech)

☑ 480μl 10% ammonium persulphate* (Pharmacia Biotech)

*Prepare this just before making the gel.

- The TEMED and ammonium persulphate should be the final components added when preparing the gel solution. Care should be taken not to introduce any air bubbles into the solution. A 50ml syringe should be used to mix and load the solution into the bottom of the gel plates, moving slowly from side to side.
- Leave to polymerise for 45 min at room temperature, then lift plates onto position on the ALFexpress instrument, add 1 litre of 1X TBE buffer in the top and bottom container and leave for 2 hours at 40°C.

8. Electrophoresis

Electrophoresis is performed in an ALFexpress automated sequencer (Pharmacia Biotech), at 30W constant power. Running times are 580 min and 300 min for HLA class I and class II respectively. The gels can be reused up to five times, but the running buffer (1X TBE) must be changed for each run. Warm the running buffer to 40°C before electrophoresis, as any slight temperature difference in the buffer and the gel may alter the mobility of the heteroduplex affecting the reproducibility in the results. The gel temperature is maintained at 40°C during electrophoresis by an external cooling system (Pharmacia Biotech).

9. Analysis of results

The mobilities of each fluorescent duplex are analysed using either Fragment Manager™ or Allele Links™ programs (Pharmacia Biotech). The apex position of each peak is assigned a value based on scales generated between markers in each lane. For HLA-A and B analysis the bottom and top markers are assigned the values of 1000 and 2000 respectively. For HLA-C and class II loci analysis, the value of 1 is assigned to the high mobility fluorescent primer signal and 1000 to the fastest duplex signal, which in all cases is the fluorescent reference homoduplex. The position of sample fluorescent heteroduplexes is computed from the mobility scales generated. These marker values are also used for alignment of tracks across each gel.

For more detailed information about how to use Fragment Manager™ and Allele Links™ programs, refer to user manual (Pharmacia Biotech).

Acknowledgements

The authors thank Andrea Pay, Mark Lowdell and Alasdair McWhinnie for helpful discussions.

References

Argüello JR, Little A-M, Pay A, Gallardo D, Rojas I, *et al.* (1998a) Mutation detection and typing of polymorphic loci through double-strand conformation analysis. *Nature Genetics* **18**:192-194

Argüello, R, Pay, AL, McDermott, A, Ross, J, Dunn, P, *et al.* (1997) Complementary strand analysis: a new approach for allelic separation in complex polyallelic genetic systems. *Nucl Acids Res* **25**: 2236-2238

Argüello, R, Avakian, H, Goldman, JM and Madrigal, JA. (1996) A novel method for simultaneous high resolution identification of HLA-A, HLA-B, and HLA-Cw alleles. *Proc Natl Acad Sci USA* **93**: 10961-10965

Argüello, JR, Little, A-M, Bohan, E, Goldman, J, Marsh, S, *et al.* (1998b) High resolution HLA class I typing by Reference Strand Mediated Conformation Analysis (RSCA). *Tissue Antigens* **52**: 57-66

Argüello, JR, Little, A-M, Bohan, E, Gallardo, D, O'Shea, J. *et al.* (1998c) A high resolution HLA class I and II matching method for bone marrow donor selection. *Bone Marrow Transpl* **22**: 527-534

Bidwell, JL (1992) Applications of the polymerase chain reaction to HLA class II typing. *Vox Sang* **63**: 81-89

Bidwell, JL and Hui, K. (1990) Human HLA-DR-Dw allotype matching by analysis of HLA-DRB gene PCR product polymorphism (PCR fingerprints). *Technique* **2**: 93-101

Blasczyk, R, van Lessen, A, Schwella, N, Huhn, D and Salama, A. (1995a) A novel HLA-DR13 allele (DRB1*1314) identified by single-strand conformation polymorphism analysis and confirmed by direct sequencing. *Hum Immunol* **43**: 309-12

Blasczyk, R, Hahn, U, Wehling, J, Huhn, D and Salama, A. (1995b) Complete subtyping of the HLA-A locus by sequence-specific amplification followed by direct sequencing or single-strand conformation polymorphism analysis. *Tissue Antigens* **46**: 86-95

Carrington, M, Miller, T, White, M, Gerrard, B, Stewart, C. *et al.* (1992) Typing of HLA-DQA1 and DQB1 using DNA single-strand conformation polymorphism. *Hum Immunol* **33**: 208-212

Cereb, N, Maye, P, Lee, S, Kong, Y and Yang, SY. (1995) Locus-specific amplification of HLA class I genes from genomic DNA: locus specific sequences in the first and third introns of HLA-A, B and C alleles. *Tissue Antigens* **45**: 1-11

Charron, D, Fauchet, R. (1996) *Twelfth International Histocompatibility Workshop Technical Handbook*

Clay, TM, Bidwell, JL, Howard, MR and Bradley BA. (1991) PCR-fingerprinting for selection of HLA matched unrelated marrow donors. *Lancet* **337**: 1049-1052

Clay, TM, Culpan, D, Howell, WM, Sage, DA, Bradley BA. *et al.* (1994) UHG crossmatching. A comparison with PCR-SSO typing in the selection of HLA-DPB1-compatible bone marrow donors. *Transplantation* **58**: 200-207

Clay, TM, Pursall, MC, Culpan, D, Bradley BA and Bidwell, JL. (1995a) DNA conformation analyses for rapid semiautomated matching of HLA class I and class II for transplantation. *Transpl Proc* **27**: 671-674

Clay, TM, Culpan, D, Pursall, MC, Bradley, BA and Bidwell, JL. (1995b) HLA-DQB1 and DQA1 matching by ambient temperature PCR-SSCP. *Eur J Immunogenet* **22**: 467-478

Dean, M and Gerrard B. (1991) Helpful hints for the detection of single-stranded conformation polymorphisms. *BioTechniques* **10**: 332-333

Hoshino, S, Kimura, A, Fukuda, Y, Dohi, K and Sasazuki, T. (1992) Polymerase chain reaction—single-strand conformation polymorphism analysis of polymorphism in DPA1 and DPB1 genes: a simple, economical, and rapid method for histocompatibility testing. *Hum Immunol* **33**: 98-107

Lo, YM, Patel, P, Mehal, WZ, Fleming, KA, Bell, JI. *et al.* (1992) Analysis of complex genetic systems by ARMS-SSCP: application to HLA genotyping. *Nucl Acids Res* **20**: 1005-1009

Martinelli, G, Farabegoli, P, Buzzi, M, Panzica, G, Zaccaria, A. *et al.* (1996) Fingerprinting of HLA class I genes for improved selection of unrelated bone marrow donors. *Eur J Immunogenet* **23**: 55-65

Orita, M, Iwahana, H, Kanazawa, H, Hayashi, K and Sekiya T. (1989) Detection of polymorphisms of human DNA by gel electrophoresis as single-strand conformation polymorphisms. *Proc Natl Acad Sci USA* **86**: 2766-2770

Parham, P, Adams, EJ and Arnett HL. (1995) The Origins of HLA-A, B, C Polymorphism. *Immunol Rev* **143**: 141-180

Pursall, MC, Clay, TM and Bidwell, JL. (1996) Combined PCR-heteroduplex and PCR-SSCP analysis for matching of HLA-A, -B and -C allotypes in marrow transplantation. *Eur J Immunogenet* **23**: 41-53

Ramon, D, Argüello, JR, Cox, ST, McWhinnie, A, Shah, A, *et al.* (1998) Application of RSCA for the typing of HLA-DPB1. *Hum Immunol* **59**: 734-747

Sheffield, VC, Beck, JS, Kwitek, AE, Sandstrom, DW and Stone, EM. (1993) The sensitivity of single-strand conformation polymorphism analysis for the detection of single base substitutions. *Genomics* **16**: 325-332

Sorrentino, R, Iannicola, C, Costanzi, S, Chersi, A and Tosi, R. (1991) Detection of complex alleles by direct analysis of DNA heteroduplexes. *Immunogenetics* **33**: 118-123

Spinardi, L, Mazars, R and Theillet, C. (1991) Protocols for an improved detection of point mutations by SSCP. *Nucl Acids Res* **19**: 4009

Wood, NAP, Clay, TM and Bidwell, JL. (1991) HLA-DR/Dw matching by PCR fingerprinting: the origin of PCR fingerprints and further applications. *Eur J Immunogenet* **18**: 147-153

Zimmerman, PA, Carrington, MN and Nutman TB. (1993) Exploiting structural differences among heteroduplex molecules to simplify genotyping the DQA1 and DQB1 alleles in human lymphocyte typing. *Nucl Acids Res* **21**: 4541-4547

CHAPTER 9

MICROSATELLITE TYPING

Anne Cambon-Thomsen and Alexandra Foissac
INSERM U 518
Faculté de Médecine
37 allées Jules Guesde
31073, Toulouse Cedex, France

Pilar Giraldo-Alvarez
Unitat d'Antropologia
Departament de Biologia Animal Biologia Vegetal i Ecologia
Facultat de Ciencies
Universitat Autonoma de Barcelona
08193 Bellaterra (Barcelona) Spain.

Brigitte Crouau-Roy
CNRS ERS 1590
Hôpital Purpan
Avenue de Grande Bretagne
31059 Toulouse Cedex, France

Introduction

Since the 1970s, the presence of DNA sequence stretches of repeated elements in the eukaryotic genomes has been demonstrated. A general term for these tandemly repeated DNA sequences is Variable Number of Tandem Repeats (VNTR); however numerous studies of such polymorphic genetic markers have allowed the definition of classes of repeat sequences according to the size and the composition of the repeated elements:

- minisatellites: often called VNTR when first described; generally greater than 6bp repeats
- microsatellites or simple sequences (Tautz, 1993); 1bp to 6bp repeats

Microsatellites

Microsatellites are also referred to as Short Tandem Repeats (STR), Simple Sequence Repeats (SSR), simple sequence length polymorphisms (SSLPs). They comprise a base motif (1-6 nucleotides) repeated in tandem up to 100 times or more and are characterised by extensive polymorphism, ubiquitous distribution all over the genome and a Mendelian co-dominant inheritance (Koreth *et al.,* 1996). The role of microsatellites in the genome and their evolutionary mechanisms are still incompletely known. Nevertheless, microsatellites are already widely used as powerful tools for genetic mapping (Dib *et al.,* 1996), population genetics (see review in Bruford and Wayne, 1993), linkage analysis (Hearne *et al.,* 1992), evolutionary studies (Rubinztein *et al.,* 1995a; 1995b; Broman *et al.,* 1998) and forensic medicine (Mayr, 1995; Weber, 1999).

Microsatellites represent a source of useful markers because of their abundance, their high allelic polymorphism and the simplicity of the methodologies involved for their typing. In the human genome, simple sequences consist of repeats of: A, CA, AAAN, AAN, or AG, in decreasing order of their frequency (Hearne *et al.,* 1992) and microsatellites seem uniformly distributed with approximately one microsatellite every 10 kb of DNA (Tautz, 1989) and one CA repeat every 30-60 kb (Hearne *et al.,* 1992; Weber and Mayr, 1989). It is thus not surprising to find a majority of CA microsatellites also in the HLA region. In humans, roughly 10,000 microsatellites have been described (Dib *et al*., 1996; Broman *et al*., 1998). Interest in such polymorphic genetic markers in linkage disequilibrium with HLA genes has provoked investigations on microsatellites in the human MHC. In this chapter, we present a summary of practical available information concerning microsatellites in the HLA region. This summary is based mainly on two previous reviews (Foissac *et al*., 1997 ; Foissac and Cambon-Thomsen, 1998) with some technical and bibliographical updates.

HLA region microsatellites

A number of microsatellites have been described and characterised within or close to the HLA region. Using literature information (1980-1998) and electronic databases (Whitehead database, **http://www-genome.wi.mit.edu/**, Genome database, **http://www.gdb.org/** and CEPH database, **http://www.cephb.fr/**, a set of 103 microsatellites with a certain degree of characterisation was published in 1998 (Foissac and Cambon-Thomsen, 1998). According to the general characteristics of short tandem repeats (STR), microsatellites located in the HLA region show allele sizes varying between 79 and 473 bp. However, allele size depends only on the primers chosen for PCR amplification; thus the size of the microsatellite allele obtained after electrophoresis does not constitute an intrinsic characteristic of the STR. The polymorphism of a microsatellite depends on variation of the number of repeats, number of alleles and their distribution. It is quantified using parameters like Polymorphism Information Content (PIC) or Percentage of Heterozygosity, calculated from the number of alleles and their frequencies in a population (Hearne *et al*., 1992). Heterozygosity is calculated as:

$Het = 1 - \Sigma i\ pi^2$, where pi = frequency of the ith allele in the population

Polymorphism information content (PIC) is:

$1 - \Sigma i\ pi^2 - \Sigma ij\ 2\ pi^2.pj^2$, where pi and pj are respectively the frequency of allele i^{th} and j^{th} in the population.

A marker is considered as reasonably informative when the number of alleles is greater than five and the PIC or heterozygosity value is above 0.75.

When evaluating the polymorphism of these microsatellites, an average number of 8.5 alleles is observed, with the number of alleles ranging from 2 to 20, associated with a mean value for polymorphism information content (PIC) of 68.5%, or a mean value for heterozygosity of 0.70. Table 9.1 shows some information about 31 of these microsatellites, chosen with the following criteria: 10 or more alleles, 80% heterozygosity and/or used in numerous or key publications about the use of microsatellites in the HLA region. However, our knowledge of microsatellites in the HLA region is increasing very rapidly: 53 among these 103 microsatellites were described between 1996 and 1998, including 29 dinucleotide repeats (mostly CA repeats,), 6 trinucleotide repeats, 8 tetranucleotide repeats, one pentanucleotide repeat and 5 complex repeat motifs. In 1999 Shiina *et al.* from the group of Inoko in Japan reported that, by systematic sequencing of 1.8kb between HLA-F to MIC-B, they found 758 microsatellites (among them, 197 dinucleotides, 134 trinucleotides, 206 tetranucleotides, 134 pentanucleotides). Among 70 of those which were polymorphic, 38 had more than 5 alleles. Apparently only two in this series had already been described previously (Shiina *et al.*, 1999). It thus becomes near impossible to maintain an updated map of such numerous markers. A Figure published in a report by Foissac and Cambon-Thomsen (1998) gives the approximate localisation of 103 microsatellites in or close to the HLA region. It is not feasible to update the printed version of the integrated map of markers in the HLA region; however, a non-exhaustive list of Web sites containing useful information which is regularly updated is given below:

http://compbio.ornl.gov/tools/channel/index.html: this site links to numerous molecular and genetic databases and is very useful and well documented;

www.citi2.fr/GENATLAS: recently updated, this site provides summary integrated maps and offers good links with other databases;

www.gdb.org: a very useful and regularly updated database. It provides a detailed map with a maximum of information on the various markers;

www.ncbi.nlm.nih.gov/genemap99: this site provides various kinds of maps;

www.généthon.fr: starts from the Genethon map with good links to other sites;

http://carbon.wi.mit.edu:8000/cgi-bin/contig/phys_map: allows access to a number of different maps, but with less information than in the first site listed;

http://star.scl.kyoto-u.ac.jp: A Japanese site very well documented for Chromosome 6. It also provides software to be downloaded in order to draw maps.

MICROSATELLITE	LOCATION	Size Range Repeat Number of alleles PIC (Het)	PCR Primers	REFERENCES
D6S1691 AFMa052vh1 z51673	6p 42.7 cM Tel. (8500 kb) / HLA-B Est Mb from telomere: 27.63	213-251 CA (Allele 215: CA_{16}) 15 85%	Pr CA: AGGACAGAATTTTGCCTC Pr GT: GCTGCTCCTGTATAAGTAATAAAC Fragment size: 215 bp	Genethon WDB Ajioka 1997
CA	6p [D6S105-D6S1260] region Tel. (480 kb) / D6S105 Centr. (140 kb) / D6S1260	195-225 CA (Allele: CA_{16}) 15 (0.88)	Pr CA: CTGGGAACTGATTTGAGAA Pr GT: AAGGGGTACGTACATTTGAAGT	Andrieux 1997
D6S105	6p22.1-p21.33 Tel. (2-3 cM) / HLA-A Tel. (1500-2500 kb) / HLA-A Tel. (4375 kb) / HLA-B Est Mb from telomere: 31.855	116-138 CA 10 - 12 81% (0.77-0.79)	Pr CA: GCCCTATAAAATCCTAATTAAC Pr GT: GAAGGAGAATTGTAATTCCG Fragment size: 131 bp	Ajioka 1997 Burt 1996 Camaschella 1996 Jazwinska 1995-1993 RahaChowdhury 1995 Worwood 1994 Weber 1991
MOGc	6p21.3-p22 Tel. (100 kb) / HLA-F Upstream MOG gene Est Mb from telomere: 34.279	122-150 CA (CA_{15}) 11 81%	Mog31: GAAATGTGAGAATAAAGGAGA Mog32: GATAAAGGGGAACTACTACA Fragment size: 132 bp	Roth 1995
RF "HLA-F"	6p21.3 Tel. (250 kb) / HLA-A 5' untranslated region of HLA-F	168-340 GAA (GAA_{22}) 19 (0.95)	RFa: CTGTCCTATTTCATATGCTCAGG RFb: ATGAACTTGTCCTGAGAATGAAG	Raha-Chowdhury 1994 Geraghty 1990

Table 9.1. Characteristics of 31informative microsatellites in the HLA region. For legend, see Page 274.

MICROSATELLITE	LOCATION	Size Range Repeat Number of alleles PIC (Het)	PCR Primers	REFERENCES
D6S273 AFM142xh6 z16657	6p 44.9 cM [Hsp70 - Bat2] region Between 2nd & 3rd exons of G6D	130-140 / 120-140 CA (Allele 135: CA_{19}) 6 - 8 75-76%	Pr CA: GCAACTTTTCTGTCAATCCA Pr GT: ACCAAACTTCAAATTTTCGG Fragment size: 135 bp	Genethon WDB Martin 1995 Ribas 1999
D6S276 AFM158ye9 z16711	6p 44.9 cM Tel. (6000 kb) / HLA-A [P5 - HLA-E] region Centr. / HLA-E Est Mb from telomere: 28.152	198-226 / 198-230 CA (Allele 205: CA_{12}) 10 - 14 83%	Pr CA: TCAATCAAATCATCCCCAGAAG Pr GT: GGGTGCAACTTGTTCCTCCT Fragment size: 205 bp	Genethon WDB Worwood 1997 Martin 1995 Bouissou 1995
D6S1666 AFMc019yc5 z54022	6p 45.4 cM Est Mb from telomere: 36.8	119-151 CA 13 86%	Pr CA: CTGAGTTGGGCAGCATTTG Pr GT: ACCCAGCATTTTGGAGTTG Fragment size: 133 bp	Genethon WDB
C3_2_12	6p21.3 MIC-C region Tel. (34 kb) / MIC-C Centr. (29 kb) / HLA-30	126-186 TG (Allele 174: TG_{37}-CG_2-CA_1) 19 0.89	Pr TG: TGTCATTCTGATCCAGGCAGGCATC Pr CA: GGAACTTGAGCAGTGAGCTCCTATG	Tamiya 1998
C3_2_11	6p21.3 [MIC-C - HLA-E] region Tel. (50 kb) / HLA-E Centr. (21 kb) / MIC-C	187-229 GA (Allele 213: GA_{22}-TA_1-GA_8) 17 0.85	Pr GA: AGATGGCATTTGGAGAGTGCAG Pr TC: TCCTTACAGCAGAGATATGTGG	Tamiya 1998
C1_4_4	6p21.3 [HLA-E - HLA-C] region Tel. (31 kb) / HLA-C Centr. (66 kb) / OTF3	364-440 GAAA (Allele 393: $GAAA_{10}$) 15 0.84	Pr GAAA: CAGCTGCTAGGTGTATCTGAATAC Pr TTTC: CAATAAGAAATTTTGCTATAAGGTAAG	Tamiya 1998
C1_4_3	6p21.3 [HLA-E - HLA-C] region Tel. (26 kb) / HLA-C Centr. (71 kb) / OTF3	413-473 GGAA (Allele 453: $GGAA_{18}$) 15 0.86	Pr GGAA: TAGAAAACGCAATCTCGGCC Pr TTCC: CTGGATTAACCTGGAGACTC	Tamiya 1998
C1_2_5	6p21.3 [HLA-C - HLA-B] region Tel. (62 kb) / HLA-B Centr. (19 kb) / HLA-C	178-220 CA (Allele 196: CA_4-AA_1-CA_{20}) 20 0.89	Pr CA: CAGTAGTAAGCCAGAAGCTATTAC Pr TG: AAGTCAAGCATATCTGCCATTTGG	Tamiya 1998

Table 9.1 (continued). Characteristics of 31informative microsatellites in the HLA region. For legend, see Page 274.

MICROSATELLITE	LOCATION	Size Range Repeat Number of alleles PIC (Het)	PCR Primers	REFERENCES
C1_2_C	6p21.3 [HLA-B - MIC-B] region Tel. (62 kb) / MIC-B Centr. (27 kb) / MIC-A	260-234 AC (Allele 108: AC_{11}) 14 0.84	Pr AC: GGATCCTAGGAACTCCCTCCTG Pr GT: GAGCAGAAGGGAGATGAAATGG	Tamiya 1998
MIB	6p21.3 Centr. (25 kb) / HLA-B Tel. (10 kb) / MIC-A	326-356 CA (CA_7 - CA_{23}) 12 83% (0.82)	Pr CA: CTACCATGACCCCCTTCCCC Pr GT: CCACAGTCTCTATCAGTCCA	Grimaldi 1996
TNFa	6p21.3 Tel. (3.5 kb) / TNF B Est Mb from telomere: 36.43	97-121 AC (AC_6 - AC_{18}) 13 0.86	IR1: GCACTCCAGCCTAGGCCACAGA IR2: GCCTCTAGATTTCATCCAGCCACA IR4: CCTCTCTCCCCTGCAACACACA	Udalova 1993 Jongeneel 1991 Nedospasov 1991
62 **TNFa - TNFb**	6p21.3 MHC Class III Tel. (7 kb) / LTA	146-197 TC-CA (TC10-CCT1-C5-TC3-C3-TGCAA1-CA15) 14 82.4% (0.821)		Hsieh 1997
82-1	6p21.3 MHC Class III G1 gene region (5' region)	86-113 CA (CA_{13}-CGCACG-CA_{15}) 13 81.3% (0.740)		Hsieh 1997
9N-3	6p21.3 MHC Class III G7 gene region	80-126 CA (CA_{17}) 13 80.6% (0.797)		Hsieh 1997
K11A	6p21.3 Region TNF - Hsp70	145-163 CA 10	Pr1: TGACTGCCCGCGTCTACTGCCTT Pr2: CCTTCACTGCCAGGCACCCCTT	D'Alfonso 1997 Colonna 1992 (HLA 1991)
R2A	6p21.3 Region TNF - Hsp70 Centr. / HLA-B	108-138 14		D'Alfonso 1997 Colonna 1992

Table 9.1 (continued). Characteristics of 31informative microsatellites in the HLA region. For legend, see Page 274.

MICROSATELLITE	LOCATION	Size Range Repeat Number of alleles PIC (Het)	PCR Primers	REFERENCES
BAT2 GT	6p21.3 [BAT1-BAT2] region Tel. / BAT2 Centr. (30 kb) / TNFa	 GT 12	BAT2A: CTCCAGCCTGGATAACAG BAT2B: ACAAGGGCTTTAGGAGGTCT	Gallagher 1997
DQ.CAR II	6p DQA1-DQB1 region Centr. (4-5 kb) / HLA-DQA1	186-218 CA 15	Pr CADQFF: TGATTCATAAGGC AAGAATCCAGCATATTGG Pr CADQR3: GCACTATCATT AAATTTGCTTTCCACAGTA	Mignot 1997
D6S2446 DQ-CAR II	6p [DQA1 - DQB1] region Tel. (7 kb) / HLA-DQB1	168 - 200 CA 13	Pr CA: GAGAATCCAGCATATTGGAG Pr GT: CACTATCATTAAATTTGCTTTCCAC	Ellis 1997
DQ.CAR	6p Centr. (10 kb) / HLA-DQA1 Tel. (2 kb) / HLA-DQB1	97-127 CA (CA_{11} - CA_{24}) 16 79%	CAR1: GAAACATATATTAACAGAGACAGACAAA CAR2: CATTTCTCTTCCTTATCACTTCATA Fragment size: 121 bp	Mignot 1997 Mignot 1995 Macaubas 1995
T16CAR	6p DQB3-DQB1 region	193-227 CA 14	Pr T16F: GATCTTGTTTGTAAAGCCATG Pr T16R: CATGACTCAGCCCCAACTC	Mignot 1997
TAP1	6p21.3 TAP region Intron 3 TAP1 gene Est Mb from telomere: 37.764	188-206 CA 6 (0.62)	Pr CA: GCTTTGATCTCCCCCCTC Pr GT: GGACAATATTTTGCTCCTGAGG	Carrington 1994
D6S1618 AFMb057yb1 z53240	6p 47.6 cM Est Mb from telomere: 35.72 - 35.85	132-164 CA 14 86%	Pr CA: GGCCTGAGCAGTGCAT Pr GT: TGATTCCTAATCTGCGGG Fragment size: 148 bp	Genethon WDB
D6S1560 AFMa205yd9 z52491	6p 47.6 cM Est Mb from telomere: 35.708	233-253 CA 11 84%	Pr CA: CTCCAGTCCCCACTGC Pr GT: CCCAAGGCCACATAGC Fragment size: 251 bp	Genethon WDB

Table 9.1 (continued). Characteristics of 31informative microsatellites in the HLA region. For legend, see Page 274.

MICROSATELLITE	LOCATION	Size Range Repeat Number of alleles PIC (Het)	PCR Primers	REFERENCES
D6S1568 AFMa222wb5 z52564	6p 47.6 cM	84-110 CA 12 87%	Pr CA: ACATGACCAGAACTTCCCAG Pr GT: AGCTAGGCCAGGCCGT Fragment size: 96 bp	Genethon WDB
D6S291 AFM203yg7 z16904	6p 49.8 cM [DPB1 - Glo] region RadHybMap: 222,75 cR	198-210 CA (Allele 199: CA_{11}) 7 70%	Pr CA: CTCAGAGGATGCCATGTCTAAAATA Pr GT: GGGGATGACGAATTATTCACTAACT Fragment size: 199-200 bp	Genethon WDB Martin 1995

Table 9.1 (continued). Characteristics of 31 informative microsatellites in the HLA region. The 31 markers have been chosen from the table published in Foissac *et al.,* (1998) and updated when new information was available, using the following criteria: 10 or more alleles, 80% heterozygosity and/or used in numerous or key publications about the use of microsatellites in the HLA region. MSAT (microsatellite; column 1): in this column, a maximum of three indicators are given: *locus symbol*, such as D6S299, which indicates the chromosome and a unique number, the *usual marker name* such as AFM217xg7 (for Genethon markers, see www.génèthon.fr) or the *original name* used in the first publication describing the marker (such as MOGa), and the *EMBL/GenBank accession number* such as Z16986, when available. LOCATION (column 2): according to available mapping data in molecular banks and publications: chromosome arm, band, distance (in cM) from the top of chromosome 6 linkage group (e.g. 41cM), more precise telomeric (tel) or centromeric (centr) localisation in respect of another marker. The physical distance in Mb (Megabases) from the telomere is also given when available in the Southampton genmap: see ftp://cedar.genetics.soton.ac.uk/pub/chrom6/gmap. INFORMATIVITY (column 3): shows several parameters regarding informativity of the markers: size range in base pairs (bp) reported to date; type of nucleotide repeat (CA, GT), if sequence available number of repeat units in the allele sequenced; number of alleles in the publications cited; polymorphism information content (PIC %) or heterozygosity values; in the markers reported by Genethon these two last parameters are estimated on 56 chromosomes. PCR PRIMERS (column 4): gives the sequence of the primers (Pr) used for the amplification of the microsatellites in the publications or database when indicated. When available, the fragment size on a reference individual is indicated. REFERENCES (column 5): for markers described in an electronically available database the following information is given: see Whitehead database (http://www-genome.wi.mit.edu/).

Clinical and research relevance

Microsatellites were first used in research applications, for example:

- genetics of diseases
- mutation rates
- various evolutionary characteristics
- recombination rate
- other population genetics parameters such as linkage disequilibrium or haplotype frequencies and structure of populations

More recently, however, they are increasingly used in a number of practical and clinical situations:

- forensic medicine
- population characteristics assessment
- diseases orientation diagnoses
- genetic instability evaluation in tumours
- chimerism evaluation in transplantation
- detection of residual leukaemic cells
- additional markers for HLA region compatibility

With respect to microsatellites in the HLA region and the genetics of diseases, a growing number of disease susceptibility studies using HLA microsatellite analysis is observed : more than 20 pathologies have been studied leading to numerous publications (see reviews: Foissac *et al.* 1997a; Foissac and Cambon-Thomsen, 1998; Foissac, 1999). Such studies involve different approaches, including:

- population genetic studies
- family studies
- association analysis
- linkage analysis
- linkage disequilibrium analysis
- genome screening
- investigations on specific disease patterns

The pathologies investigated using microsatellite analysis alone or in addition to HLA polymorphisms include:

- haemochromatosis
- insulin-dependent diabetes mellitus

- celiac disease
- Behçet's disease
- idiopathic nephrotic syndrome
- multiple sclerosis
- inflammatory bowel disease
- Crohn's disease
- asthma
- autosomal dominant cerebellar ataxia
- porphyria cutanea tarda
- rheumatoid arthritis (Singal *et al.,* 1998a, 1998b)
- early-onset pauciarticular juvenile chronic arthritis
- systemic lupus erythematosus
- ankylosing spondylitis (Yabuki *et al.,* 1999)
- IgA deficiency (Vorechovsky *et al.,* 1999)
- narcolepsy-cataplexy
- Hodgkin's disease
- schizophrenia
- clozapine-induced agranulocytosis
- follicular centre cell lymphoma
- colorectal cancer
- nasopharyngeal carcinoma

Several conclusions about the benefits provided by HLA microsatellite study can be drawn, including:

- the refinement of disease susceptibility locus mapping (e.g. haemochromatosis)
- the description or exclusion of additional genetic susceptibility or protection factors in the HLA region (e.g. celiac disease, Behçet disease, multiple sclerosis, early onset pauciarticular juvenile chronic arthritis, schizophrenia, agranulocytosis, colorectal cancer, nasopharyngeal carcinoma)
- a further knowledge of HLA region involvement in the genetic susceptibility or pathophysiology of the disease (insulin-dependent diabetes mellitus, rheumatoid arthritis, systemic lupus erythematosus, narcolepsy-cataplexy, follicular centre cell lymphoma)
- the detection of disease expression specificity (rheumatoid arthritis)
- the report of new syndromes (subtype of Crohn's disease)
- the discovery of disease association pattern through susceptibility similarity (haemochromatosis, porphyria cutanea tarda)

Some examples of new knowledge gained from HLA microsatellite studies include:

- perhaps the most famous example, the intensive studies involving a large panel of microsatellites that resulted in the localisation of the potential haemochromatosis gene, HFE (Feder *et al.*, 1996).
- more recently, the remarkable reduction of the Behçet disease critical region to a 46 kb segment centromeric to HLA-B, close or identical to the MIC-A gene, by association analysis using refined microsatellite mapping (Ota *et al.*, 1999)
- the correlation sometimes observed between functional properties and microsatellites such as a higher in vitro production of TNFα by macrophages from individuals having certain TNFa alleles (Pociot *et al* 1993), or a correlation between TNFa and CTLp frequencies in unrelated bone marrow donor-recipient pairs (Hanifi Moghaddam *et al.*, 1998).
- in insulin-dependent diabetes mellitus, the heterozygosity for TNFa is an additional risk factor and a second region within the MHC, in addition to the class II region, was shown to contribute to IDDM susceptibility, mapped in an interval of 200kb around the microsatellite locus D6S273 centromeric of TNF (Hanifi Moghaddam *et al.*, 1997; 1998 ; Lie *et al.* 1999)
- the association of given profiles of TNFa microsatellites with various degrees of severity of rheumatoid arthritis through interaction with HLA-DRB1 (Mu *et al* 1999).

These examples, as well as haplotype information merging microsatellites and HLA genes, may be particularly useful with regards to the HLA/disease component proposed and co-ordinated by E. Thorsby for the 13th International Histocompatibility Workshop (see Web site http://www.ihwc.org/components/). Here, the main ideas are to consider HLA associated diseases where one HLA component is sufficiently well known and where the direct involvement of HLA molecules in the pathophysiology of the disease is verified or highly probable; to select in various populations, cases and controls perfectly matched for the HLA markers known to be involved directly in the disease; and to type them for other markers of the HLA region, especially microsatellites, in order to detect additional susceptibility factors.

Various other applications of microsatellites of the HLA region have been reported in the following domains:

Genetic mapping (Crouau-Roy *et al.*,1993a; Lin *et al.*, 1998; Guillaudeux *et al.*, 1998)

Population studies (Bergstrom *et al.*, 1999; Grote *et al.*, 1998; Lin *et al.*, 1997; Ota *et al.*, 1997; Crouau-Roy *et al.*, 1993b; Worwood *et al.,* 1997; Ramsbottom *et al.*, 1997)

Recombination studies (Thomsen *et al.*, 1996; 1997; Martin *et al.*, 1995; Barmada *et al.*, 1997; Malfroy *et al.*, 1997; Cullen *et al.*, 1997; Carrington, 1999; Ajioka *et al.,* 1997b).

Transplantation studies (Asano *et al.*, 1997; Carrington and Wade, 1996; Foissac *et al.*, 1997; Ketheesan *et al.*, 1999). A promising application seems to be the value of microsatellites in establishment of haplotypes from unrelated individuals, by increasing the number of markers per haplotype. Two consequent possible uses are:

- a pre-screening of new volunteer donors for bone marrow donors registries, in order to quickly pin-point those having the most classical frequent haplotypes and to discard them from further expensive HLA typing runs
- a final test to choose between several HLA-A, -B, DR-typed donors for a given patient. Here, it may be more informative and less expensive to type for HLA region microsatellite polymorphisms, than to test other genetic markers for which the clinical usefulness has not yet been fully documented

Methods

Two features must be noted concerning the nomenclature and analysis of microsatellites:

- due to the lack of an official nomenclature system for names of microsatellite loci and alleles, ambiguities may emerge when comparing results from different sources;
- discrepancies are sometimes observed between laboratories and when different experimental protocols are used (Abraham *et al.*, 1993; Thomsen *et al.*, 1997).

This shows the urgent necessity of reaching a sufficient level of standardisation in the procedures and in the interpretation of results obtained by microsatellite analysis. Such a standardisation process both for nomenclature of loci and alleles, and for allele size assignment, commenced during the 12th International Histocompatibility Workshop (IHW), especially within the recombinant families component. The various ways of naming microsatellite alleles are based upon:

- a simple serial order of alleles from the shortest to the longest (used with manual methods where "by eye" comparisons are made with previously typed controls used as references)
- the number of base pairs (used in semi-automated methods which quantify the fragment size by comparison with a size marker)
- more complex information including the number of repeats, for example TNFa5 or TNFa -105 or TNFa $(AC)_{10}$ or TNFa $(AC)_{10}$-105-a5.

Furthermore, there is no universally accepted way of naming the microsatellite loci: the most frequently used system is the "DXS" system where X represents the number of the chromosome (e.g. D6S in case of HLA): however, this gives no idea about the precise location, or the neighbouring genes where known (for example, TNFa). A good compromise is to combine the two types of information, for example D6S-TNFa.

From a technical point of view (Koreth *et al.*, 1996), the major characteristics of methods involved in the analysis of microsatellites (i.e. PCR, gel electrophoresis), are simplicity, rapidity, and low typing costs for multiple samples. In parallel with the increasing use of microsatellite markers, equipment and technologies are also improving. Thanks to specialist software and the use of automatic DNA sequencers, semi-automated genotyping of microsatellites is now available, which increases the accuracy and the reproducibility of experiments (Foissac *et al.*, 1997). For large scale testing, special technology for microsatellites analysis has been developed, which includes sophisticated allele-calling software, high capacity water bath thermal cyclers, and instruments for the automated sizing of fluorescent PCR products. The introduction of such technology has reduced the current cost for testing 400 microsatellites (over the entire human genome) to around US$150 per person (Weber, 1999 and personal communication).

Below are described characteristic protocols for microsatellite analysis, currently used in our laboratories.

DNA extraction

DNA is extracted and purified from cell line pellets by an enzyme method (extraction by proteinase K on a column according to the specifications provided with the kit, QIAmp (Qiagen)). The optical density is measured spectrophotometrically and the DNA is adjusted to a concentration of 100ng/µl.

For DNA extraction directly from blood samples, a chemical method based on perchlorate usage is alternatively used.

PCR amplification and labelling of primers

PCR is performed in 10µl reaction volumes containing 10pmol of each primer (see Table 9.2 for an example of 8 microsatellites, ranging telomeric to HLA-A to

Msat	Primers	Labelling system
D6S105	D6S105A D6S105B	Tet (Green)
MOGc	MOG31 MOG32	6-Fam (Blue)
D6S265	D6S265A D6S265B	6-Fam (Blue)
MIB	MIBA MIBB	6-Fam (Blue)
TNFa	IR2 IR4	6-Fam (Blue)
TNFb	IR1 IR2	Tet (Green)
DQ-CAR	CAR1 CAR2	Tet (Green)
D6S291	D6S291A D6S291B	Tet (Green)

Table 9.2. Primers and labelling system for 8 examples of HLA region microsatellites

centromeric to HLA-DP: D6S105, MOGc, D6S265, MIB, TNFa, TNFb, DQ CAR, D6S291), standard PCR buffer, 50-100ng of DNA and 0.25-0.50U of *Taq* DNA polymerase (Thermophilic DNA Polymerase, Promega). The reaction is performed in an automated thermal cycler (Thermolyne Amplitron^{R} II, Barnstead I Thermolyne Corp.). One of the primers is fluorescently marked (Carrano *et al.* 1989; Edwards *et al.* 1991). In order to use a laser for fluorescence detection, it is necessary for one of the primers to be fluorescently labelled at the 5' end. The fluorochrome labelling used may include Tamra, Rox, C6Fam, Tet, Hex, Joe and the classical fluorescein and rhodamine.

	D6S105	MOGc	D6S265	MIB	TNFa	TNFb	DQ-CAR	D6S291
DNA	10 ng/µl	10 ng/µl	10 ng/µl	10 ng/µl	10 ng/µl	10 ng/µl	10 ng/µl	10 ng/µl
Primer 1	1 µM	0.25 µM	1 µM	0.8 µM	0.025 µM	0.025 µM	1 µM	1 µM
Primer 2	1 µM	0.25 µM	1 µM	0.8 µM	0.025 µM	0.025 µM	1µM	1µM
dNTP	250 µM	200 µM	250 µM	100 µM	200 µM	200 µM	125 µM	125 µM
Taq	0.5 U	0.5 U	0.5 U	0.5 U	0.25 U	0.25 U	0.5 U	0.5 U
Buffer*	1X	1X	1X	1X	1X	1X	1X	1X
$MgCl_2$	2.5 mM	1.5 mM	2.5 mM	1.5 mM	1.5 mM	1.5 mM	1.5 mM	1.5 mM

Table 9.3. *Composition of the Thermophilic DNA Polymerase Reaction Buffer (Promega): Tris-HCl (10 mM, pH9), KCl (50 mM), EDTA (0.1 mM), Triton X-100 (0.1%).

Standard PCR mixes

Compositions of standard PCR mixes are shown in Table 9.3.

PCR amplification conditions

The parameters used for PCR amplification are shown in Table 9.4

	MOGc	D6S265 D6S105	MIB	TNFa TNFb	DQ-CAR D6S291
Predenaturation	94°C - 3 min	94°C - 3 min	95°C - 3 min	95°C - 5 min	94°C - 3 min
Denaturation	94°C - 30 s	94°C - 60 s	95°C - 60 s	95°C - 300 s	94°C - 30 s
Hybridisation	50°C - 30 s	55°C - 60 s	55°C - 30 s	58°C - 30 s	57°C - 60 s
Extension	72°C - 30 s	72°C - 60 s	72°C - 60 s	72°C - 10 s	72°C - 60 s
Final Extension	72°C - 10 min	72°C - 10 min	72°C - 10 min	72°C - 5 min	72°C - 10 min
Number of cycles	22	19	21	31	21

Table 9.4. Conditions shown are optimised for the Amplitron II (Thermolyne)

Electrophoresis

Following PCR, the reaction mixture was mixed with formamide-Dextran blue in order to insure an optimal migration and with an internal-lane size standard (Tamra 2500: restriction digestions of phage Lambda; Applied Biosystems, Perkin-Elmer Corp.), labelled with a different coloured dye from that on the DNA sample. This was used to calibrate sizes from lane to lane and from gel to gel.

After denaturation (95°C - 5 min) and cooling on ice, samples were submitted to electrophoresis on a standard 6% to 9% denaturing polyacrylamide gel, using a voltage of 1100V, in 1X migration buffer (Tris Borate EDTA (TBE), see below) using an automated DNA sequencer (373 ABI sequencer, Perkin-Elmer Corp.).

Final composition of samples :

- ☑ PCR product 0.4 µl-2 µl
- ☑ Size marker (Tamra 2500) 0.4 µl
- ☑ Formamide- dextran blue buffer 3 µl

Sample volume per well: 3.5 µl

For certain microsatellites, multiplexing or loading more than one microsatellite test per lane (co-migration) is possible. This permits simultaneous analysis of several microsatellites of different sizes. For example, co-migration of

TNFa/TNFb; DQ-CAR/MIB; D6S105/D6S265 and DQ-CAR/D6S291 may be performed.

Composition of migration buffer

TBE buffer (10X):

- ☑ Tris 107.8 g
- ☑ Boric Acid 55 g
- ☑ EDTA 8.2 g
- ☑ Distilled water to 1 litre

Electrophoresis conditions

These are shown in Table 9.5

Parameter	Value
Voltage	1100 V
Amperage	40 mA
Power	30 W
Migration duration	120 min - 300 min

Table 9.5. Electrophoresis conditions used.

Interpretation

During the electrophoretic migration, fluorescent signals are produced, resulting from laser excitation of labelled PCR products. These are collected and quantified, for example using the Genescan Collection Software (Genescan 672, Perkin-Elmer Applied Biosystems). This provides a graphical representation of the gel and determines the microsatellite allele band size. The allelic bands are directly distinguished by computer analysis, which automatically determines the size of each PCR-generated fragment and the amount of fluorescent signal. Most automated sequencers now have equivalent genotyping software. The calculations are based on the "local method" (Southern, 1979). This calculation method uses the reciprocal mathematical relationship between the electrophoretic mobility of a fragment and its length. According to an equation based on the empirical relation between fragment length and mobility of alleles and internal size marker, the size (in number of base pairs) of each microsatellite allele is established by using two successive fitting curves. This uses groups of points including the unknown size microsatellite allele, and 3 fragments adjacent to the size marker Tamra 2500, whose sizes are predefined.

Variants

When using a non semi-automated method, a number of other systems for "by-eye" reading of sizes can be used, as follows:

1. *Radioactive labelling*

This can be incorporated at the amplification level, using radioactive internal labelling of the microsatellite itself, by incorporation of a radioactive nucleotide (α^{32}P dCTP), or by end labelling by using a 5' radioactive primer (γ^{32}P dATP), or at the step of post-resolution stage by specific hybridisation of a 5' radioactively labelled probe (usually a PCR primer). The latter is followed by autoradiography, though this type of labelling has been widely superseded by fluorescence.

2. *Staining*

Ethidium bromide for direct visualisation of fragments under UV transillumination, or silver staining, can also be used.

Some difficulties and pitfalls in microsatellite analysis

A knowledge of the following potential difficulties assists the interpretation of results in family studies and in studies of unrelated individuals.

Nomenclature: see the discussion above

Secondary polymorphisms: these can occasionally prevent efficient annealing of PCR primers to the template, resulting in weak or even null alleles; and is responsible for a number of typing ambiguities (Weber, 1999).

Strand slippage: this increases as the repeat length decreases. This is a severe problem with one nucleotide repeats, which consequently are never used in practise. It requires attention for dinucleotide repeats, but is not a major problem for tri- and tetra-nucleotide repeats.

Mutation rate: this varies according to the locus, the genes in the locality, and the size of the microsatellite (Jin *et al.*, 1996). Thus, it is difficult to assess a common status for all microsatellites. Further, an apparent mutation can be due to slippage in the course of *in vitro* culture of a cell line, and does not necessarily represent a true *in vivo* phenomenon.

Homoplasy: sometimes, two amplified fragments of a microsatellite with the same fragment size do not correspond to the same allele of the microsatellite because of a difference in sequences or other complexity in the repeat. This has been described outside the MHC (Jin *et al.*, 1996; Brinkmann *et al.*, 1997) and within the MHC, for example in the MIB microsatellite close to HLA-B (Grimaldi and Crouau-Roy, 1997). Only sequencing of the fragment can discriminate between such alleles.

Conclusion

As the areas of application of microsatellites in the HLA region become more widely investigated, so interest in HLA microsatellites continues to increase. The future of HLA microsatellite applications has various potentials, for example as a transition tool before a complete elucidation of the HLA region sequence, or the development of long-term microsatellite analysis strategy. Against the background of polymorphism in the HLA region, microsatellite markers may prove to be of transitional use, before contemplation of sequencing all of the alleles of the functionally relevant HLA genes. Since the structural and evolutionary characteristics of microsatellite markers are of interest, long-term use of microsatellites is foreseeable in a global approach to characterisation of human MHC polymorphism. It may also be of interest to couple the study of microsatellites to that of a number of single nucleotide polymorhisms (SNPs) in the same region.

Acknowledgements. This chapter is based on work supported by the following sources: EU "HCM": ERBCHBGCT 920090 and 920032, Conseil régional Midi-Pyrénées: 9407538 and 9507784, an INSERM/AFS grant Number 5FS5, an ART grant 02-1996 and EFG 1997. A. Foissac was the recipient of a Fellowship from CNRS and from Fondation de France.

References

Abraham, LJ, Marley, JV, Nedospasov, SA, Cambon-Thomsen, A, Crouau-Roy, B, *et al.* (1993) Microsatellite, restriction fragment-length polymorphism, and sequence-specific oligonucleotide typing of the tumor necrosis factor region. Comparisons of the 4AOHW cell panel *Hum Immunol* **38**: 17-23

Ajioka, RS, Jorde, LB, Gruen, JR, Yu, P, Dimitrova, D, *et al.* (1997a) Haplotype analysis of hemochromatosis: evaluation of different linkage-disequilibrium approaches and evolution of disease chromosomes *Amer J Hum Genet* **60**: 1439-1447

Ajioka, RS, Yu, P, Gruen, JR, Edwards, CQ, Griffen, LM, *et al.* (1997b) Recombinations defining centromeric and telomeric borders for the hereditary haemochromatosis locus *J Med Genet* **34**: 28-33

Andrieux, N, Jouanolle, AM, Gandon, G, Mosser, J (1997) A highly informative dinucleotide repeat polymorphism telomeric to HLA-F *Immunogenetics* **46**: 355-356

Asano, H, Kobayashi, T, Uchida, K, Hayashi, S, Yokoyama, I, *et al.* (1997) Significance of tumor necrosis factor microsatellite polymorphism in renal transplantation *Tissue Antigens* **50**: 484-488

Barmada, N, Delaney, NL, Bias, WB, Schmeckpeper, BJ (1997) Recombination hot spots in the HLA region of chromosome 6: Refinement of localization using microsatellite markers. In: *Genetic diversity of HLA: Functional and medical implication* Vol I (Ed. Charron, D), pp.109-112. EDK, Paris, France

Bergstrom, T, Engkvist, H, Erlandsson, R, Josefsson, A, Mack, S, *et al.* (1999) Tracing the origin of HLA-DRB1 alleles by microsatellite polymorphism *Amer J Hum Genet* **64**: 1709-1718

Bouissou, C, Pontarotti, P and Crouau-Roy, B (1995) A precise meiotic map in the class I region of the human major histocompatibility complex *Genomics* **30**: 486-492

Brinkmann, B, Klintschar, M, Neuhuber, F, Huhne, J and Rolf, B (1998) Mutation rate in human microsatellites: influence of the structure and length of the tandem repeat *Amer J Hum Genet* **62**: 1408-1415

Broman, K, Murray, J, Sheffield, V, White, R and Weber, J (1998) Comprehensive human genetic maps: individual and sex-specific variation in recombination *Amer J Hum Genet* **63**: 861-869

Bruford, MW and Wayne, RK (1993) Microsatellites and their application to population genetic studies *Curr Opin Genet Dev* **3**: 939-943

Burt, MJ, Smit, DJ, Pyper, WR, Powell, LW and Jazwinska, EC (1996) A 45-megabase YAC contig and physical map over the hemochromatosis gene region *Genomics* **33**: 153-158

Camaschella, C, Roetto, A, Gasparini, P, Piperno, A, Fortina, P, *et al.* (1996) Allelic association of microsatellites of 6p in Italian hemochromatosis patients *Hum Genet* **97**: 476-481

Carrano, A, Lamerdin, J, Ashworth, L, Watkins, B, Branscomb, E, *et al.* (1989) A high-resolution, fluorescence-based, semiautomated method for DNA fingerprinting *Genomics* **4**: 129-136

Carrington, M (1999) Recombination within the human MHC *Immunol Rev* **167**: 245-256

Carrington, M and Dean, M (1994) A polymorphic dinucleotide repeat in the third intron of TAP1 *Hum Molec Genet* **3**: 218

Carrington, M and Wade, J (1996) Selection of transplant donors based on MHC microsatellite data—correction to previously published material *Hum Immunol* **51**: 106-109

Colonna, M, Ferrara, GB, Strominger, JL and Spies, T (1992) Hypervariable microsatellites in the central region of the MHC class III region. In: *HLA - Proceedings of the 11th International Histocompatibility Workshop and Conference* Vol II (Ed. Tsuji, K, Aizawa, M, Sasazuki, T), pp 179-181. Oxford University Press, Oxford

Crouau-Roy, B, Bouissou, C, Sommer, E, Pontarotti, P and Thomsen, M (1993a) Analysis of HLA-A/B recombinant families with new polymorphic markers *Hum Immunol* **38**: 132-136

Crouau-Roy, B, Briant, L, Bouissou, C, Stravropoulos, C, Pociot, F, *et al.* (1993b) Tumor necrosis factor microsatellites in four European populations *Hum Immunol* **38**: 213-216

Cullen, M, Noble, J, Erlich, H, Thorpe, K, Beck, S, *et al.* (1997) Characterization of recombination in the HLA class II region *Amer J Hum Genet* **60**: 397-407

D'Alfonso, S, Cappello, N, Carcassi, C, Fasano, ME and Momigliano-Richiardi, P (1997) Microsatellites in the HLA central region are markers of HLA conserved haplotypes. In: *Genetic diversity of HLA: Functional and medical implication* Vol I (Ed. Charron, D), pp.125-127 EDK, Paris, France

Dib, C, Faure, S, Fizames, C, Samson, D, Drouot, N, *et al.* (1996) A comprehensive genetic map of the human genome based on 5,264 microsatellites *Nature* **380**: 152-154

Edwards, A, Hammond, H, Jin, L, Caskey, C and Chakraborty, R (1992) Genetic variation at five trimeric and tetrameric tandem repeat loci in four human population groups *Genomics* **12**: 241-253

Ellis, MC, Hetisimer, AH, Ruddy, DA, Hansen, SL, Kronmal, GS, *et al.* (1997) HLA class II haplotype and sequence analysis support a role for DQ in narcolepsy *Immunogenetics* **46**: 410-417

Feder, JN, Gnirke, A, Thomas, W, Tsuchihashi, Z, Ruddy, DA, *et al.* (1996) A novel MHC class I-like gene is mutated in patients with hereditary haemochromatosis *Nature Genetics* **13**: 399-408

Foissac, A (1999) Analyse de microsatellites et génétique humaine Utilisations en immunogénétique et étude du chromosome 6 : potentialités d'applications en transplantation de moelle osseuse. Doctoral thesis: Université Paul Sabatier (Toulouse III)

Foissac, A and Cambon-Thomsen, A (1998) Microsatellites in the HLA region: 1998 update *Tissue Antigens* **52**: 318-352

Foissac, A, Crouau-Roy, B, Faure, S, Thomsen, M, Cambon-Thomsen, A (1997a) Microsatellites in the HLA region: an overview *Tissue Antigens* **49**: 197-214

Foissac, A, Fort, ML, Giraldo, P, Abbal, M, Raffoux, C, *et al.* (1997b) Microsatellites in the HLA region: potential applications in bone marrow transplantation *Transpl Proc* **29**: 2374-2375

Gallagher, G, Eskdale, J and Miller, S (1997) A highly polymorphic microsatellite marker in the human MHC class III region, close to the BAT2 gene *Immunogenetics* **46**: 357-358

Geraghty, DE, Wei, XH, Orr, HT and Koller, BH (1990) Human leukocyte antigen F (HLA-F) An expressed HLA gene composed of a class I coding sequence linked to a novel transcribed repetitive element *J Exp Med* **171**: 1-18

Grimaldi, M and Crouau-Roy, B (1997) Microsatellite allelic homoplasy due to variable flanking sequences *J Mol Evol* **44**: 336-340

Grimaldi, MC, Clayton, J, Pontarotti, P, Cambon-Thomsen, A and Crouau-Roy, B (1996) New highly polymorphic microsatellite marker in linkage disequilibrium with HLA-B *Hum Immunol* **51**: 89-94

Grote, M, Klitz, W and Thomson, G (1998) Constrained disequilibrium values and hitchhiking in a three-locus system *Genetics* **150**: 1295-1307

Guillaudeux, T, Janer, M, Wong, G, Spies, T and Geraghty, D (1998) The complete genomic sequence of 424,015 bp at the centromeric end of the HLA class I region: gene content and polymorphism *Proc Nat Acad Sci USA* **95**: 9494-9499

Hanifi Moghaddam, P, de Knijf, P, Roep, BO, Van der Auwera, B, Naipal, A, *et al.* (1998a) Genetic structure of IDDM1: two separate regions in the major histocompatibility complex contribute to susceptibility or protection Belgian Diabetes Registry *Diabetes* **47**: 263-269

Hanifi Moghaddam, P, Zwinderman, A, Kazemi, M, Van der Voort Maarschalk, M, Ruigrok, M, *et al.* (1998b) TNFa microsatellite locus correlates with CTLp frequency in unrelated bone marrow donor-recipient pairs *Hum Immunol* **59**: 295-301

Hanifi Moghaddam, P, Zwinderman, AH, de Knijff, P, Roep, BO, Schipper, RF, *et al.* (1997) TNFa microsatellite polymorphism modulates the risk of IDDM in Caucasians with the high-risk genotype HLA DQA1*0501-DQB1*0201/DQA1*0301-DQB1*0302 Belgian Diabetes Registry *Diabetes* **46**: 1514-1515

Hearne, CM, Ghosh, S and Todd, JA (1992) Microsatellites for linkage analysis of genetic traits *Trends Genet* **8**: 288-294

Hsieh, SL, March, RE, Khanna, A, Cross, SJ and Campbell, RD (1997) Mapping of 10 novel microsatellites in the MHC class III region: application to the study of autoimmune disease *J Rheumatol* **24**: 220-222

Jazwinska, EC, Lee, SC, Webb, SI, Halliday, JW and Powell, LW (1993) Localization of the hemochromatosis gene close to D6S105 *Amer J Hum Genet* **53**: 347-352

Jazwinska, EC, Pyper, WR, Burt, MJ, Francis, JL, Goldwurm, S, *et al.* (1995) Haplotype analysis in Australian hemochromatosis patients: evidence for a predominant ancestral haplotype exclusively associated with hemochromatosis *Amer J Hum Genet* **56**: 428-433

Jin, L, Macaubas, C, Hallmayer, J, Kimura, A, Mignot, E (1996) Mutation rate varies among alleles at a microsatellite locus: phylogenetic evidence *Proc Nat Acad Sci USA* **93**: 15285-15288

Jongeneel, CV, Briant, L, Udalova, IA, Sevin, A, Nedospasov, SA, *et al.* (1991) Extensive genetic polymorphism in the human tumor necrosis factor region and relation to extended HLA haplotypes *Proc Nat Acad Sci USA* **88**: 9717-9721

Ketheesan, N, Gaudieri, S, Witt, C, Tay, G, Townend, D, *et al.* (1999) Reconstruction of the block matching profiles *Hum Immunol* **60**: 171-176

Koreth, J, Leary, JJ and McGee, J (1996) Microsatellites and PCR genomic analysis *J Pathol* **178**: 239-248

Lie, B, Todd , J, Pociot, F, Nerup, J, Akselsen, H, *et al.* (1999) The predisposition to type 1 diabetes linked to the human leukocyte antigen complex includes at least one non-class II gene *Amer J Hum Genet* **64**: 793-800

Lin, L, Jin, L, Kimura, A, Carrington, M and Mignot, E (1997) DQ microsatellite association studies in three ethnic groups *Tissue Antigens* **50**: 507-520

Lin, L, Jin, L, Lin, X, Voros, A, Underhill, P, *et al.* (1998) Microsatellite single nucleotide polymorphisms in the HLA-DQ region *Tissue Antigens* **52**: 9-18

Macaubas, C, Hallmayer, J, Kalil, J, Kimura, A, Yasunaga, S, *et al.* (1995) Extensive polymorphism of a (CA)n microsatellite located in the HLA-DQA1/DQB1 class II region *Hum Immunol* **42**: 209-220

Malfroy, L, Roth, MP, Carrington, M, Borot, N, Volz, A, *et al.* (1997) Heterogeneity in rates of recombination in the 6-Mb region telomeric to the human major histocompatibility complex *Genomics* **43**: 226-231

Martin, M, Mann, D, Carrington, M (1995) Recombination rates across the HLA complex: use of microsatellites as a rapid screen for recombinant chromosomes *Hum Molec Genet* **4**: 423-428

Mayr, WR (1995) DNA markers in forensic medicine *Transfusion Clinique et Biologique* **2**: 325-328

Mignot, E, Kimura, A, Abbal, M, Thorsby, E, Lin, X, *et al.* (1995) DQCAR microsatellite polymorphisms in three selected HLA class II-associated diseases *Tissue Antigens* **46**: 299-304

Mignot, E, Kimura, A, Lattermann, A, Lin, X, Yasunaga, S, *et al.* (1997) Extensive HLA class II studies in 58 non-DRB1*15 (DR2) narcoleptic patients with cataplexy *Tissue Antigens* **49**: 329-341

Mu, H, Chen, J, Jiang, Y, King, M, Thomson, G, *et al.* (1999) Tumor necrosis factor a microsatellite polymorphism is associated with rheumatoid arthritis severity through an interaction with the HLA-DRB1 shared epitope *Arthritis and Rheumatism* **42**: 438-442

Nedospasov, SA, Udalova, IA, Kuprash, DV and Turetskaya, RL (1991) DNA sequence polymorphism at the human tumor necrosis factor (TNF) locus Numerous TNF/lymphotoxin alleles tagged by two closely linked microsatellites in the upstream region of the lymphotoxin (TNF-beta) gene *J Immunol* **147**: 1053-1059

Ota, M, Katsuyama, Y, Mizuki, N, Ando, H, Furihata, K, *et al.* (1997) Trinucleotide repeat polymorphism within exon 5 of the MICA gene (MHC class I chain-related gene A): allele frequency data in the nine population groups Japanese, Northern Han, Hui, Uygur, Kazakhstan, Iranian, Saudi Arabian, Greek and Italian *Tissue Antigens* **49**: 448-454

Ota, M, Mizuki, N, Katsuyama, Y, Tamiya, G, Shiina, T, *et al.* (1999) The critical region for Behcet disease in the human major histocompatibility complex is reduced to a 46-kb segment centromeric of HLA-B, by association analysis using refined microsatellite mapping *Amer J Hum Genet* **64**: 1406-1410

Pociot, F, Briant, L, Jongeneel, CV, Molvig, J, Worsaae, H, *et al.* (1993) Association of tumor necrosis factor (TNF) and class II major histocompatibility complex alleles with the secretion of TNF-alpha and TNF-beta by human mononuclear cells: a possible link to insulin-dependent diabetes mellitus *Eur J Immunol* **23**: 224-231

Raha-Chowdhury, R, Bowen, DJ, Stone, C, Pointon, JJ, Terwilliger, JD, *et al.* (1995) New polymorphic microsatellite markers place the haemochromatosis gene telomeric to D6S105 *Hum Molec Genet* **4**: 1869-1874

Raha-Chowdhury, R, Tigue, NJ, Worwood, M (1994) Trinucleotide repeat microsatellite in the 5' untranslated region of HLA-F *Hum Molec Genet* **3**: 2084

Ramsbottom, D, Carcassi, C, de Solages, H, Abbal, M, Crouau-Roy, B, *et al.* (1997) MHC haplotypes including eight microsatellites in French Basques and in Sardinians In: *Genetic diversity of HLA: Functional and medical implication* Vol II (Ed. Charron, D), pp.178-180 EDK, Paris, France

Ribas, G, Neville, M, Wixon, J, Cheng , J and Campbell, R (1999) Genes encoding three new members of the leukocyte antigen 6 superfamily and a novel member of Ig superfamily, together with genes encoding the regulatory nuclear chloride ion channel protein (hRNCC) and a nomega-nomega-dimethylarginine dimethylaminohydrolase homologue, are found in a 30-kb segment of the MHC class III region *J Immunol* **163**: 278-287

Roth, MP, Dolbois, L, Borot, N, Amadou, C, Clanet, M, *et al.* (1995) Three highly polymorphic microsatellites at the human myelin oligodendrocyte glycoprotein locus, 100 kb telomeric to HLA-F Characterization and relation to HLA haplotypes *Hum Immunol* **43**: 276-282

Rubinsztein, DC, Amos, W, Leggo, J, Goodburn, S, Jain, S, *et al.* (1995a) Microsatellite evolution—evidence for directionality and variation in rate between species *Nature Genetics* **10**: 337-343

Rubinsztein, DC, Leggo, J and Amos, W (1995b) Microsatellites evolve more rapidly in humans than in chimpanzees *Genomics* **30**: 610-612

Shiina, T, Tamiya, G, Takashima, N, Makino, S, Kikkawa, E, *et al.* (1999) Large-scale genome sequencing of the entire HLA Class I region and disease association *Hum Immunol* **60 suppl 1**: S3

Singal, DP, Li, J and Ye, M (1998a) DQCAR microsatellite polymorphism and susceptibility to rheumatoid arthritis *Tissue Antigens* **51**: 613-617

Singal, DP, Li, J, Ye, M and Lei, K (1998b) D6S273 microsatellite polymorphism and susceptibility to rheumatoid arthritis *Tissue Antigens* **52**: 353-358

Southern, EM (1979) Measurement of DNA length by gel electrophoresis *Anal Biochem* **100**: 319-323

Tamiya, G, Ota, M, Katsuyama, Y, Shiina, T, Oka, A, *et al.* (1998) Twenty-six new polymorphic microsatellite markers around the HLA-B, -C and -E loci in the human MHC class I region *Tissue Antigens* **51**: 337-346

Tautz, D (1989) Hypervariability of simple sequences as a general source for polymorphic DNA markers *Nucl Acids Res* **17**: 6463-6471

Tautz, D (1993) Notes on the definition and nomenclature of tandemly repetitive DNA sequences. In: *DNA fingerprinting: State of the science* (Ed. Pena, SDJ, Chakraborty, R, Epplen, JT, Jeffreys, AJ), pp.21-28. Birkhauser Verlag, Basel, Switzerland

Thomsen, M, Alcalay, D, Barmada, M, Borelli, I, Breda-Coimbra, H, *et al.* (1997) MHC recombinant families. In: *Genetic diversity of HLA: Functional and medical implication* Vol I (Ed. Charron, D), pp.188-195 EDK, Paris, France

Thomsen, M, Cullen, M, Carrington, M, Foissac, A, Abbal, M, *et al.* (1996) Localization of the recombination points in a family with two DR/DP recombinations *Tissue Antigens* **47**: 492-497

Udalova, IA, Nedospasov, SA, Webb, GC, Chaplin, DD and Turetskaya, RL (1993) Highly informative typing of the human TNF locus using six adjacent polymorphic markers *Genomics* **16**: 180-186

Vorechovsky, I, Webster, A, Plebani, A and Hammarstrom, L (1999) Genetic linkage of IgA deficiency to the major histocompatibility complex: evidence for allele segregation distortion, parent-of-origin penetrance differences, and the role of anti-IgA antibodies in disease predisposition *Amer J Hum Genet* **64**: 1096-1109

Weber, J (1999) Biology of microsatellites In: *La diversité du génome et son impact en santé publique VIIème Congrès Annuel de Génétique Humaine* (Ed. CEPH), pp.91-93. SmithKline Beechman, Paris

Weber, JL, Kwitek, AE, May, PE and Zoghbi, HY (1991) Dinucleotide repeat polymorphism at the D6S105 locus *Nucl Acids Res* **19**: 968

Weber, JL and May, PE (1989) Abundant class of human DNA polymorphisms which can be typed using the polymerase chain reaction *Amer J Hum Genet* **44**: 388-96

Worwood, M, Raha Chowdhury, R, Robson, KJ, Pointon, J, Shearman, JD, *et al.* (1997) The HLA A1-B8 haplotype extends 6 Mb beyond HLA-A: associations between HLA-A, B, F and 15 microsatellite markers *Tissue Antigens* **50**: 521-526

Worwood, M, Raha-Chowdhury, R and Darke, C (1994) Distribution of alleles at D6S105 and D6S265 with possible HLA haplotype associations *Tissue Antigens* **44**: 322-325

Yabuki, K, Ota, M, Goto, K, Kimura, T, Nomura, E, *et al.* (1999) Triplet repeat polymorphism in the MICA gene in HLA-B27 positive and negative caucasian patients with ankylosing spondylitis *Hum Immunol* **60**: 83-86

CHAPTER 10

ON-LINE HLA SEQUENCE ALIGNMENTS

G. J. Laundy
University of Bristol
Division of Transplantation Sciences
Southmead Hospital
Bristol BS10 5NB, England

J. L. Bidwell
University of Bristol
Department of Pathology & Microbiology
Homoeopathic Hospital Site
Cotham, Bristol BS6 6JU, England

Introduction

Extensive DNA studies during the last ten to fifteen years have established the molecular basis for the extreme diversity of HLA class I and class II alleles both within and between ethnic groups. They have further revealed that clinical outcome following transplantation may be compromised by subtle differences between donor and recipient MHC nucleotide sequences which may not be reliably identified by classical serological techniques.

Sequence similarity search programs, multiple sequence alignments and the availability of electronically transferable nucleotide and amino acid sequence data have revolutionised access to molecular biological data, particularly in the field of HLA. As a result:

- The study of the relationship between primary sequence, molecular structure and function has been simplified;
- The speed with which sequence-specific oligonucleotides (allele-specific, group-specific or locus-specific PCR primers) can be designed and synthesized has improved dramatically;
- Establishing the biological relevance of different HLA polymorphisms in transplantation and disease has been simplified by the speed and accuracy with which such polymorphisms can be identified.

Since 1968 the *WHO Nomenclature Committee for Factors of the HLA System* have published regular comprehensive reports. Initially these were produced following International Histocompatibility Workshops (every two to four years) but are now compiled on an annual basis (Bodmer *et al.,* 1997). These reports are valuable key references to the enormous diversity of the HLA system. They provide details of all known HLA class I and class II specificities defined by serological and/or molecular techniques. Of particular value to the molecular biologist is the inclusion of sequence accession numbers. With this information the user can rapidly access nucleotide and amino acid sequence details, from any one of a number of sources (for example GenBank or EMBL). Monthly updates of newly assigned HLA alleles, confirmatory sequences, withdrawn sequences, accession numbers and submitting authors are published in *Human Immunology*, *Tissue Antigens* and the *European Journal of Immunogenetics* (see, for example, Marsh, 1998) and on the World Wide Web (WWW).

Producing nucleotide sequence alignments by manual means alone is labour intensive. In the past the HLA community has been well served by the efforts of Zemmour and Parham (1993) who constructed and published HLA nucleotide sequence alignments spanning exons 2, 3 and 4 for all known class I genes. Subsequently, a comprehensive analysis of the nucleotide and protein sequences for exons 5-8 of the HLA-A, B and C alleles provided hitherto unavailable information on transmembrane and cytoplasmic domains (Crew, 1997). Summers and colleagues (1993) published a useful compilation of HLA class I non-coding nucleotide sequences spanning the 5'and 3' untranslated regions and introns 1-7. This unique series of sequence reports was completed with the publication of comprehensive class II nucleotide sequence alignments for HLA-DRA, DRB, DQA, DQB and DP (Marsh and Bodmer, 1993; 1994). A useful computer-readable sequence alignment database was distributed by the *European Journal of Immunogenetics* on 3.5-inch and 5.25-inch computer diskettes, entitled *Genes On Disk*. The database included HLA class I (Marsh and Bodmer, 1993) and class II (Zemmour and Parham, 1993) nucleotide sequence alignments, protein alignments and associated references in ASCII format. The data could also be acquired electronically either by mail message or by *ftp* (file transfer protocol). The most recently published databases (Table 10.1) cover HLA class I region nucleotide (exons 2, 3 and 4) and amino acid (α_1 and α_2 domain) sequence alignments (Mason and Parham, 1998) and HLA class II region nucleotide and amino acid sequence alignments (Marsh, 1998).

On-line sequences

Given the appropriate *accession number* the interested user can rapidly access the nucleotide and protein sequence for individual HLA alleles: however, a lag time often exists between publication of the accession number and availability of the associated sequence. There are various routes through which these sequences can be downloaded.

The European Bioinformatics Institute (EBI) maintains Europe's primary nucleotide database, the European Molecular Biology Laboratory (EMBL) Nucleotide Sequence Database (2.7 x 10^6 entries as of October 1998) and the University of Geneva SWISS-PROT Protein Sequence Database (Rodriguez-

Locus	Nucleotide sequences	Locus	Nucleotide sequences
HLA-A	86	HLA-DRB8	1
HLA-B	185	HLA-DRB9	1
HLA-C	45	HLA-DQA1	19
HLA-DRA	2	HLA-DQB1	35
HLA-DRB1	197	HLA-DPA1	13
HLA-DRB2	1	HLA-DPB1	83
HLA-DRB3	17	HLA-DMA	4
HLA-DRB4	7	HLA-DMB	5
HLA-DRB5	14	TAP1	5
HLA-DRB6	3	TAP2	4
HLA-DRB7	2		

Table 10.1. HLA Class I and Class II nucleotide sequences (Mason and Parham, 1998; Marsh, 1998)

Tomé *et al.,* 1996). This is a primary information site incorporating more than fifty specialist molecular biology databases, software and useful documentation.

GenBank (Benson *et al.,* 1998) is the National Institutes of Health Genetic Sequence Database of all publicly available nucleotide and protein sequences. It is based at the National Center for Biotechnology Information (NCBI) and is part of the International Nucleotide Sequence Database Collaboration which includes EMBL and the DNA Databank of Japan (DDBJ). As of August 1998 the database included approximately 1.8×10^9 bases in 2.5×10^6 records covering 2.5×10^6 loci (release 108.0). All entries are supplemented with bibliographical (MEDLINE) and scientific data. GenBank data is accessible through NCBI's integrated retrieval system, *Entrez*. New sequences, revisions and updates can be reported to GenBank by direct electronic submission using either a WWW form *BankIt* or by using stand-alone submission software *Sequin*, currently available in a beta-test version from the NCBI.

The SWISS-PROT database of protein sequences (Rodriguez-Tomé *et al.,* 1996, 7.5×10^4 entries as of September 1998) and the supplementary TrEMBL database (1.6×10^5 entries) are the result of collaboration between the University of Geneva and EMBL (Bairoch and Apweiler, 1997). The data have been derived from various sources including direct author submission and DNA sequence translation from the EMBL Nucleotide Sequence Database.

The *PIR* (Protein Information Resource) is the result of a global collaboration between centres involved in the collection of macromolecular sequence data (Barker *et al.,* 1993) and is maintained by the National Biomedical Research Foundation (NBRF). The PIR-International Protein Sequence Database has 1.1×10^5 entries (release 58.0, September 1998). An alignment database and a 3D-sequence database can also be accessed from this site.

On-Line Sequence Alignments

HLA class I nucleotide and amino acid sequence alignments can be accessed through the WWW at a public *ftp* site:

ftp://cmgm.stanford.edu/pub/NMDP

(Mason and Parham, 1998). Alignments may be downloaded in text (*.txt) format which can readily be viewed by setting word processor parameters to Courier 8 point font, A4 portrait orientation; or in spreadsheet format allowing direct import into a package such as Microsoft® Excel™. Sequence information can also be downloaded in PIR format allowing manual alignments using *GeneDoc* or similar software packages (see below). This information can also be accessed through the Anthony Nolan Laboratories HLA Informatics site at:

http://www.anthonynolan.com/HIG/data.html

HLA class II region data, including non-classical and pseudogene alignments (Marsh, 1998) are also available from this site which is further enhanced by a user-friendly graphical interface, an extensive reference section and an on-line version of the current *Nomenclature for Factors of the HLA system*. An alternative route to these sequence alignment databases is via the extensive American Society for Histocompatibility and Immunogenetics (ASHI) web site at:

http://www.swmed.edu/home_pages/ASHI

The ImMunoGeneTics (IMGT) database provides extensive information on immunoglobulins (Ig), T cell receptors (TcR) and the MHC of all species. The HLA database (IMGT/HLA) provides a specialist database for all HLA class I and class II molecules. Among the facilities available are allele sequences and alignments, protein translations and alignments and various tools for alignment and sequence retrieval. Extensive details of reference cells associated with each officially recognised HLA sequence are included. Visit this site at your earliest opportunity.

http://www.ebi.ac.uk/imgt/hla/intro.html

Other On-line Resources

There are numerous integrated on-line resources which will aid navigation through the plethora of information available. Examples of such sites include:

- The *BCM Search Launcher*, a World Wide Web server that organizes molecular biology related remote search and analysis services by function and provides a single point-of-entry for related searches.

- The *Bionet Electronic Newsgroup Network for Biology (BIOSCI)* is a major electronic communications forum with both US (Stanford University) and UK (Daresbury Laboratory) nodes.

Shareware and freeware computer applications

The following is not intended to be an exhaustive survey of what is available to the user. All packages have advantages and disadvantages and need to be examined carefully to identify individual suitability.

GeneDoc

GeneDoc is a freeware multiple sequence alignment editor and analysis package for Microsoft® Windows, Microsoft® Windows for Workgroups™ version 3.1 or greater, Microsoft® Windows 95™ or Microsoft® Windows NT™. The user can import sequence data in several formats including MSF (*.msf), PIR (*.pir), Clustal (*.aln) and Pearson Fasta (*.ssq). The GeneDoc program files are available for download either from the GeneDoc Home Page:

http://www.cris.com/~Ketchup/genedoc.shtml

or perhaps more conveniently from the American Society for Histocompatibility and Immunogenetics (ASHI) HLA Sequences page at:

http://www.swmed.edu/home_pages/ASHI/sequences/a_p.html.

HLA class I and class II sequences are available in GeneDoc format (PIR) via the ASHI web site.

MACAW

MACAW (Multiple Alignment Construction & Analysis Workbench, version 2.0.5) is an interactive freeware program that allows the manipulation and alignment (Figure 10.1) of imported nucleotide sequences (in plain text or FASTA format) through a user-friendly interface (Schuler *et al.,* 1991). The program will run on Win16, Win32i and Win32a platforms using Microsoft® Windows™, Microsoft® Windows for Workgroups™ version 3.1 or greater, Microsoft® Windows 95™ or Microsoft® Windows NT™. System requirements include 8Mb memory (16Mb recommended), a Windows-supported graphics display card and mouse. The Apple Macintosh® Mac68k platform is also supported using system software 7.0 or later. The application is available as a self-extracting file, MACAWZ.EXE, from the NCBI anonymous FTP server:

ftp://ncbi.nlm.nih.gov/pub/macaw/

Copy MACAWZ.EXE into a new directory and RUN the program. The self-extracted files include 16 and 32-bit versions of the MACAW program together

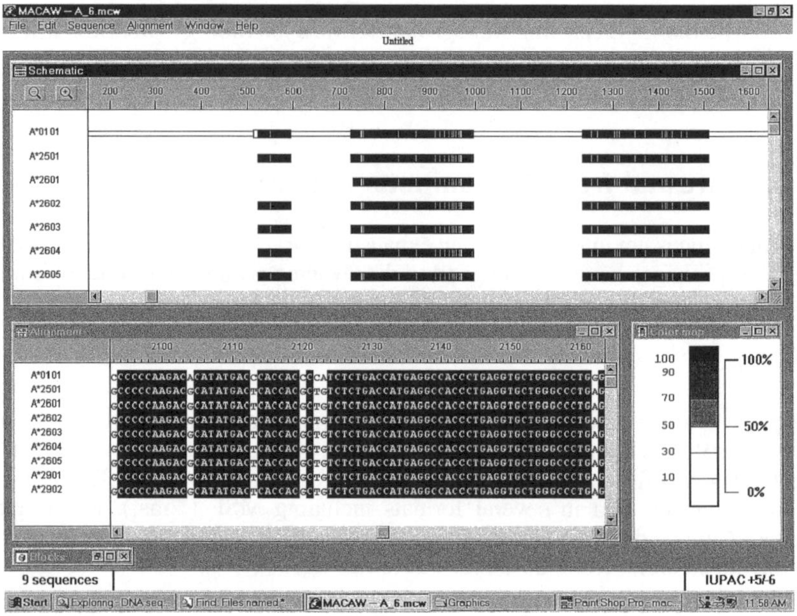

Figure 10.1. MACAW alignment of HLA-A nucleotide sequences. Upper window: schematic alignment of a genomic DNA clone for HLA-A*0101 (top line) and six cDNA clones. Lower (left) window: nucleotide sequence details of nine HLA-A alleles at position 2093-2163, polymorphic sequences blocked in white.

with comprehensive instructions in a Microsoft® Word for Windows™ document. Note that MACAW has a limit on the number of sequences which can be compared and therefore multiple files may need to be generated: however, use of a consensus sequence at the head of each file will permit interfile comparisons. Although not used extensively for HLA alignments to date, the interested reader will find extensive examples of the use of MACAW for human cytokine gene nucleotide sequence alignments at:

http://www.pam.bris.ac.uk/services/cytokine.htm

ProMSED2

ProMSED2 (Protein multiple sequence editor) is a Microsoft® Windows™ package written in C++ (Borland® C++ 4.0) which facilitates protein and nucleotide alignment and is available for a small charge from the authors (see Appendix). ProMSED2 reads data in the following main sequence formats: EMBL/SWISS (*.ref), Pearson, ClustalV, Intelligenetics (*.ig) and PIR and, using the ClustalV algorithm, allows flexible interactive and automatic sequence alignments in a user-friendly Microsoft® Word for Windows™ environment.

Program*	Operating System
Alignment search software	
BCM Search launcher	Mac
BESTSCOR	All
BLASTINC	Mac
BLASTLIB	Mac
CLUSTAL W	Mac, MS-DOS
ClustalX	Mac, MS-Windows
FSAP	Mac, MS-DOS
GAP	MS-DOS
SIM2	Mac, MS-Windows
Alignment editing and display	
ALSCRIPT	MS-DOS
DNA Stacks	Mac
LALNVIEW	Mac, MS-DOS
Sequin	Mac, MS-Windows (3.x, 95)
SeqVu	Mac
Sequence format conversion tools	
BCM Search launcher	Mac
DataMinder	Mac
DnaSP	MS-Windows (3.x, 95)
DNA Stacks	Mac
SEQIO	MS-Windows NT
Sequin	Mac, MS-Windows (3.x, 95)

Table 10.2. Examples of alignment search, edit and conversion software for Macintosh and Microsoft operating systems. * Further details of programs: consult the Biocat Home Page via the EBI URL.

Other software

During recent months there has been a huge increase in the number of DNA-alignment associated software packages described on the World Wide Web. The European Bioinformatics Institute *BioCatalog* resource:

http://www.ebi.ac.uk/biocat/biocat.html

provides details of numerous packages covering DNA and protein alignment, mapping, genetics, molecular evolution and graphics. The DNA domain of the BioCatalog describes software (Table 10.2) suitable for sequence search, alignment, display, sequence format conversion (for example from GenBank format to FASTA) and RNA analysis.

Appendices

Internet Sites

- ASHI (American Society for Histocompatibility and Immunogenetics)
http://www.swmed.edu/home_pages/ASHI/
- BCM Search Launcher
http://gc.bcm.tmc.edu:8088/search-launcher/ launcher.html
- BioCatalogue
http://www.ebi.ac.uk/biocat/ biocat.html
- BioMedNet
http://biomednet.com/
- Bionet Electronic Newsgroup Network for Biology
http://www.bionet.com
- Bone Marrow Donors Worldwide (BMDW)
http://www.BMDW.ORG/
- BSHI (British Society for Histocompatibility and Immunogenetics)
http://www.umds.ac.uk/tissue/bshi1.html
- Dictionary of HLA Serological & DNA Equivalents
http://bmdw.org/wmda/FormA.html
- EBI (European Bioinformatics Institute, EMBL outstation)
http://www.ebi.ac.uk/
- European Molecular Biology Laboratory (EMBL)
http://www.embl-heidelberg.de/
- GenBank (National Center for Biotechnology Information)
http://www.ncbi.nlm.nih.gov/Web/Genbank/
- Gene Cards (Weizmann Institute of Science)
http://bioinformatics.weizmann.ac.il/cards/
- Genome Database
http://www.gdb.org/gdb/gdbtop.html
- HLA class I and II Sequence Alignments
http://www.anthonynolan.com/HIG/data.html
- HLA class II Sequence Alignments
ftp://cmgm.stanford.edu/pub/NMDP/
- Human Cytokine Gene Nucleotide Sequence Alignments
http://www.pam.bris.ac.uk/services/ cytokine.htm
- ImMunoGeneTics Database
http://www.ebi.ac.uk/imgt/
- Immunology Links
http://www.immunologylink.com

- MEDLINE
  http://www.ncbi.nlm.nih.gov/PubMed/
- NCBI Entrez Browser
  http://www.ncbi.nlm.nih.gov/Entrez/
- OMIM (Online Mutations in Man)
  http://www3.ncbi.nlm.nih.gov/omim/
- PIR-International Protein Sequence Database
  http://www-nbrf.georgetown.edu/pir/
- Sequence Retrieval System SEQNET (SRSWWW) at Hinxton
  http://srs.hgmp.mrc.ac.uk/
- SWISS-PROT
  http://www.expasy.ch/sprot/
- World Wide Web Virtual Library: Immunology
  http://mcb.harvard.edu/BioLinks.html

Software

- ClustalW
  http://www.no.embnet.org/clustalw.html
- GeneDoc
  http://www.cris.com/~Ketchup/genedoc.shtml
- Microsoft Internet Explorer
  http://microsoft.com/
- MACAW FTP site (Win 16/32)
  ftp://ncbi.nlm.nih.gov/pub/macaw/win16/
- MACAW FTP site (other platforms)
  ftp://ncbi.nlm.nih.gov/pub/macaw/
- Netscape Navigator
  http://home.netscape.com/
- ProMSED2
  ftp://iubio.bio.indiana.edu/molbio/ibmpc/promsed2.exe
- Sequin
  ftp://ncbi.nlm.nih.gov/sequin/

Contact E-mail addresses

MACAW	Gregory D Schuler (schuler@ncbi.nlm.nih.gov)
ProMSED	Alexey M Eroshkin (eroshkin@vector.nsk.su)

References

Bairoch, A and Apweiler, R (1997). The SWISS-PROT protein sequence data bank and its supplement TREMBL. *Nucl Acids Res* **25:** 31-36

Barker, WC, George, DG, Mewes, HW, Pfeiffer, F and Tsugita A. (1993). The PIR-International Databases 1993. *Nucl Acids Res* **21:** 3089-3092

Benson, DA, Boguski, MS, Lipman, DJ, Ostell, J and Ouellette, BF (1998). GenBank. *Nucl Acids Res* **26**: 1-7.

Bodmer, JG, Marsh, SGE, Albert, ED, Bodmer, WF, Bontrop, RE. *et al.* (1997). Nomenclature for Factors of the HLA system, 1996. *Eur J Immunogenet* **24:** 105-151

Crew, MD (1997). Compilation of distinct HLA-A, -B and -C transmembrane and cytoplasmic domain-encoding sequences. *Eur J Immunogenet* **24:** 443-449

Marsh, SGE and Bodmer, JG (1993). HLA class II nucleotide sequences, 1992. *Eur J Immunogenet* **20:** 47-49

Marsh, SGE and Bodmer, JG (1994). HLA class II nucleotide sequences, 1994. *Eur J Immunogenet* **21:** 519-551

Marsh, SGE (1998) Nomenclature for factors of the HLA system, update February 1998. *Hum Immunol* **59:** 323

Marsh, SGE (1998). HLA class II region sequences, 1998. *Tissue Antigens* **51:** 467-507

Mason, PM and Parham, P (1998). HLA class I region sequences, 1998. *Tissue Antigens* **51:** 417-466

Rodriguez-Tomé, P, Stoehr, PJ, Cameron, GN and Flores, P (1996). The European Bioinformatics Institute (EBI) databases. *Nucl Acids Res* **24:** 6-13

Schuler, GD, Altschul, SF and Lipman, DJ (1991). A workbench for multiple alignment construction and analysis. *Proteins: Structure, Function and Genetics* **9:** 180-190

Summer, CW, Hampson, VJ and Taylor, GM (1993). HLA class I non-coding nucleotide sequences, 1992. *Eur J Immunogenet* **20:** 201-240

Zemmour, J and Parham, P (1993). HLA class I nucleotide sequences, 1992. *Eur J Immunogenet* **20:** 29-45

PART 3

CELL-BASED HISTOCOMPATIBILITY TESTING

PART 3 OVERVIEW

CELL-BASED HISTOCOMPATIBILITY TESTING

C. Navarrete
NBS - London & The South East
North London Centre
Colindale Avenue
London NW9 5BG

HLA compatibility between a transplant recipient and a potential donor is one of the main factors that contributes to the successful outcome of the transplant. Major and minor differences in the HLA antigens between donor and recipient cells can be detected by T cells with a high degree of sensitivity.

Throughout the years a number of in vitro cellular assays have been developed to assess these differences. In the following section (Chapter 11), Ed Kaminsky provides a comprehensive account of the standard methodology and of the more recently described techniques currently in use.

The majority of these techniques have been derived from the observation that lymphocytes from two unrelated individuals could stimulate each other when cultured in vitro for a period of time (Bain *et al.,* 1964). This stimulation which was due primarily to differences in the HLA-Dw antigens coded for genes within the HLA class II region, resulted in cellular activation accompanied by blast transformation. The technique that was soon developed to identify the determinants involved became known as the mixed lymphocyte culture (MLC) (Bach and Hirschhorn, 1964).

During the MLC period both CD4+ proliferating and CD8+ cytotoxic T cells are generated, therefore most techniques involve the measurement of either cell proliferation or cell killing. Cell proliferation can be assessed by determining the ^{3}H-Thymidine incorporated by the dividing cells or by identifying the type and levels of cytokines secreted by MLC activated cells. An example of the latter is the limiting dilution analysis (LDA) to determine the frequency of IL-2 secreting (helper) T cell precursors (HTLp).

On the other hand, cell cytotoxicity has traditionally been assessed by determining the amount of ^{51}Chromium released by the lysed target cells in a test known as cell mediated lympholysis (CML). An extension of this technique is the LDA to quantitate the frequency of cytotoxic T lymphocyte precursors (CTLp) generated during the culture period. The percentage of cells killed by these effectors is then assessed by the ^{51}Cr release assay or by the release of fluorescent dyes.

Although HLA class I incompatibility primarily stimulates the generation of cytotoxic effectors and HLA class II incompatibility results in the activation of CD4+ helper T cells, optimum generation of CD8+ effector cells can be achieved by the activation of CD4+ cells in the first instance. These CD4+ cells can then contribute to the generation and differentiation of cytotoxic effector cells via the direct secretion of cytokines or via the activation of dendritic cells (Ridge *et al.*, 1998).

Experimental data has shown that although HLA-DR, -DQ and -DP molecules can all contribute to the strong cellular proliferation obtained in the primary mixed lymphocyte culture (MLC), HLA -DR seems to play a more prominent role.

With respect to HLA class I incompatibilities, LDA used to quantitate the CTLp frequency against HLA class I incompatibilities have shown that all HLA class I molecules (HLA-A, -B and -Cw) can induce the generation of CTLp. However, HLA-B antigens can generate a higher frequency of these effectors than HLA-A molecules.

The clinical relevance of the cellular techniques has been investigated in a number of studies involving bone marrow and renal transplant recipients. In the case of the MLC test, the results obtained showed no correlation between the in vitro reactivity and the incidence and severity of graft versus host disease (GVHD) observed in bone marrow transplant recipients.

However, techniques involving LDA of the frequency of IL-2 secreting alloreactive helper T cells (HTLp) seem to provide a better correlation with the incidence and severity of GVHD in transplants between HLA identical siblings.

Although the frequency CTLp has a strong correlation with the presence of HLA class I disparities, analysis performed prior to bone marrow transplantation using unrelated donors have failed to consistently demonstrate a correlation between donor anti-recipient CTLp frequencies and the incidence and severity of GVHD.

With our current knowledge on the influence of both pro-inflammatory and regulatory cytokines in the development of both humoral and cellular responses, techniques which can allow a combined analysis of both cells and cytokines produced in response to alloantigen (and to nominal antigen), stimulation will become more and more relevant (Murray, 1998). In this respect the analysis of cytokine secretion in bone marrow transplant patients has shown a good correlation between secretion of TNFα and the development of GVHD.

More recently, by using the ELISPOT technique (a modification of the ELISA test involving the detection and enumeration of cytokine secreting cells), it has been demonstrated that the level of cytokines secreted (such as IFNγ and IL-5) by mitogen stimulated peripheral blood lymphocytes are highly predictive of allograft function in these patients (Tary-Lehmann *et al.,* 1998).

With the current availability of high resolution DNA typing for most HLA alleles, and the increased use of T cell depletion in bone marrow transplantation, the clinical relevance of these techniques has sometimes been questioned. However, information regarding the degree of cellular alloreactivity between HLA matched unrelated individuals may be useful for the post transplant management of the patient. Furthermore, in cases where more than one donor is available this information may also be used to select the most suitable donors.

More recently, soluble MHC molecules loaded with fluorescently labelled viral or tumour derived peptides, are being used for the quantitation of antigen specific CD8+ T cells (Altman *et al.,* 1996). In the future a similar approach may be developed to allow the identification of alloreactive T cells (Romero *et al.,* 1998) and donor selection.

References

Altman, JD, Moss, PAH, Goulder, PJR, Barouch, DH, McHeyzer--Williams, MG, *et al.* (1996) Phenotypic analysis of antigen-specific T lymphocytes. Science, **274**, 94-96

Bain, B, Vas, MR and Lowestein, L (1964) The development of large immature mononuclear cells in mixed leuykocyte cultures. *Blood* **23:** 108

Bach, FH and Hirschhorn, K (1964) Lymphocyte interactions: a potential histocompatibility test in vitro. *Science* **142:** 183

Murray, JS (1998) How the MHC selects Th1/Th2 immunity. *Immunol Today* **19:** 157-163

Ridge, JR, Di Rosa, F and Matzinger, P (1998) A conditioned dendritic cell can be a temporal bridge between a $CD4^+$ T-helper and a T-killer cell. *Nature* **394:** 474-478

Romero, P, Dunbar, PR, Valmori, D, Pittet, M, Ogg, GS, *et al.* (1998) Ex vivo straining of metastic lymph nodes by class I major histocompatibility complex tetramers reveals high numbers of antigen-experienced tumor-specific cytotoxic T lymphocytes. *J Exp Med* **188:** 1-10

Tary-Lehmann, M, Hricik, DE, Justice, AC, Potter, NS and Heeger, PS (1998) Enzyme-linked immunosorbent assay splot detection of interferon-_ and interleukin 5-producing cells as a predictive marker for renal allograft failure. *Transplantation* **66:** 219-224

CHAPTER 11

CELL-BASED HISTOCOMPATIBILITY TESTING

E. Kaminski
Derriford Combined Laboratories
Level 7
Derriford Hospital
Plymouth PL6 8DH, England

Introduction

Normal individuals do not react against their own (autologous) tissue. However, a vigorous response, termed alloreactivity, can be mounted against foreign (allogeneic) tissue leading to graft rejection or graft-versus-host disease (GVHD). It is now known that the cellular basis for alloreactivity is the recognition, by alloreactive T lymphocytes, of cell surface alloantigens (HLA in humans) encoded for by the MHC. In view of the importance of HLA matching for transplantation outcome, highly sophisticated HLA typing methods have been developed which, for fortunate recipients, will identify a well matched donor. However, due to a limited donor pool, there will be a proportion of recipients where the typing techniques identify a 'major' or 'minor' degree of HLA incompatibility. It is recognized that successful transplants can occasionally be performed against 'major' HLA mismatches. However, a 'minor' HLA mismatch at the level of a single amino acid difference between donor and recipient can lead to severe GVHD (Keever *et al.,* 1994) or rejection (Fleischhauer *et al.,* 1990) after unrelated donor bone marrow transplantation. There is thus clearly a need for *in vitro* assays for quantifying alloreactivity and defining the significance of HLA mismatching. A series of cellular functional assays, based on simple mixed lymphocyte cultures, have been developed and will be discussed below.

Mixed Lymphocyte Reaction (MLR) / Mixed Lymphocyte Culture (MLC)

Introduction

When a mixture of two populations of mononuclear cells are cultured together this is termed a mixed lymphocyte culture (MLC) or mixed lymphocyte reaction (MLR) (Bain *et al.,* 1964, Bach *et al.,* 1964). Whilst cells from HLA-identical individuals do not respond against each other, cells from HLA-mismatched individuals undergo DNA synthesis, blast transformation, and proliferation, which peaks at 4-6 days. In such a culture, the lymphocytes from both individuals recognize the other as foreign, giving rise to a two-way MLR. The most important modification of this technique is the so-called 'one-way' MLR in which the stimulator cells are treated with irradiation or mitomycin C to prevent them from responding (Bach *et al.,* 1966). Such a one-way MLR can be set up in either the graft-versus-host (GVH) or host-versus-graft (HVG) directions. In an MLR, the cells are cultured together and then [^{3}H] thymidine is added to the cultures. Thymidine only incorporates into the DNA of dividing cells and thus will radiolabel the responding population. Finally, the cells are harvested and the amount of thymidine uptake measure by a β counter. The test response is compared to a positive control (response to HLA-mismatched cells) and a negative control (response to autologous cells). When the test reactivity is significantly above the autologous control, the MLR is considered positive.

It was soon recognized that, during mixed lymphocyte culture, two distinct populations of lymphocytes are stimulated, a proliferating and a cytotoxic population, and that these are stimulated by different MHC differences (Bach *et al.,* 1973, 1976). In an MLR, the responding cells are mainly alloreactive, $CD4^+$, helper T lymphocytes recognizing HLA class II differences on the foreign stimulatory cells. However, there is also a very weak component attributable to proliferating $CD8^+$ lymphocytes recognizing HLA class I antigens. The stimulatory cells are antigen presenting monocytes or B lymphocytes which, unlike resting T lymphocytes, have HLA class II antigens on their surface. Originally it was thought that the HLA determinants responsible for the MLR were encoded by a distinct HLA locus, HLA-*D*, but this is no longer tenable. HLA-DR mismatches predominate in the MLC (Al-Daccak *et al.,* 1990a, Baxter-Lowe *et al.,* 1992) and HLA-DR and DQ mismatches defined by RFLP correlate with a positive MLR (Clay *et al.,* 1989). However, positive MLCs can occur in HLA-DR and DQ matched pairs suggesting a role for other antigens such as HLA-DP (Clay *et al.,* 1989) and HLA A & B (Termijtelen *et al.,* 1981a). The contribution of DP has long been controversial, early studies indicating both no influence of DP on the MLR (Pawelec *et al.,* 1982) and an influence (Termijtelen *et al.,* 1981b) but more recent studies demonstrate that, although DP does not give rise to such a strong proliferative response as DR and DQ, some DP mismatches can indeed induce proliferation in MLC (Al-Daccak *et al.,* 1990b, Cesbron *et al.,* 1990, Olerup *et al.,* 1990, Moreau *et al.,* 1993, Awdeh *et al.,* 1995). Either, particular HLA-DP antigens are stimulatory or HLA-DP plays a role when priming has occurred, eg after multiple transfusions. Finally, *in vitro* responses to non HLA or minor Histocompatibility antigens can usually only be detected after *in vivo* sensitization by transfusion, transplantation, or pregnancy (Ting and Simpson 1989).

Clinical relevance

The MLR is a semiquantitative HLA matching test for confirming HLA class II identity between donor and recipient. Although it has played an important role in the selection of unrelated donors for bone marrow transplantation (BMT), it is now accepted that it is relatively imprecise and does not predict GVHD and/or clinical outcome after BMT from identical sibling (Lim *et al.,* 1988, DeGast *et al.,* 1992), unrelated (Hows *et al.,* 1986, Al-Daccak *et al.,* 1990b, Mickelson *et al.,* 1993 & 1996, Segall *et al.,* 1996) or related haploidentical donors (Mickelson *et al.,* 1994).

In the case of renal transplantation, there is evidence for (Langhoff *et al.*, 1985, Harmon *et al.*, 1982) and against (Cullen *et al.*, 1977, Burke *et al.*, 1993, Steinmann *et al.*, 1994) the MLR predicting rejection and clinical outcome. The reasons for the MLR not predicting clinical outcome may be that it mainly detects $CD4^+$ class II reactive lymphocytes and not $CD8^+$ class I reactive lymphocytes, which are an important effector cell population, and/or the fact that it is only semiquantitative.

Methods

There is a standardized MLC technique proposed during the Eighth International Histocompatibility Workshop (Dupont *et al.*, 1980).

1. *Samples*

- Patient, donor & third party control.
- 20 ml of peripheral blood in 400iu/20ml preservative free heparin.
- The blood should ideally be fresh but can be kept overnight at room temperature or the
- mononuclear cells isolated (see below) and cryopreserved in liquid nitrogen.

2. *Method* (all steps to be performed in a class II cabinet under aseptic conditions):

Patient cells = stimulator (S)
Donor cells = responder (R)
Control cells = third party control of known HLA phenotype (X)

2.1. *Preparation of cells*

- Isolate peripheral blood mononuclear cells (PBMC) by density gradient centrifugation. Dilute peripheral blood 1:1 with culture medium, layer onto Ficoll-Hypaque and centrifuge at 2,000 rpm for 20 min.
- Harvest interface cells, resuspend in culture medium and wash at 1,800 rpm for 10 min, followed by two further washes at 1,200 rpm for 5 min.
- Resuspend cells in an exact quantity of culture medium.
- Count cell numbers using a haemocytometer and adjust concentrations to 1.0×10^6.
- Divide the responder (R), stimulator (S) and 3rd party (X) cells into two aliquots. Label one aliquot R, S and X and the other §R, §S and §X.
- Irradiate the aliquots of cells marked §R, §S and §X with 3,000 rads.

2.2. *Plating-out cells*

- Plate out, using a repeating microtitre pipette, 50μl aliquots of cells in triplicate to sterile 96 well roundbottom microtitre plates to achieve 5 x 10^4 of responders and 5 x 10^4 of stimulators per well, using the following combinations:

  R + §S; S + §R; R + §R; R + §X; X + §S

- As controls, plate out R cells and 50μl medium only, and §R cells and 50μl culture medium only, as follows:

  R + O; §R + O

2.3. *Cell culture and assay*

- Incubate at 37°C in a humidified atmosphere of 5% CO_2 in air for five days.
- Add 1.0 μCi of tritiated thymidine to each well, and incubate at 37° C for 18 h.
- Harvest the cells onto filter discs or mats and count in a β counter. There are currently a number of different harvesting machines and counting systems available. Consult the manufacturer's instruction manual for the appropriate procedures to follow.

3. *Analysis of MLR data*

- Calculate the mean count for each triplicate.
- Calculate the relative response index (RRI) and stimulation index (SI) as follows:

$$RRI = \frac{(R + \S S) - (R + \S R)}{(R + \S X) - (R + \S R)} \times 100\ \%$$

$$SI = \frac{(R + \S S)}{(R + \S R)}$$

- The test response is compared to a positive (response to 3rd party cells) and a negative (response to autologous cells) control.

4. *Interpretation of results*

When the test reactivity is significantly above the autologous control, the MLR is considered positive. The exact cutoff to define positivity has to be determined by each laboratory and this should take into account background proliferation which can be affected by the patient's disease; e.g. chronic myeloid leukaemia gives higher backgrounds. The results are usually expressed as a relative response index (RRI). A positive RRI or a stimulation index of 2 suggests HLA mismatching.

Internal & external QC

The internal controls consist of:

- responder cells plus irradiated third party cells (R + §X) to confirm that the responder cells are capable of proliferating
- third party cells plus irradiated stimulator cells (X + §S) to confirm that the stimulator cells are capable of stimulating.

There is no external QC scheme available.

Specialist equipment or reagents required

Culture Medium:

☑ 1x RPMI 1640 (Gibco)

☑ Penicillin 100iu/ml (Flow Labs)

☑ Streptomycin 100iu/ml (Flow Labs)

☑ L-Glutamine 200mM (Flow Labs)

☑ Human heat inactivated pooled 10% AB serum (AB serum is only required for cultures - not for washing)

Other reagents:

☑ ^{3}H (tritiated) thymidine (Amersham)

☑ Ficoll-Hypaque (Pharmacia)

Equipment:

☑ Radiation source (usually a gamma irradiator)

☑ Cell harvester

☑ Laminar flow hood

☑ β-counter

Modifications of Mixed Lymphocyte Cultures

Mixed epidermal cell-lymphocyte reaction

In this assay, responder PBMCs are incubated with irradiated stimulator epidermal cells, derived from suction blisters, for 6 days. Proliferation is then measured as in a standard MLC (Bagot *et al.,* 1986a). The mixed epidermal cell-lymphocyte reaction has been shown to predict acute GVHD after identical sibling, MLR negative BMT (Bagot *et al.,* 1986a, 1986b, 1988), suggesting recognition of minor histocompatibility antigens.

Skin explant assay

In this assay, responder PBMCs are incubated with irradiated stimulator PBMCs for 7-8 days - primary mixed lymphocyte culture. The primed cells are then added to skin explants for 3 days, and the secondary response evaluated by grading, histopathologically, the graft-versus-host activity in the skin (Berkman *et al.,* 1985). It has been demonstrated that the effector cells in this assay are CD3, CD4 and CD8+ve lymphocytes (Dickinson *et al.,* 1988, Sviland *et al.,* 1990). More recently, Dickinson *et al.,* demonstrated the role of cytokines in the skin-explant assay (see section on cytokines later). The skin explant assay has been shown to correlate with acute GVHD after identical sibling BMT (Berkman *et al.,* 1985, Vogelsang *et al.,* 1985, Sviland *et al.,* 1990, Dickinson *et al.,* submitted), suggesting recognition of minor histocompatibility antigens.

T-cell activation molecule gene expression in MLC

In this assay, responder PBMCs are incubated with unirradiated PBMCs for 2 days - a two-way MLC. A T-cell mitogen (Con A) is then added for 12 h, followed by semiquantitative analysis of IL-2R (CD25), CD28, CTLA-4, ICAM-1, and CD44 mRNA by PCR. One study has demonstrated increased CD28, CTLA-4 and CD44 mRNA in those patients with severe GVHD after identical sibling BMT (Tanaka *et al.,* 1995a).

Addition of cytokines to the MLC

It has been demonstrated that the addition of cytokines to a standard MLC enables the prediction of acute GVHD after identical sibling BMT (Bishara *et al.,* 1994).

Cell Mediated Lympholysis (CML)

Introduction

If, after a one-way MLC between HLA-mismatched individuals, "target" cells from the original stimulator are added to the culture, these cells will be killed. The target cells are lysed by responder T lymphocytes which were "primed" during the MLC to recognize foreign antigens on the stimulator cells. This is termed cell mediated lympholysis (CML) or cytotoxicity. In a CML assay the responding cells are mainly alloreactive, $CD8^+$ cytotoxic T lymphocytes recognizing HLA class I (A, B, and C) differences on the foreign stimulatory cells (Kristensen 1978), but there is also a minority population of $CD4^+$ cytotoxic T lymphocytes recognising HLA class II (DR, DQ, and DP) antigens (Breuning *et al.,*. 1984). Although primary *in vitro* responses by cytotoxic T cells to minor Histocompatibility antigens cannot be detected by CML, primed responses to minor Histocompatibility antigens, due to sensitization by blood transfusion, between HLA identical siblings can be detected (Parkman *et al.,* 1976).

Clinical relevance

CML is a semiquantitative HLA matching test which confirms HLA class I and, to a lesser extent, class II identity between donor and recipient. It can also be used to detect previous sensitization to minor Histocompatibility antigens. High pretransplant CML activity has been shown to predict rejection after renal allografting (Harmon *et al.,*. 1982) and graft rejection after BMT from HLA-identical siblings sensitized by blood transfusions to minor histocompatibility antigens (Warren *et al.,* 1976, 1980, Voogt *et al.,* 1990). Cytotoxic T cells are thought to be an important effector cell population in both graft rejection and GVHD, and the CML may well be a more complete in vitro correlate of the allograft reaction than the MLR. The clinical potential of the CML assay is becoming increasingly recognized but is limited by the fact that it is a semiquantitative test.

Methods

There is now a standardised CML technique which was proposed during the Third European CML Workshop (Kristensen 1980) and the methodology will be only briefly summarised here. Responder mononuclear cells are cultured with irradiated (3000 rads) or mitomycin treated, stimulator, mononuclear cells in microtiter plates. Target cells are prepared by culturing stimulator mononuclear cells with phytohaemagglutinin (PHA), a T cell mitogen. After 4-5 days incubation, ^{51}Cr-labeled "targets" are added to the cultures and incubated for a further 3-4 h. When targets are lysed they release their ^{51}Cr into the supernatant. The supernatant is then harvested and the amount of ^{51}Cr release measured. The test response is compared to a positive (maximal or total ^{51}Cr release obtained by lysing targets with detergent) and to a negative (spontaneous ^{51}Cr release) control. The degree of lysis is measured as the percentage of ^{51}Cr release in the specific target cells compared to the total ^{51}Cr release.

Cytotoxic T Lymphocyte Precursor (CTL-p) frequency analysis

Introduction to limiting dilution analysis (LDA)

For detailed reviews of LDA see the following: Lefkovits and Waldmann 1984, Waldmann and Lefkovits 1984, Waldmann *et al.,* 1987, Sharrock *et al.,* 1990. The aim of limiting dilution analysis (LDA) is to determine the frequency of precursors (cells with the potential to become mature cells upon stimulation) of alloreactive lymphocytes within a population of mononuclear cells. Precursors of both cytotoxic T lymphocytes (CTL-p) or helper T lymphocytes (HTL-p) can be measured. LDA involves partitioning the mononuclear cell population containing the precursor cell of interest into multiple wells at different concentrations by serial dilutions. At high concentrations there will be, on average, more than one precursor per well and at low concentrations there will be, on average, no CTL-p per well. The responder mononuclear cells are then cultured with irradiated allogeneic stimulator mononuclear cells, as in a primary MLC, until sufficient progeny of the precursor have been generated to be detected by an appropriate assay. In the case of CTL-p this will entail a cytotoxic assay and, in the case of HTL-p, a proliferative assay. In order to decide which wells initially contained one or more precursors (positive wells) or in which there were no precursors (negative wells), an arbitrary control is selected from which to score all other wells for positivity or negativity. In order for the system to be limiting, the only limiting factor in an individual culture must be the input number of mononuclear cells containing the precursor. Thus, all necessary growth factors and nutrients must be added in excess.

The theory of LDA is that, provided the initial cell of interest in the responder population is randomly distributed, the proportion of negative cultures is unequivocally defined by the zero term of the Poisson distribution. The proportion of cultures which are negative at any given cell input is defined by the expression: $F_0 = e^{-u}$ where F_0 is the fraction of negative cultures per total number of cultures; ie, the base of the natural logarithm, and u the average number of precursor cells per culture. The above expression can be converted to its logarithmic form as follows: $u = -\text{Ln}\ (F_0)$. This can be represented graphically as a straight line in a semilogarithmic plot. In other words, the negative logarithm of the fraction of nonresponding cultures is linearly proportional to the mean number of precursors per culture. The resulting straight line can be used for an estimation of frequency. If $u = 1$ is substituted in the zero term of the Poisson formula: $F_0 = e^{-1} = 1/e = 1/2.7 = 0.37 = 37\%$.

Therefore, by interpolating at the level of 37% nonresponding cultures, the concentration of responder cells containing an average of one precursor cell can be estimated (Fig 11.1).

The line can also be used to act as an internal control to verify that the system is measuring the activity of a single limiting cell type. A straight line means that the cultures are in accordance with "single hit" kinetics. Validity testing to detect deviations from single hit has been discussed by Taswell (1984). The lines can be

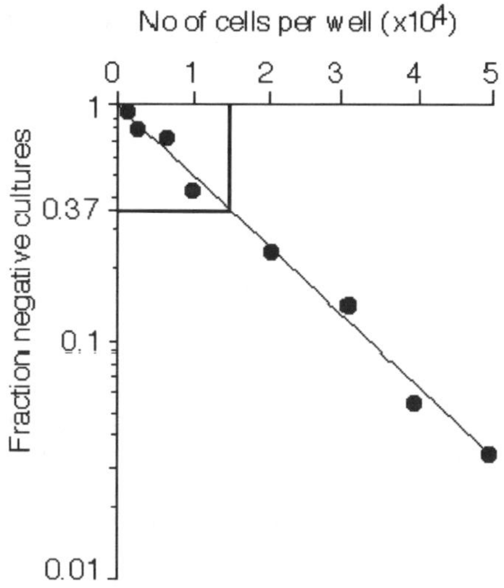

Figure 11.1. Semi-logarithmic plot of mononuclear cell input against the fraction of nonresponding cultures. In this single-hit curve the frequency of CTL-p / HTL-p for allo-MHC can be interpolated from $F_0 = 0.37$. the estimated frequency is about 1:14 x 10^3.

fitted using the least squares method which determines the best line through the origin; χ^2 values can then be used to determine goodness of fit, ie, how well the experimental data fits the line. There are several statistical methods for estimating the frequency of responding cells: least squares, weighted mean, maximum likelihood, and minimum χ^2 (Taswell 1981). Maximum likelihood estimation is a commonly used method because it uses experimental data and has been shown to be more statistically valid than frequency estimation from fitted lines (Fazekas de St. Groth 1982).

Introduction to CTL-p

An alloreactive cytotoxic T lymphocyte precursor (CTL-p) is a naive T cell which has the potential to differentiate into a mature CTL after encountering the specific alloantigen recognised by its T cell receptor. The frequency of allo-reactive CTL-p was shown to be high in humans (van Oers *et al.,* 1978) and varies between different individuals (Kabelitz *et al.,* 1985, Sharrock *et al.,* 1987), this variation being related to the degree of HLA matching between donor and recipient (Kaminski *et al.,* 1988). The CTL-p response detected by LDA has been attributed to a predominance of alloreactive $CD8^+$ CTLs recognising HLA class I differences on the foreign stimulatory cells, with a minor contribution by $CD4^+$ CTLs (Moretta *et al.,* 1983; Kabelitz *et al.,* 1985). However, there is now evidence that, although in vitro the bulk of the CTL-p response is due to $CD8^+$ CTLs, there is also a significant contribution due to $CD4^+$ CTLs recognising HLA class II antigens, which can be more easily detected if the $CD8^+$ response is negated by matching for HLA class I antigens or by depletion of the $CD8^+$ subset (Man *et al.,* 1990).

HLA class I mismatches predominate in CTL-p assays, HLA-A and -B (Zhang *et al.,* 1989, 1990a; Breur-Vriesendorp *et al.,* 1990, 1991), and HLA-C (Barnardo *et al.,* 1996) mismatches being detected. However, CTL-p assays can also detect HLA class II differences, including DR and DQ, (Man *et al.,* 1990; Busca *et al.,* 1995), but the contribution of DP is unclear (Sage, personal communication). Finally, it has also been demonstrated that CTL-p frequencies against HLA-B antigens are higher than against HLA-A (Zhang *et al.,* 1990b) and this may explain why matching for HLA-B is more important for good allograft survival than matching for HLA-A.

As in the CML assay, primary *in vitro* CTL-p responses to minor histocompatibiilty antigens cannot be detected by LDA (Kaminski *et al.,* 1988; Irschick *et al.,* 1992), and this is thought to be due to the extremely low frequency of minor histocompatibility-specific T cells. However, high CTL-p responses between HLA-identical siblings have been demonstrated in patients sensitized by blood transfusions, and these are probably directed at minor histocompatibility antigens (Kaminski *et al.,* 1990).

Clinical relevance

CTL-p frequency analysis is a quantitative HLA matching test which confirms HLA class I and class II identity between donor and recipient. In unrelated donor/patient pairs prior to BMT, CTL-p can recognise very fine antigenic variants indistinguishable by serological methods, including HLA class I antigens: HLA-A, HLA-B (Zhang *et al.,*. 1990a; Kaminski *et al.,* 1991a, Rufer *et al.,* 1993, 1995, Slavcev *et al.,* 1995, Cukrova *et al.,* 1995, Spencer *et al.,* 1995a, Speiser *et al.,* 1996), HLA-C (Barnardo *et al.,* 1996, Speiser *et al.,* 1996) and HLA class II antigens: HLA-DR and DQ (Kaminski *et al.,* 1991a; Busca *et al.,* 1995). The importance of fine antigenic variants is demonstrated by two cases of unrelated donor BMT in which the patients and donors differed only by subtypes of HLA B44 (B44.1 and B44.2) due to a single amino acid difference at position 156 of the B44 molecule. In one case this resulted in GVHD (Keever *et al.,* 1994) and in the other in rejection (Fleischhauer *et al.,* 1990); in both cases, CTLs specific for the mismatched B44 antigen were demonstrated. CTL-p frequency analysis can also provide a pretransplant measure of both GVH and HVG reactivity. High CTL-p frequency has been shown to predict severe acute GVHD after HLA matched unrelated donor BMT (Kaminski *et al.,* 1989; Roosnek *et al.,* 1993; Schwarer *et al.,* 1994; Spencer *et al.,* 1995a,b; Speiser *et al.,* 1996) and after haploidentical BMT (Roosnek *et al.,* 1993). However, two groups have not demonstrated a correlation between pretransplant CTL-p and GVHD after unrelated donor BMT (Fussell *et al.,* 1994; Montagna *et al.,* 1996). In the case of identical sibling BMT, no correlation has been shown between pretransplant CTL-p and GVHD (Irschick *et al.,* 1992, Dickinson *et al.,* submitted). Thus CTL-p frequency analysis may be useful in aiding final donor selection before unrelated or mismatched related donor BMT, particularly in situations where there is a choice of more than one donor.

In the case of organ allografts, it has proved difficult to correlate pretransplant CTL-p reactivity with graft rejection. No correlation has been demonstrated between pretransplant CTL-p and rejection after renal transplantation (Steinmann *et al.,* 1994; Bouma *et al.,* 1995; Mestre *et al.,* 1996); liver transplantation (Eberspacher *et al.,* 1994) or heart transplantation (Reader *et al.,* 1990). One study however did show a correlation between pretransplant CTL-p and rejection after heart transplantation (Hu *et al.,* 1994).

Methods

The protocol described here is based on that developed by Kaminski (1991b), and uses radiolabelled chromium-51. For an alternative labeling method using Europium, see Bouma *et al.,* (1992).

1. *Samples*

Patient, donor & third party control: 20 ml of peripheral blood in 400iu/20ml preservative free heparin.

The blood should ideally be fresh but can be kept overnight at room temperature or the mononuclear cells isolated (see below) and cryopreserved in liquid nitrogen.

2. *Method*

All steps should be performed in a class II cabinet under aseptic conditions.

Patient cells = stimulator (S)
Donor cells = responder (R)
Control cells = 3rd party control of known HLA phenotype (X)

2.1. *Preparation of cells:*

- Isolate peripheral blood mononuclear cells (PBMC) by density gradient centrifugation. Dilute peripheral blood 1:1 with culture medium, layer onto Ficoll-Hypaque and centrifuge at 2,000 rpm for 20 min.
- Harvest interface cells, resuspend in culture medium and wash at 1,800 rpm for 10 mins, followed by two further washes at 1,200 rpm for 5 min.
- Resuspend cells in an exact quantity of culture medium.
- Count cell numbers using a haemocytometer and adjust concentrations to 1.0×10^6/ml. The total number of responder cells required for a full assay is 7.0×10^6 and the number of stimulator cells is 19×10^6.
- Divide the stimulator (S) and 3rd party (X) cells into two aliquots. Label one aliquot, S and X and the other §S and §X. Label responder cells (R).
- Irradiate the aliquots of cells marked §S and §X with 3,000 rads.

2.2. *Responder cell dilutions:*

Prepare dilutions by taking aliquots of the responder cells (R), at an initial concentration of 1.0 x 10^6/ml, and diluting in culture medium so as to achieve the following concentrations: 1.0, 0.8, 0.6, 0.4, 0.2, 0.1, 0.05 and 0.025 x 10^6/ml.

2.3. *Plating out responder cells:*

Plate out, using a repeating microtitre pipette, 50µl aliquots of 30 replicates per dilution (if there is a shortage of cells, 24 replicates can be used) of responder cells (R) to sterile 96 well roundbottom microtitre plates. This will achieve the following number of responder cells per well:

Cell concentration	**No of cells per well**
1.0 x 10^6/ml	5 x 10^4/ml
0.8 x 10^6/ml	4 x 10^4/ml
0.6 x 10^6/ml	3 x 10^4/ml
0.4 x 10^6/ml	2 x 10^4/ml
0.2 x 10^6/ml	1 x 10^4/ml
0.1 x 10^6/ml	0.5 x 10^4/ml
0.05 x 10^6/ml	0.25 x 10^4/ml
0.025 x 10^6/ml	0.125 x 10^4/ml

2.4. *Plating out stimulator cells:*

Add 50µl aliquots of irradiated stimulator cells (§S) to all the above wells

2.5. *Plating out controls:*

50µl §S + 50µl culture medium	(§S + 0)
50µl R (1.0 x 10^6/ml) + 50µl §X	(R + §X)
50µl X + 50µl §S	(X + §S)

Use 15 replicates per control.

2.6. *Cell culture:*

- Add 50 µl of culture medium to ALL the above wells to achieve a final volume of 150µl per well.
- Incubate at 37°C in a humidified atmosphere of 5% CO_2 in air for ten days.
- On days 3 and 6, feed cultures with 25 µl culture medium containing rIL-2 to give a final concentration of 5 U/ml rIL-2 per well.

2.7. *Preparation of targets for cytotoxicity assays (PHA blasts):*

- On day 0, plate out five 1ml aliquots of stimulator cells (S) and one 1ml aliquot of third party cells (X) at a concentration of 1.0 x 10^6/ml in sterile 24-well flat-bottomed tissue culture plates. Add phytohaemagglutinin (PHA) to each well to achieve a concentration of 2 µg/ml and incubate at 37°C in a humidified atmosphere of 5% CO_2 in air for ten days.
- The cultures will require splitting and feeding with fresh culture medium containing 10 U/ml rIL-2 when the medium turns yellow; ie every 2 or 3 days.

2.8. *Radiolabelling of targets for cytotoxicity assay:*

- On the day of assay, harvest the "PHA-blasts", wash twice in medium at 1,200 rpm for 5 mins and resuspend in 2 mls of medium. Count the cell concentration using a haemocytometer and aliquot a volume of cells sufficient to give 5 x 10^6 into a fresh tube. Centrifuge at 1,200 rpm for 5 mins, discard supernatant, and resuspend pellet by flicking the tube gently.
- Add sodium chromate (^{51}Cr) at an activity of 200 µCi/10^7 cells, to the cells in a total volume of 50 µl (including AB serum) and incubate at 37°C for 1h. Add culture medium and wash the cells three times by centrifuging at 1,200 rpm for 5 min. Count cell numbers and adjust concentration to 1 x 10^5/ml. The total number of targets (S) required for a full assay is 3 x 10^6.

2.9. *Cytotoxicity assay:*

- On the day of assay, remove 100 µl of supernatant from all the wells. Add 100µl (1 x 10^4) of the ^{51}Cr-labelled targets (S) to each well except R + §X, where 100µl (1 x 10^4) of the ^{51}Cr-labelled targets (X) are added. Shake plates gently for 1 min on a plate shaker. For the spontaneous ^{51}Cr release, add 100µl of targets to 100µl of medium and for the total ^{51}Cr release, add 100µl of targets to 100µl of 1% Triton X. Incubate the plates for 4 h at 37°C.
- Centrifuge plates in a plate centrifuge at 1000 rpm for 5 min. Transfer 100µl of supernatant to 2 -3 ml tubes. Seal with wax and count irradiation using a gamma counter.

2.10. *Scoring wells for positivity or negativity*

Calculate the mean ^{51}Cr release of the background control wells §S + 0 (irradiated stimulators only). Wells are scored as positive if their ^{51}Cr release is greater than the mean + 3 SD of the background control ^{51}Cr release, otherwise they are scored as negative. On this basis the number of negative cultures for each dilution is calculated.

3. *Analysis of Limiting Dilution Data*

The frequency of responding cells is routinely determined by maximum likelihood estimation. However, it is first necessary to validate the curve as single hit, prior to an estimation of frequency. A number of computer programmes have been developed to perform validity testing and estimate frequencies. These are generally based on Taswell formulae (1981), including Taswell (1984), Stribosch *et al.,* (1987) and Waldmann *et al.,* (1987). Interested readers would be recommended to directly contact laboratories routinely performing LDA. CTL-p frequency results are usually expressed as the number of PBMC containing 1 precursor; eg 1: 14,000 (Fig 11.1), and the variance as 95% confidence limits.

4. *Interpretation of CTL-p results*

Each laboratory must determine its own definition of positive and negative CTL-ps. An arbitrary cut-off of 1: 100,000 is often used for defining 'high / low' CTL-p responses, i.e. a high CTL-p = 1:1,000 - 1:100,000 and a low CTL-p = 1:100,000 - 1:1,000,000. In general, a 'high' CTL-p response is suggestive of HLA mismatching, and a 'low' CTL-p response, particularly one below 1:200,000, of good HLA matching. CTL-p responses between 1:100,000 and 1:200,000 could suggest a mismatch of lesser clinical significance.

Internal & external QC

The internal controls consist of:

- responder cells plus irradiated third party cells (R + §X) tested against third party (X) targets, to confirm that the responder cells are capable of cytotoxicity
- third party cells plus irradiated stimulator cells (X + §S) tested against stimulator (S) targets, to confirm that the stimulator cells are capable of stimulating

There is no external QC scheme available.

Specialist equipment or reagents required

Culture Medium

- ☑ 1x RPMI 1640 (Gibco)
- ☑ Penicillin 100iu/ml (Flow Labs)
- ☑ Streptomycin 100iu/ml (Flow Labs)
- ☑ L-Glutamine 200mM (Flow Labs)
- ☑ Human heat inactivated pooled 10% AB serum (AB serum is only required for cultures - not for washing)

Reagents

- ☑ Ficoll-Hypaque (Pharmacia)
- ☑ rIL-2 (Boehringer-Mannheim)
- ☑ Phytohaemagglutinin (Wellcome)
- ☑ ^{51}Cr sodium chromate (Amersham)

Equipment

- ☑ Radiation source (usually a gamma irradiator)
- ☑ Laminar flow hood
- ☑ γ-counter
- ☑ Plate shaker

Modified CTL-p assays

In these assays, anti-CD8 monoclonal antibodies, CSA or FK506 are added to standard CTL-p assays in order to differentiate between naive & primed CTLs. Using such systems, it has been demonstrated that CTLs directed against HLA class I antigens, towards which the patient has formed anti-HLA class I antibodies, were more 'primed' than CTLs directed to HLA class I antigens towards which no antibodies have been formed (Roelen *et al.*, 1993). In addition, it has been shown that CTL-p against HLA-B are more 'primed' than CTL-p against HLA-A (Roelen *et al.*, 1994). Such assays may be of value in highly sensitized patients awaiting a renal transplant.

Helper T Lymphocyte Precursor (HTL-p) frequency analysis for the enumeration of IL-2 secreting-cell frequencies

Introduction

For a more general introduction to limiting dilution analysis, see under CTL-p frequency analysis, above.

An alloreactive helper T lymphocyte precursor (HTL-p) is a naive T cell which has the potential to differentiate into a mature helper T lymphocyte after encountering the specific alloantigen recognised by its T cell receptor. In this case, we are interested in the frequencies of HTL-p with the potential to secrete interleukin-2 (IL-2). Several limiting dilution assays for quantifying numbers of IL-2 secreting HTL-p have been described (Vie and Miller 1986; Orosz *et al.,* 1987, Theobald *et al.,* 1989, 1990, Deacock *et al.,* 1992a, Young *et al.,* 1996, Hornick *et al.,* 1997). As is the case with CTL-p, the frequency of allo-reactive HTL-p has been shown to be high in humans (Moretta *et al.,* 1985) and varies between different individuals (Orosz *et al.,* 1987), this variation being related to the degree of HLA matching between donor and recipient (Deacock *et al.,* 1992a). The HTL-p response detected by LDA is attributable to a predominance of alloreactive $CD4^+$ HTLs recognising HLA class II differences on the foreign stimulatory cells, but also to a significant contribution of $CD8^+$ HTLs recognising HLA class I (Joos *et al.,* 1989). HTL-p assays recognise both HLA class I and class II antigens (Joos *et al.,* 1989, Theobald *et al.,* 1993, Schwarer *et al.,* 1994), including HLA-DP (Potolicchio *et al.,* 1996, Sage personal communication). Finally, two studies have demonstrated high HTL-p frequencies between HLA identical siblings, suggesting recognition of minor Histocompatibility antigens (Theobald *et al.,* 1992, Schwarer *et al.,* 1993), however, two more recent studies were unable to confirm this (Freidel *et al.,* 1996, Dickinson *et al.,* submitted).

Clinical relevance

HTL-p assays have been shown to have similar predictive value to CTL-p and predict acute GVHD after unrelated donor BMT (Schwarer *et al.,* 1994). In addition, correlations have been demonstrated between HTL-p and acute GVHD after identical sibling BMT (Theobald *et al.,* 1992, Schwarer *et al.,* 1993; Weston *et al.,* 1997) and chronic GVHD after identical sibling BMT (Bunjes *et al.,* 1995), however two more recent studies were unable to confirm this (Freidel *et al.,* 1996, Dickinson *et al.,* submitted). Thus HTL-p frequency analysis may be useful in aiding final donor selection before unrelated or mismatched related donor BMT, particularly in situations where there is a choice of more than one donor.

In the case of organ transplantation, no correlation has been demonstrated between pretransplant HTL-p and rejection after renal transplantation (Bouma *et al.,* 1995, Beik *et al.,* 1997). One study however did show a correlation between HTL-p and T cell sensitization in patients with chronic renal failure (Deacock *et al.,* 1992b).

Methods

The protocol described here is based on that developed by Deacock *et al.,* (1992a) and Hornick *et al.,* (1997), and is reproduced here with kind permission of the Clinical Immunology Laboratory, Imperial College, Hammersmith Hospital.

1. *Samples*

☑ Patient, donor & third party control.

☑ 20 ml of peripheral blood in 400iu/20ml preservative free heparin. The blood should ideally be fresh but can be kept overnight at room temperature or the mononuclear cells isolated (see below) and cryopreserved in liquid nitrogen.

2. *Method*

All steps should be performed in a class II cabinet under aseptic conditions

Patient cells = stimulator (S)
Donor cells = responder (R)
Control cells = 3rd party control of known HLA phenotype (X)

2.1. *Preparation of cells*

- Isolate peripheral blood mononuclear cells (PBMC) by density gradient centrifugation. Dilute peripheral blood 1:1 with culture medium, layer onto Ficoll-Hypaque and centrifuge at 2,000 rpm for 20 min.
- Harvest interface cells, resuspend in culture medium and wash at 1,800 rpm for 10 min, followed by two further washes at 1,200 rpm for 5 min.
- Resuspend cells in an exact quantity of culture medium.
- Divide the third party cells (X) into two aliquots marked (X) and (§X). Label responder cells (R) and stimulator cells (§S).
- Count cell numbers using a haemocytometer and adjust cell concentrations as follows:

Responder (R)	= 1.0×10^6/ml
Third party (X)	= 1.0×10^6/ml
Stimulator (§S)	= 0.5×10^6/ml
Third party (§X)	= 0.5×10^6/ml

- The total number of responder cells required for a full assay is 11.0×10^6 and the number of stimulator cells is 12.0×10^6.
- Irradiate the aliquots of cells marked §S and §X with 3,000 rads

2.2. *Responder cell dilutions:*

Prepare dilutions by taking aliquots of the responder cells (R), at an initial concentration of 1.0 x 10^6/ml, and diluting in culture medium so as to achieve the following concentrations: 1.0, 0.8, 0.6, 0.4, 0.2, 0.1, 0.05 and 0.025 x 10^6/ml.

2.3. *Plating out responder cells:*

Plate out, using a repeating microtitre pipette, 50µl aliquots of 24 replicates per dilution of responder cells (R) to sterile 96 well roundbottom microtitre plates. This will achieve the following number of responder cells per well:

Cell concentration	**No of cells per well**
1.0 x 10^6/ml	5 x 10^4/ml
0.8 x 10^6/ml	4 x 10^4/ml
0.6 x 10^6/ml	3 x 10^4/ml
0.4 x 10^6/ml	2 x 10^4/ml
0.2 x 10^6/ml	1 x 10^4/ml
0.1 x 10^6/ml	0.5 x 10^4/ml
0.05 x 10^6/ml	0.25 x 10^4/ml
0.025 x 10^6/ml	0.125 x 10^4/ml

2.4. *Plating out stimulator cells:*

Add 100µl aliquots of irradiated stimulator cells (§S) to all the above wells

2.5. *Plating out controls:*

100µl §S + 50 µl culture medium	(§S + 0) in 24 wells
50µl R (1.0 x 10^6/ml) + 100µl §X	(R + §X) in 12 wells
50µl X + 100µl §S	(X + §S) in 12 wells
50µl R (all dilutions) + 100µl culture medium	(R + 0) in 24 wells

Incubate at 37°C in a humidified atmosphere of 5% CO_2 in air for 64 h.

2.6. *Preparation of CTLL cell line:*

- Grow cell line in culture medium containing 10% FCS and 10 - 20 U/ml rIL-2 at 37°C in a humidified atmosphere of 5% CO_2 in air. The cultures will require splitting and feeding with fresh culture medium containing rIL-2 three times a week.
- After 64 hours incubation, irradiate plates with 2,500 rads.

2.7. *IL-2 controls:*

- Prepare doubling dilutions of rIL-2, starting at 2 iu/ml to achieve the following concentrations (shown approx):

  2, 1, 0.5, 0.25, 0.125, 0.0625, 0.03, 0.015, 0.0078, 0.004 iu/ml

- Include a medium only control (ie no IL-2)
- Plate out 100µl of each IL-2 dilution to 6 wells, including the medium only control, commencing with the lowest concentration to prevent contamination.

2.8. *Assay:*

- Harvest CTLL cells, centrifuge once at 1000rpm for 10 min, wash twice at 1200 rpm for 5 min and adjust CTLL cell concentration to 1 x 10^5/ml.
- Add 25µl of CTLL cells to all wells (ie 2.5 x 10^3 per well).
- Incubate plates at 37°C in a humidified atmosphere of 5% CO_2 in air for 36 h.
- Add 1µCi/well of Tritiated [^{3}H] thymidine and incubate at 37°C for 18 h.
- Harvest the cells onto filter discs or mats and count in a β-counter. There are currently a number of different harvesting machines and counting systems available. Consult the manufacturer's instruction manual for the appropriate procedures to follow

2.9. *Scoring wells for positivity or negativity*

Calculate the mean CPM of the background control wells §S + 0 (irradiated stimulators only). Wells are scored as positive if their CPM is greater than the mean + 3 SD of the background control CPM, otherwise they are scored as negative. On this basis the number of negative cultures for each dilution is calculated.

3. *Analysis of limiting dilution data*

The frequency of responding cells is routinely determined by maximum likelihood estimation. However, it is first necessary to validate the curve as single hit, prior to an estimation of frequency. A number of computer programmes have been developed to perform validity testing and estimate frequencies. These are generally based on Taswell formulae (1981), including Taswell (1984), Stribosch *et al.,* (1987) and Waldmann *et al.,* (1987). Interested readers would be recommended to directly contact laboratories routinely performing LDA. HTL-p frequency results are usually expressed as the number of PBMC containing 1 precursor; eg 1: 14,000 (Fig 11.1), and the variance as 95% confidence limits.

4. *Interpretation of HTL-p results*

Each laboratory must determine its own definition of positive and negative HTL-p frequency. An arbitrary cut-off of 1: 100,000 is often used for defining 'high / low' HTL-p responses. ie a high HTL-p = 1:1,000 - 1:100,000 and a low HTL-p = 1:100,000 - 1:1,000,000. In general, a 'high' HTL-p response is suggestive of HLA mismatching, and a 'low' HTL-p response, particularly one below 1:200,000, of good HLA matching.

Internal & external QC

The internal controls consist of:

- responder cells plus irradiated third party cells (R + §X), to confirm that the responder cells are capable of secreting IL-2
- third party cells plus irradiated stimulator cells (X + §S), to confirm that the stimulator cells are capable of stimulating.

There is no external QC scheme available.

Specialist equipment or reagents required

Culture Medium

☑ 1x RPMI 1640 (Gibco)

☑ Penicillin 100iu/ml (Flow Labs)

☑ Streptomycin 100iu/ml (Flow Labs)

☑ L-Glutamine 200mM (Flow Labs)

☑ Human heat inactivated pooled 10% AB serum (AB serum is only required for cultures - not for washing)

Reagents

☑ Ficoll-Hypaque (Pharmacia)

☑ rIL-2 (Boehringer-Mannheim)

☑ ^{3}H (tritiated) thymidine (Amersham)

☑ Foetal calf serum (FCS) (Globepharm)

☑ CTLL-2 cell line (European Collection of Animal Cultures, Salisbury)

Equipment

- ☑ Radiation source (usually a gamma irradiator)
- ☑ Cell harvester
- ☑ Laminar flow hood
- ☑ β-counter

Combined CTL-p & HTL-p assays

There are two published methods for a combined limiting dilution assay for measuring both CTL-p and HTL-p at the same time (Wang *et al.,* 1996, van der Meer *et al.,* 1997).

Helper T Lymphocyte Precursor (HTL-p) frequency analysis for the enumeration of IL-4 secreting cell frequencies

In this assay, the frequency of HTL-p with the potential to secrete IL-4 are measured by limiting dilution analysis (Imami *et al.,* in press). For an introduction to limiting dilution analysis, see CTL-p above. Frequency analysis of IL-4 secreting HTL-p has been shown to inversely correlate with CTL-p, and high frequencies were shown to be associated with a decreased risk of GVHD after unrelated donor BMT (Imani *et al.,* in press).

Cytokine Profiles

Introduction

Cytokines are a group of proteins, secreted particularly by T lymphocytes and macrophages, which regulate immune responses. In the last few years, murine and human studies have shown that helper T lymphocytes can be divided into functional subpopulations on the basis of cytokine secretion (Mosmann and Sad 1996). Th1 cells mainly produce interleukin-2 (IL-2), interferon-gamma (IFNγ) and tumour necrosis factor-α (TNFα), while Th2 cells produce interleukin-4 (IL-4), interleukin-5 (IL-5) and interleukin-10 (IL-10). The Th1 subpopulation is associated with inflammation and cell-mediated immunity, while the Th2 subpopulation is associated with humoral immunity and is anti-inflammatory. In transplantation, Th1 cytokines are implicated in rejection and acute graft-versus-host disease, while Th2 cytokines may be implicated in tolerance (Nickerson *et al.,* 1994, Dallman 1995, Piccotti *et al.,* 1997). In view of this, 'cytokine 'profiling' has become a new tool with which to attempt to dissect alloreactivity.

Cytokine profiling can be performed *in vitro* in a number of different ways:

- precursor frequencies of cytokine-secreting helper T lymphocytes can be measured by limiting dilution analysis (see HTL-p above);
- numbers of cells expressing intracytoplasmic cytokines can be quantified by flow cytometry;
- cytokine mRNA in cells can be detected by PCR or by *in situ* hybridization;
- cytokine protein secretion can be quantified by stimulating lymphocytes *in vitro* and measuring the concentration of cytokines in culture supernatants by ELISA.

Limiting dilution analysis of cytokine-secreting cells has demonstrated large interindividual variations in frequencies of alloreactive IL-2 and IL-4 secreting HTL-p (see HTL-p above). Flow cytometric analysis of lymphocytes expressing intracytoplasmnic cytokines has shown large interindividual variations in numbers of IL-2 and IFNγ secreting lymphocytes (Ferry *et al.,* 1997). Measurement of cytokine protein secretion in culture supernatant following mitogen stimulation, has demonstrated large interindividual variations in the amount of IL-2, IL-4 and IFNγ secreted (Kaminski *et al.,* 1995). At this point it should be stressed that different stimuli (eg mitogens, antigens, antibodies, etc) may have different effects on the cytokine profile (Imada *et al.,* 1995). Several studies have looked at cytokines secreted during mixed lymphocyte culture (MLC), including IFNγ (Manger *et al.,* 1981), IL-2 (Ilonen *et al.,* 1984), IL-2 and IL-3 (Bishara *et al.,* 1991, 1993), TNFα and IL-6 (Toungouz *et al.,* 1993) and IL-10 (Toungouz *et al.,* 1996). Finally, for a number of cytokines there is now evidence for genetic polymorphisms which may determine the amount of protein secreted (Daser *et al.,* 1996).

Clinical relevance

Measurement of cytokine secretion in MLC can detect HLA-DRB1 and DQB1 mismatches (Danzer *et al.,* 1994) and DR4 polymorphisms (Toungouz *et al.,* 1994). Quantitation of IL-2 and IFNγ protein secretion and/or detection of IL-2, IL-5 and IFNγ gene expression in MLC, has been shown to predict acute GVHD after identical sibling or mismatched BMT (Tanaka *et al.,* 1994,1995b). Studies using the skin explant assay (see modifications of MLC above) have demonstrated the role of the cytokines TNFα and IFNγ as important mediators of the *in vitro* cellular damage seen in the skin (Dickinson *et al.,* 1991,1994a, 1994b). In addition, high levels of TNFα and IFNγ in MLR supernatants correlated with the severity of acute GVHD after identical sibling BMT (Dickinson *et al.,* 1994b), suggesting recognition of minor Histocompatibility antigens.

In renal transplantation, cytokine secretion in mitogen-stimulated cultures has been measured pretransplant - one study demonstrated a correlation between high levels of IFNγ and a high risk of acute rejection (Kaminski *et al.,* 1995), while another did not confirm this finding, but showed an unexpected correlation between low levels of IL-10 and a low risk of rejection (Weimer *et al.,* 1996). It is now known that genetic polymorphisms of TNFα and IL-10 determine the high / low secretory status of these cytokines. Families who are low TNFα and high IL-10 secretors have been shown to be at high risk of fatal meningococcal disease (Westendorp *et al.,* 1997). Cytokine gene polymorphisms have been studied with relevance to cardiac transplantation - TNFα and IL-10 polymorphisms have been shown to correlate with the amount of protein secreted (Turner *et al.,* 1995, 1997), and high TNFα / low IL-10 secretor genotypes appear to be associated with rejection (Turner *et al.,* 1997).

Methods to determine cytokine protein secretion profiles (IL-2, IL-4, IL-10 and IFNγ)

The protocol described here is based on that developed by Kaminski *et al.,* (1995).

1. *Samples*

☑ Patient **or** donor (depending on which is to be studied)

☑ 20 ml of peripheral blood in 400iu/20ml preservative-free heparin. The blood should ideally be fresh but can be kept overnight at room temperature or the

☑ mononuclear cells isolated (see below) and cryopreserved in liquid nitrogen.

2. *Method*

All steps to be performed in a class II cabinet under aseptic conditions

Patient or donor cells = responder (R)

2.1. *Cell preparation:*

- Isolate peripheral blood mononuclear cells (PBMC) by density gradient centrifugation. Dilute peripheral blood 1:1 with culture medium, layer onto Ficoll-Hypaque and centrifuge at 2,000 rpm for 20 mins.
- Harvest interface cells, resuspend in culture medium and wash at 1,800 rpm for 10 min, followed by two further washes at 1,200 rpm for 5 min.
- Resuspend cells in an exact quantity of culture medium. Count cell numbers using a haemocytometer and adjust the cell concentrations to 1.0×10^6/ml.

2.2. *Plating out responder cells:*

- Plate out several 1ml aliquots of cells (1.0 x 10^6) to sterile 24 well flat-bottom plates.
- Label equal numbers of wells as follows:

Background controls	R + 0
Mitogen-stimulated cultures	R + PHA

- Add PHA only to the wells marked (R + PHA), to give a final concentration of 1μg/ml.
- Incubate at 37°C in a humidified atmosphere of 5% CO_2 in air for 48 h.
- At the end of the incubation period, harvest the supernatants and centrifuge at 1,200 rpm for 5 min. Decant the cell-free supernatants to a freezing tube and store at -20°C until required.
- When convenient, thaw out the supernatants and measure the concentrations of cytokines of interest (eg IL-2, IL-4, IL-10, IFNγ, etc) in both the background and PHA-stimulated supernatants, in triplicate, using commercial ELISA assays.

3. *Analysis and interpretation of cytokine data:*

- Calculate the means of each triplicate for the background and PHA-stimulated cytokine concentrations.
- The significance of such estimations is still being evaluated

Specialist equipment or reagents required

Culture Medium

☑ 1x RPMI 1640 (Gibco)

☑ Penicillin 100iu/ml (Flow Labs)

☑ Streptomycin 100iu/ml (Flow Labs)

☑ L-Glutamine 200mM (Flow Labs)

☑ Human heat inactivated pooled 10% AB serum (AB serum is only required for cultures - not for washing)

Reagents

- ☑ Ficoll-Hypaque (Pharmacia)
- ☑ Phytohaemagglutinin (PHA) (Sigma-Aldrich Ltd).
- ☑ IL-2 ELISA kits (R&D Systems)
- ☑ IL-4, IL-10 & IFNγ ELISA kits (Eurogenetics)

Equipment

- ☑ ELISA plate reader
- ☑ Laminar flow hood

References

Al-Daccak, R, Loiseau, P, Miramont, P, Rabian, C, Raffoux, C, *et al.* (1990a). Evaluation of HLA-Class II identity between unrelated individuals by serological typing, DNA-RFLP method, and mixed lymphocyte reaction. *Hum Immunol* **29**: 189-201

Al-Daccak, R, Loiseau, P, Rabian, C, Devergie, A, Bourdeau, H, *et al.* (1990b). HLA-DR, DQ, and/or DP genotypic mismatches between recipient-donor pairs in unrelated bone marrow transplantation and transplant clinical outcome. *Transplantation* **50**: 960-964

Awdeh, ZL, Alper, CA, Fici, DA, Ronco, II P and Yunis EJ (1995). Predictability of alloreactivity among unrelated individuals: role for HLA-DPB1. *Tissue Antigens* **46**: 180-186

Bach, F and Hirschhorn, K (1964). Lymphocyte interaction: a potential histocompatibility test in vitro. *Science* **143:** 813-814

Bach, FH and Voynow, NK (1966). One-way stimulation in mixed leukocyte cultures. *Science* **153**: 545-547

Bach, FH, Segall, M, Zier, KS, Sondel, PM and Alter, BJ (1973). Cell mediated immunity: separation of cells involved in recognitive and destructive phases. *Science* **180**: 403-406

Bach, FH, Bach, ML and Sondel, PM (1976). Differential function of major histocompatibility complex antigens in T-lymphocyte activation. *Nature* **259**: 273-281

Bagot, M, Cordonnier, C, Tilkin, A-F, Heslan, M, Vernant, J-P, *et al.* (1986a). A possible predictive test for graft-versus-host disease in bone marrow graft recipients: the mixed-epidermal cell-lymphocyte reaction. *Transplantation* **41:** 316-319

Bagot, M, Cordonnier, C, Vernant, J-P, Dubertret, L, Rochant H, *et al.* (1986b). Mixed epidermal cell-lymphocyte reaction in prediction of acute graft-versus-host disease in bone marrow recipients. *JNCI* **76**: 1317-1319

Bagot, M, Mary, J-Y, Hesland, M, Kuentz, M, Cordonnier, C, *et al.* (1988). The mixed epidermal cell lymphocyte-reaction is the most predictive factor of acute graft-versus-host disease in bone marrow graft recipients. *Brit J Haem* **70:** 403-409

Bain, B, Vas, MR and Lowenstein, L (1964). The development of large immature mononuclear cells in mixed leukocyte cultures. *Blood* **23**: 108-116

Barnardo, MC, Davey, NJ, Bunce, M, Brookes, PA, Lechler, RI, *et al.* (1996). A correlation between HLA-C matching and donor antirecipient CTL precursor frequency in bone marrow transplantation. *Transplantation* **61**: 1420-1423

Baxter-Lowe, LA, Eckels, DD, Ash, R, Casper, J, Hunter, JB, *et al.* (1992). The predictive value of HLA-DR oligotyping for MLC responses. *Transplantation* **53**: 1352-1357

Beik, AI, Higgins, RM, Lam, FT and Morris, AG (1997). Clinical significance of selective decline of donor-reactive IL-2-producing T lymphocytes after renal transplantation. *Transpl Immunol* **5**: 89-96

Berkman, A, Farmer, E, Tutschka, P, Hess, A and Santos, G (1985). Skin explant culture as a model for cutaneous graft-versus-host disease. *Exp Hematol* **10 (Suppl. 12)**: 33-40

Bishara, A, Kedar, E, Leshem, B, Rosenkovitch, E and Brautbar, C (1991). A short human and mouse MLR assay utilising lymphokine (IL-2, IL-3) secretion as an early activation event. *Transplantation* **51:** 1104-1109

Bishara, A, Kedar, E, Leshem, B, Slavin, S, Cohen, I, *et al.* (1993). A 2-day MLR procedure for marrow donor selection for allogeneic bone marrow transplantation. *Eur J Immunogenet* **20:** 289-292

Bishara, A, Brautbar, C, Nagler, A, Slavin, S, Leshem, B, *et al.* (1994). Prediction by a modified mixed leukocyte reaction assay of graft-versus-host disease and graft rejection after allogeneic bone marrow transplantation. *Transplantation* **57**: 1474-1479

Bouma, GJ, van der Meer-Prins, PMW, van Bree, FPMJ, van Rood, JJ and Claas, FHJ (1992). Determination of cytotoxic T-lymphocyte precursor frequencies using Europium labeling as a nonradioactive alternative to labeling with chromium-51, *Hum Immunol* **35**: 85-92

Bouma, GJ, van der Meer-Prins, EMW, van der Woude, FJ, van Rood JJ, and Claas FHJ (1995). Relevance of pretransplant donor-specific T cell allorepertoire for human kidney graft survival. *Transplantation* **59**: 969-976

Breuning, MH, Breur, BS, Engelsma, MY and Ivanyi P (1984). Activation of cytotoxic T lymphocytes in HLA-A, -B and -C-identical responder-stimulator pairs I. *Tissue Antigens* **24**: 81-89

Breur-Vriesendorp, BS, Vingerhoed, J, Schaasberg, WP and Ivanyi, P (1990). Variations in the T-cell repertoire against HLA antigens in humans. *Hum Immunol* **27**: 1-15

Breur-Vriesendorp, BS, Vingerhoed, J, van Twuyver, E, de Waal, LP and Ivanyi, P (1991). Frequency analysis of HLA-specific cytotoxic T lymphocyte precursors in humans. *Transplantation* **51**: 1096-1103

Bunjes, D, Theobald, M, Nierle, T, Arnold, R and Heimpel, H (1995). Presence of host-specific interleukin 2-secreting T helper cell precursors correlates closely with active primary and secondary chronic graft-versus-host disease. *Bone Marrow Transpl* **15**: 727-732

Burke, GW, Alouch, M, Cirocco, R, Markou, M, Gomez, C, *et al.* (1993). Rejection in HLA-identical living related donor kidney transplants: lack of predictive immunologic parameters. *Transplantation* **57**: 750-751

Busca, A, Attisano, C, Miniero, R, Vassallo, E, Amoroso, A, *et al.* (1995). Usefulness of frequency analysis of cytotoxic T-lymphocyte precursors (CTL-p). for selection of HLA matched unrelated marrow donors. *Panminerva Med* **37**: 168-170

Cesbron, A, Moreau, P, Milpied, N, Muller, JY, Harousseau, JL, *et al.* (1990). Influence of HLA-DP mismatches on primary MLR responses in unrelated HLA-A, B, DR, DQ, DW identical pairs in allogeneic bone marrow transplantation. *Bone Marrow Transpl* **6**: 337-340

Clay, TM, Jones, HP, Bidwell, JL, Darke, C, Harvey, J, *et al.* (1989). A comparison of DNA-RFLP typing with serology and mixed lymphocyte reaction in the selection of matched unrelated bone marrow donors. *Bone Marrow Transpl* **4**: 493-499

Cukrova, V, Dolezalova, L, Loudova, M, Matejkova, E, Korinkova, P, *et al.* (1995). Frequency analysis of cytotoxic T-lymphocyte precursors in search for donors in bone marrow transplantation. *Neoplasma* **42**: 3-8

Cullen, PR, Lester ,S, Rouch, J and Morris, PJ (1977). Mixed lymphocyte reaction and graft survival in forty cadaveric renal transplants. *Clin Exp Immunol* **28**: 218-222

Dallman, MJ (1995). Cytokines and transplantation: Th1/Th2 regulation of the immune response to solid organ transplants in the adult. *Curr Opin Immunol* **7**: 632-638

Danzer, SG, a Campo, C, Kunze, B, Kirchner, H and Rink, L (1994). Identification of HLA-DRB1 and HLA-DQB1 identical individuals by a cytokine-based mixed lymphocyte culture. *Lymphokine Cytokine Res* **13:** 303-308

Daser, A, Mitchison, H, Mitchison, A and Müller, B (1996). Non-classical-MHC genetics of immunological disease in man and mouse. The key role of pro-inflammatory cytokine genes. *Cytokine* **8**: 593-597

Deacock, S, Schwarer, A, Batchelor, R, Goldman, J and Lechler, R (1992a). A rapid limiting dilution assay for measuring frequencies of alloreactive, interleukin-2-producing T cells in humans. *J Immunol Methods* **147**: 83-92

Deacock, SJ and Lechler, RI (1992b). Positive correlation of T cell sensitization with frequencies of alloreactive T helper cells in chronic renal failure patients. *Transplantation* **54**: 338-343

DeGast, GC, Mickelson, EM, Beatty, PG, Amos, D, Sullivan, KM, *et al*. (1992). Mixed leukocyte culture reactivity and graft-versus-host disease in HLA-identical marrow transplantation for leukemia. *Bone Marrow Transplantation* **9**: 87-90

Dickinson, AM, Sviland, L, Carey, P, Reid, MM, Hamilton PJ, *et al*. (1988). Skin explant culture as a model for cutaneous graft-versus-host disease in humans. *Bone Marrow Transpl* **3:** 323-329

Dickinson, AM, Sviland, L, Dunn, J, Carey, P and Proctor, SJ (1991). Demonstration of direct involvement of cytokines in graft-versus-host reactions using an in vitro human skin explant model. *Bone Marrow Transplantation* **7**: 209-216

Dickinson, AM, Sviland, L, Jackson, G, Dunn, J, Stephens, S. *et al*. (1994a). Monoclonal anti-TNF-α suppresses graft vs host disease reactions in an in vitro human skin model. *Cytokine* **6**: 141-146

Dickinson, AM, Sviland, L, Hamilton, PJ, Usher, P, Taylor, P. *et al*. (1994b). Cytokine involvement in predicting clinical graft-versus-host disease in allogeneic bone marrow transplant recipients. *Bone Marrow Transpl* **13:** 65-70

Dickinson, AM, Sviland, L, Wang, XN, Jackson, G, Taylor, PRA, *et al.* Predicting graft-versus-host disease in HLA identical bone marrow transplants - a comparison of T cell frequency analysis and a human skin explant model. (Submitted)

Dupont, B, Brown, DW, Yunis, EJ and Carpenter, CB (1980). HLA-D by cellular typing. In: *Histocompatibility Testing* (Ed. Terasaki, PI), pp.229-267. UCLA Typing Laboratory, Los Angeles

Eberspacher, MLL, Otto, G, Herfarth, C and Kabelitz, D (1994). Frequency analysis of donor-reactive cytotoxic T lymphocyte precursors in liver allograft recipients. *Transplantation* **57**: 1746-1752

Fazekas de St. Groth S (1982). The evaluation of limiting dilution assays. *J Immunol Methods* **49**: R11-R23

Ferry, B, Antrobus, P, Huzicka, I, Farrell, A, Lane, A, *et al.* (1997). Intracellular cytokine expression in whole blood preparations from normals and patients with atopic dermatitis. *Clin Exp Immunol* **110**: 410-417

Fleischhauer, K, Kernan, NA, O'Reilly, RJ, Dupont, B and Yang, SY (1990). Bone marrow-allograft rejection by T lymphocytes recognising a single amino acid difference in HLA-B44. *N Engl J Med* **323**: 1818-1822

Freidel, AC, Mauricette, M, Gebuhrer, L, Farre, A, Collet, M, *et al.* (1996). Study of HLTp in adult patients receiving bone marrow transplantation from HLA geno-identical sibs. *Hum Immunol* **42**: 84

Fussell, ST, Donnellan, M, Cooley, MA and Farrell, C (1994). Cytotoxic T lymphocyte precursor frequency does not correlate with either the incidence or severity of graft-versus-host disease after matched unrelated donor bone marrow transplantation. *Transplantation* **57**: 673-676

Harmon, WE, Parkman, R, Lavin, PT, Grupe, WE, Ingelfinger, JR. *et al.* (1982). Comparison of cell-mediated lympholysis and mixed lymphocyte culture in the immunologic evaluation for renal transplantation. *J Immunol* **129**: 1573-1577

Hornick, PI, Brookes, PA, Mason, PD, Taylor, KM, Yacoub, MH, *et al.* (1997). Optimising a limiting dilution culture system for quantifying the frequency of IL-2 producing alloreactive T helper lymphocytes. *Transplantation* **64:** 472-479

Hows, JM, Yin, JL, Marsh, J, Swirsky, D, Jones, L, *et al.* (1986). Histocompatible unrelated volunteer donors compared with HLA nonidentical family donors in marrow transplantation for aplastic anaemia and leukemia. *Blood* **68:** 1322-1328

Hu, H, Robertus, M, de Jonge, N, Gmelig-Meyling, FH, van der Meulen, A, *et al.* (1994). Reduction of donor-specific cytotoxic T lymphocyte precursors in peripheral blood of allografted heart recipients. *Transplantation* **58**: 1263-1268

Ilonen, J and Karttunen, R (1984). The production of interleukin 2 as a measure of reactivity in mixed lymphocyte culture. *Immunobiol* **167**: 399-403

Imada, M, Simons, FER, Jay, FT and HayGlass, KT (1995). Antigen mediated and polyclonal stimulation of human cytokine production elicit qualitatively different patterns of cytokine gene expression. *Int Immunol* **7**: 229-237

Imami, N, Brookes, PA, Lombardi, G, Hakooz, B, Johns, M, *et al.* (1998). Association between IL-4 producing T lymphocyte frequencies and reduced graft-versus-host disease. *Transplantation* (in press)

Irschick, EU, Hladik, F, Niederwieser, D, Bußbaumer, W, Holler, E, *et al.* (1992). Studies on the mechanism of tolerance or graft-versus-host disease in allogeneic bone marrow recipients at the level of cytotoxic T-cell precursor frequencies. *Blood* **79:** 1622-1628

Jooss, J, Eiermann, TH, Wagner, H and Kabelitz, D (1989). Interleukin 2 Production by Alloantigen-Stimulated $CD4^+$ and $CD8^+$ human T cell subsets: Frequency of HLA class I or Class II - reactive precursor cells and clonal specificity of activated T cells. *Immunobiol* **179**: 366-381

Kabelitz, D, Herzog, WR, Zanker, B and Wagner, H (1985). Human cytotoxic T lymphocytes I. Limiting-dilution analysis of alloreactive cytotoxic T-lymphocyte precursor frequencies. *Scand J Immunol* **22**: 329-335

Kaminski, E, Sharrock, C, Hows, J, Ritter, M, Arthur, C. *et al.* (1988). Frequency analysis of cytotoxic T lymphocyte precursors - possible relevance to HLA-matched unrelated donor bone marrow transplantation. *Bone Marrow Transpl* **3**: 149-165

Kaminski, E, Hows, J, Man, S, Brookes, P, Mackinnon, S. *et al.* (1989). Prediction of graft versus host disease by frequency analysis of cytotoxic T cells after unrelated donor bone marrow transplantation. *Transplantation* **48**: 608-613

Kaminski, ER, Hows, JM, Goldman, JM and Batchelor, JR (1990). Pretransfused patients with severe aplastic anaemia exhibit high numbers of cytotoxic T lymphocyte precursors probably directed at non-HLA antigens. *Brit J Haem* **76:** 401-405

Kaminski, ER, Hows, JM, Bridge, J, Davey, NJ, Brookes, PA, *et al.* (1991a). Cytotoxic T lymphocyte precursor (CTL-p) frequency analysis in unrelated donor bone marrow transplantation; two case studies. *Bone Marrow Transpl* **8**: 47-50

Kaminski, E, Hows, J, Goldman, J and Batchelor, R (1991b). Optimising a limiting dilution culture system for quantitating frequencies of alloreactive cytotoxic T lymphocyte precursors. *Cellular Immunol* **137**: 88-95

Kaminski, ER, Kaminski, A, Bending, MR, Chang, R, Heads, A, *et al*. (1995). In vitro cytokine profiles and their relevance to rejection following renal transplantation. *Transplantation* **60:** 703-706

Keever, CA, Leong, N, Cunningham, I, Copelan, EA, Avalos, BR, *et al*. (1994). *Bone Marrow Transpl* **14:** 137-145

Kristensen, T (1978). Cell-mediated lympholysis in man: CML specificities and their possible relevance. *Transplant Proc* **10**: 319-325

Kristensen, T (1980) Human histocompatibility testing by T cell-mediated lympholysis: a European standard CML technique. *Tissue Antigens* **16**: 335-367

Langhoff, E, Jakobsen, BK, Platz, P, Ryder, LP and Svejgaard, A (1985). The impact of low donor-specific MLR versus HLA-DR compatibility on kidney graft survival. *Transplantation* **39**: 18-21

Lefkovits, I, and Waldmann, H (1984). Limiting dilution analysis of cells of the immune system. I. The clonal basis of the immune response. *Immunol Today* **5**: 265-268

Lim, SH, Patton, WN, Jobson, S, Gentle, TA, Baynham, MID, *et al*. (1988). Mixed lymphocyte reactions do not predict severity of graft versus host disease (GVHD) in HLA-DR compatible, sibling bone marrow transplants. *J Clin Pathol* **41**: 1155-1157

Man, S, Lechler, RI, Batchelor, JR and Sharrock, CEM (1990). Individual variation in the frequency of HLA class II-specific cytotoxic T lymphocyte precursors. *Eur J Immunol* **20**: 847-854

Manger, B, Kalden, JR, Zawatzky, R and Kirchner, H (1981). Interferon production in the human mixed lymphocyte culture, *Transplantation* **32**: 149-152

Mestre, M, Massip, E, Bas, J, Alsina, J, Romeu, A. *et al*. (1996). Longitudinal study of the frequency of cytotoxic T cell precursors in kidney allograft recipients. *Clin Exp Immunol* **104:** 108-114

Mickelson, EM, Bartsch, GE, Hansen, JA and Dupont, B (1993). The MLC assay - a test for HLA-D region compatibility between patients and unrelated donors: results of a national marrow donor program involving multiple centres. *Tissue Antigens* **42:** 465-72

Mickelson, EM, Guthrie, LA, Etzioni, R, Anasetti, C, Martin, PJ, *et al.* (1994). Role of the mixed lymphocyte culture (MLC) reaction in marrow donor selection: matching for transplants from related haploidentical donors. *Tissue Antigens* **44:** 83-92

Mickelson, EM, Longton, G, Anasetti, C, Petersdorf, E, Marin, P, *et al.* (1996). Evaluation of the mixed lymphocyte culture (MLC) assay as a method for selecting unrelated donors for marrow transplantation. *Tissue Antigens* **47:** 27-36

Montagna, D, Maccario, R, Comoli, P, Prete, L, Zecca, M, *et al.* (1996). Frequency of donor cytotoxic T cell precursors does not correlate with occurrence of acute graft-versus-host disease in children transplanted using unrelated donors. *Journal of Clinical Immunology* **16**: 107-114

Moretta, A, Pantaleo, G, Moretta, L, Mingari, MC and Cerottini, JC (1983). Quantitative assessment of the pool size and subset division of cytolytic T lymphocytes within human resting or alloreactive peripheral blood populations. *J Exp Med* **158:** 571-585

Moretta, A (1985). Frequency and surface phenotype of human T lymphocytes producing interleukin-2: Analysis by limiting dilution and cell cloning. *Eur J Immunol.* **15**: 148-155

Moreau, P, Milpied, N, Cesbron, A, Mahe, B, Bignon, JD. *et al.* (1993). Mixed leukocyte culture reactivity, HLA-DP typing and GVHD. *Bone Marrow Transpl* **11:** 85-86

Mosmann, TR and Sad, S (1996). The expanding universe of T-cell subsets: Th1, Th2 and more. *Immunol Today* **17:** 138-146

Nickerson, P, Steurer, W, Steiger, J, Zheng, X, Steele, AW, *et al.* (1994). Cytokines and the Th1/Th2 paradigm in transplantation. *Curr Opin Immunol* **6:** 757-764

Olerup, O, Moller, E and Persson, U (1990). HLA-DP incompatibilities induce significant proliferation in primary mixed lymphocyte cultures in HLA-A, -B, -DR and -DQ identical individuals: implications for allogeneic bone marrow transplantation. *Tissue Antigens* **36:** 194-202

Orosz, CG, Adams, PW and Ferguson, RM (1987). Frequency of human alloantigen-reactive T lymphocytes. II Method for limiting dilution analysis of alloantigen-reactive helper T cells in human peripheral blood. *Transplantation* **43**: 718-724

Parkman, R, Rosen, FS, Rappaport, J, Camitta, B, Levey, RL, *et al.* (1976). Detection of genetically determined histocompatibility antigen differences between HLA-identical and MLC non reactive siblings. *Transplantation* **21**: 110-116

Pawelec, CG, Shaw, S, Schneider, M, Blaurock, M, Frauer, M, *et al.* (1982). Population studies of the HLA-linked SB antigens and their relative importance in MLC typing: analysis of HLA-D homozygous typing cells and normal heterozygous populations. *Hum Immunol* **5**: 215-223

Piccotti, JR, Chan, SY, van Buskirk, AM, Eichwald, EJ and Bishop, DK (1997). Are the Th2 helper T lymphocytes beneficial, deleterious, or irrelevant in promoting allograft survival? *Transplantation* **63**: 619-624

Potolicchio, I, Brookes, PA, Madrigal, A, Lechler, RI and Sorrentino, R (1996). HLA-DPB1 mismatch at position 69 is associated with high helper T lymphocyte precursor frequencies in unrelated bone marrow transplant pairs. *Transplantation* **62**: 1347-1352

Reader, JA, Burke, MM, Counihan, P, Kirby, JA, Adams, S, *et al.* (1990). Noninvasive monitoring of human cardiac allograft rejection. *Transplantation* **50**: 29-33

Roelen, DL, van Bree, FPMJ, Schanz, U, van Rood, JJ and Claas, FHJ (1993). Differential inhibition of primed alloreactive CTLs in vitro by clinically used concentrations of cyclosporine and FK506. *Transplantation* **56**: 190-195

Roelen, DL, van Bree, SPMJ, van Beelen, E, Schanz, U, van Rood, JJ, *et al.* (1994). Cytotoxic T lymphocytes against HLA-B antigens are less naive than cytotoxic T lymphocytes against HLA-A antigens. *Transplantation* **57**: 446-450

Roosnek, E, Hogendijk, S, Zawadynski, S, Speiser, D, Tiercy, J-M, *et al.* (1993). The frequency of pretransplant donor cytotoxic T cell precursors with anti-host specificity predicts survival of patients transplanted with bone marrow from donors other than HLA-identical siblings. *Transplantation* **56**: 691-696

Rufer, N, Breur-Vriesendorp, BS, Tiercy, J-M, Slavcev, S, Lardy, NM, *et al.* (1993). High-resolution histocompatibility testing of a group of 16 B44-positive, ABD serologically matched unrelated donor-recipient pairs. *Hum Immunol* **38**: 235-239

Rufer, N, Tiercy, J-M, Breur-Vriesendorp, B, Gauchat-Feiss, D, Shi, X, *et al.* (1995). Histoincompatibilities in ABDR-matched unrelated donor recipient combinations. *Bone Marrow Transpl* **16**: 641-646

Schwarer, AP, Zheng Jiang, Y, Brookes, PA, Barrett, AJ, Batchelor, JR, *et al.* (1993). Frequency of anti-recipient alloreactive helper T-cell precursors in donor blood and graft-versus-host disease after HLA-identical sibling bone marrow transplantation. *Lancet* **341**: 203-205

Schwarer, AP, Zheng Jiang, Y, Deacock, S, Brookes, PA, Barrett, AJ. *et al.* (1994). Comparison of helper and cytotoxic antirecipient T cell frequencies in unrelated bone marrow transplantation. *Transplantation* **58**: 1198-1203

Segall, M, Noreen, H, Edwins, L, Haake, R, Xo, S. *et al.* (1996). Lack of correlation of MLC reactivity with acute graft-versus-host disease and mortality in unrelated donor bone marrow transplantation. *Hum Immunol* **49:** 49-55

Sharrock, CEM, Man, S, Wanachiwanawin, W and Batchelor, JR (1987). Analysis of the alloreactive T cell repertoire in man. I. Differences in precursor frequency for cytotoxic T cell responses against allogeneic MHC molecules in unrelated individuals. *Transplantation* **43:** 699-703

Sharrock, CEM, Kaminski, E and Man, S (1990). Limiting dilution analysis of human T cells: a useful clinical tool. *Immunol Today* **11:** 281-286

Slavcev, AS, Breur-Vriesendorp, BS and Ivanyi, P (1995). Estimates of cytotoxic T-lymphocyte precursor frequencies against HLA class I antigens in responder-stimulator pairs with a negative mixed lymphocyte culture reaction. *Hum Immunol* **44**: 97-102

Speiser, DE, Loliger, CC, Siren, MK and Jeannet, M (1996). Pretransplant cytotoxic donor T-cell activity specific to patient HLA class I antigens correlating with mortality after unrelated BMT. *Brit J Haem* **93**: 935-939

Spencer, A, Szydlo, RM, Brookes, PA, Kaminski, E, Rule, S, *et al.* (1995a). Bone marrow transplantation for chronic myeloid leukemia with volunteer unrelated donors using ex vivo or in vivo T-cell depletion: major prognostic impact of HLA Class I identity between donor and recipient. *Blood* **86**: 3590-3597

Spencer, A, Brookes, PA, Kaminski, E, Hows, JM, Szydlo, RM, *et al.* (1995b). Cytotoxic T lymphocyte precursor frequency analyses in bone marrow transplantation with volunteer unrelated donors. *Transplantation* **59**: 1302-1308

Steinmann, J, Kaden, J, May, G, Schroder, K, Herwartz, C, *et al.* (1994). Failure of in vitro T-cell assays to predict clinical outcome after human kidney transplantation. *J Clin Lab Anal* **8**: 157-162

Strijbosch, LWG, Buurman, WA, Does, RJMM, Zinken, PH and Groenewegen, G (1987). Limiting dilution assays. Experimental design and statistical analysis. *J Immunol Methods* **97**: 133-140.

Sviland, L, Dickinson, AM, Carey, PJ, Pearson, ADJ and Proctor, SJ (1990). An in vitro predictive test for clinical graft-versus-host disease in allogeneic bone marrow transplant recipients. *Bone Marrow Transpl* **5:** 105-109

Tanaka, J, Imamura, M, Kasai, M, Kobayashi S, Hashino, S, *et al.* (1994). Cytokine gene expression in the mixed lymphocyte culture in allogeneic bone marrow transplants as a predictive method for transplantation-related complications. *Brit J Haem* **87**: 415-418

Tanaka, J (1995a). Possible role of T-cell surface molecule gene expression in the mixed lymphocyte culture for predicting transplantation-related complications after allogeneic bone marrow transplantation. *Eur J Haem* **55**: 282-284

Tanaka, J, Imamura, M, Kasai, M and Sakurada, K (1995b). Transplantation-related complications predicted by cytokine gene expression in the mixed lymphocyte culture in allogeneic bone marrow transplants. *Leukemia and Lymphoma* **19**: 27-32

Taswell, C (1981). Limiting dilution assays for the determination of immunocompetent cell frequencies. I Data analysis. *J Immunol* **126**: 1614-1619

Taswell, C (1984). Limiting dilution assays for the determination of immunocompetent cell frequencies. III Validity tests for the single-hit Poisson model. *J Immunol Methods* **72:** 29-40

Termijtelen, A and van Rood, JJ (1981a). Complexity of stimulation in MLC and the influence of matching for HLA-A and -B. *Scan J Immunol* **14**: 459-466

Termijtelen, A and van Rood, JJ (1981b). The role in primary MLC of the non HLA D/DR determinant PL3A. *Tissue Antigens* **17**: 57-63

Theobald, M, Hoffmann, T and Heit, W (1989). Assessment of human allospecific IL-2 secreting helper T lymphocytes in limiting dilution cultures using restimulation and split well analysis. *J Immunol Methods* **121**: 19-32

Theobald, M, Hoffmann, T, Bunjes, D and Heit, W (1990). Frequency, specificity, and phenotype of clonally growing human alloreactive interleukin-2 secreting helper T lymphocyte precursors. *Transplantation* **50**: 850-856

Theobald, M, Nierle, T, Bunjes, D, Arnold, R and Heimpel, H (1992). Host-specific interleukin-2 secreting donor T-cell precursors as predictors of acute graft-versus-host disease in bone marrow transplantation between HLA-identical siblings. *New Engl J Med* **327**: 1613-1617

Theobald, M and Bunjes, D (1993). Pretransplant detection of human minor histocompatibility antigen-specific naive and memory interleukin-2-secreting T cells within class I major histocompatibility complex (MHC)-restricted CD8+ and class II MHC-restricted CD4+ T-cell subsets. *Blood* **82**: 298-306

Ting, A and Simpson, E (1989). Major and minor histocompatibility antigens. In: *Organ Transplantation: current clinical and immunological concepts* (Ed. Brent, L and Sells, RA), pp.1-8. Bailliere-Tindall, London

Toungouz, M, Denys, CH, De Groote, D, Andrien, ME and Dupont, EC (1993). Alloactivation induced during mixed lymphocyte reaction provokes release of tumour necrosis factor α and interleukin-6 by macrophages and primes them to lipopolysaccharides. *Hum Immunol* **38:** 221-225

Toungouz, M, Denys, CH, Andrien, ME, de Groote, D and Dupont, EC (1994). Tumor necrosis factor -α and interleukin-6 production induced by variations of DR4 polymorphism during the primary mixed lymphocyte reaction. *Transplantation* **58:** 1393-1398

Toungouz, M, Denys, C, de Groote, D, Andrien, M and Dupont, E (1996). Optimal control of interferon-α and tumor necrosis factor-α by interleukin-10 produced in response to one HLA-DR mismatch during the primary mixed lymphocyte reaction. *Transplantation* **61**: 497-502

Turner, DM, Grant, SCD, Lamb, WR, Brenchley, PEC, Dyer, PA, *et al.* (1995). A genetic marker of high TNF-α production in heart transplant recipients. *Transplantation* **60**: 1113-1117

Turner, D, Grant, SCD, Yonan, N, Sheldon, S, Dyer, PA, *et al.* (1997). Cytokine gene polymorphism and Heart Transplant Rejection. *Transplantation* **64:** 776-779

Van der Meer, Joosten I, Ruiter, J and Allebes, WA (1997). A single [3H] thymidine-based limiting dilution analysis to determine HTLp and CTLp frequencies for bone marrow donor selection. *Bone Marrow Transpl* **20:** 149-155

Van Oers, MHJ, Pinkster, J and Zeijlemaker, WP (1978). Quantification of antigen reactive cells among human T lymphocytes. *Eur J Immunol* **8:** 477-484

Vie, H and Miller, RA (1986), Estimation by limiting dilution analysis of human IL2-secreting T cells: detection of IL2 produced by single lymphokine-secreting T cells. *J Immunol* **136:** 3292-3297

Vogelsang, GB, Hes, AD, Berkman, AW, Tutschka, PJ Farmer, ER, *et al.* (1985). An in vitro predictive test for graft versus host disease in patients with genotypic HLA-identical bone marrow transplants. *New Eng J Med* **313**: 645-650

Voogt, PJ, Fibbe, WE, Marijt, WAF, Goulmy, E, Veenhof, WFJ, *et al.* (1990). Rejection of one-marrow graft by recipient-derived cytotoxic T lymphocyte against minor histocompatibility antigens. *Lancet* **335**: 131-134

Waldmann, H and Lefkovits, I (1984). Limiting dilution analysis of the immune response. II. What can be learnt? *Immunol Today* **5**: 295-298

Waldmann, H, Cobbold, S and Lefkovits, I (1987). Limited dilution analysis. In: *Lymphocytes a practical approach* (Ed. Klaus, GGB), pp.163-188. IRL Press, Oxford

Wang, XN, Proctor, SJ and Dickinson, AM (1996). Frequency analysis of recipient-reactive helper and cytotoxic T lymphocyte precursors using a combined single limiting dilution assay. *Transpl Immunol* **4:** 247-251

Warren, RP, Storb, R, Weiden, PL, Mickelson, EM and Thomas, ED (1976). Direct and antibody-dependent cell-mediated cytotoxicity against HLA identical sibling lymphocytes. *Transplantation* **22**: 631-635

Warren, RP, Storb, R, Weiden PL, Su, PJ and Thomas, ED (1980). Prediction of marrow graft rejection by the lymphocyte-mediated cytotoxicity and antibody-dependent cell-mediated cytotoxicity assays. *Transplantation* **30:** 118-121

Weimer, R, Zipperle, S, Daniel, V, Carl, S, Staehler, G, *et al.* (1996). Pretransplant CD4 helper function and interleukin 10 response predict risk of acute kidney graft rejection. *Transplantation* **62**: 1606-1614

Westendorp, RGJ, Langermans, JAM, Hulzinga, TWJ, Elouali, AH, Verweij, CL, *et al.* (1997). Genetic influence on cytokine production and fatal meningococcal disease. *Lancet* **349**: 170-173

Weston, LE, Geczy, AF and Farrell, C (1997). Donor T-cell frequencies as predictors of acute graft-versus-host disease in bone marrow transplantation between HLA-identical siblings. *Transplantation* **64**: 836-841

Young, NT, Roelen, DL, Dallman, MJ, Wood, KJ, Morris, PJ, *et al.* (1996). Enumeration of human alloreactive helper T lymphocyte precursor frequencies by limiting dilution analysis of interleukin-2 production. *J Immunol Methods* **195:** 33-41

Zhang, L, Li, SG, Vandekerckhove, B, Termijtelen, A, van Rood, JJ, *et al.* (1989). Analysis of cytotoxic T cell precursor frequencies directed against individual HLA-A and -B alloantigens. *J Immunol Methods* **121**: 39-45

Zhang, L, Rinke de Wit, TF, Li, SG, van Rood, JJ and Claas, FHJ (1990a). Subtypes of HLA-A1 defined on the basis of CTL precursor frequencies. *Hum Immunol* **27**: 80-89

Zhang, L, van Bree, S, van Rood, JJ and Claas, FHJ (1990b). The effect of individual HLA-A and -B mismatches on the generation of cytotoxic T lymphocyte precursors. *Transplantation* **50**: 1008-1010

PART 4

DONOR SELECTION

PART 4 OVERVIEW

DONOR SELECTION

C. Darke
Regional Tissue Typing Laboratory
Welsh Blood Service
Ely Valley Road, Talbot Green
Pontyclun, Cardiff CF72 9WB, Wales

In this speciality there are primary differences in donor origin, the procurement, supply, storage and histocompatibility requirements of donor material and the urgency and availability of substitute and alternative patient treatments. These make the distinction between *organ allocation* (the case for all cadaveric donor derived solid organs, except corneas) and *donor selection* apparent.

Thus, the scarce cadaveric donor organ is allocated to an eligible patient after applying complex algorithms, often controlled by central agencies, to ensure fairness and maximum clinical benefit. However, when donor material is more naturally available, as in the case of unrelated stem cell donors and HLA typed platelet donors, warranted donor selection is highly dependent on genetic chance (e.g. HLA phenotype frequency and ethnic background) and the financial resources controlling the quality and size of the donor panels available. Further, there may be a genetic or emotional relationship between the patient and their living donor.

Thus, devoting solid organs for transplantation and identifying suitable donors for stem cell transplantation or platelet transfusion is highly complex being influenced collectively by considerations of immunogenetics, ethics, legislation and medical and social policy. The first advocate of donor selection on the basis of immunogenetics was probably Hektoen (1907) who advised selection founded on crossmatching and the recipient's blood group. Compatibility for ABO blood group blood, attempted histocompatibility for the HLA system and the outcome of *in vitro* donor/recipient crossmatching tests have always played a dominant role in organ allocation and donor selection. However, there are still fundamental uncertainties in this area, including the influence of detailed HLA matching, the role of other genetic systems and the clinical utility of donor/recipient crossmatching methods. That these uncertainties still exist is a measure of the biological and logistic intricacy of these procedures.

In Chapters 12 to 14 the fundamentals of allocation of solid organs for transplantation and the selection of donors for haemopoietic stem cell transplantation and HLA matched platelet transfusion are described including:

- Principles of allocation and histocompatibility in solid organ transplantation
- Allocation of kidneys, livers, thoracic organs, corneas, and multi-organ transplants
- Problems of waiting times and clinical urgency in solid organ transplantation
- Sources of haemopoietic stem cells
- Clinical effects of HLA matching in stem cell transplantation
- Donor selection procedures for potential family and unrelated stem cell donors
- Non-immunological and immunological refractoriness to platelet transfusions
- Management of immunological platelet refractoriness
- Recruitment and selection of platelet donors
- Prevention of platelet refractoriness and HLA alloimmunisation

The HLA system unquestionably plays a pivotal role in recipient/donor histocompatibility. Thus, HLA-A,B,DR specificity matching reduces transplant failure and sensitisation in solid organ transplant recipients. HLA identity, at three class I loci and up to six class II loci, is probably required for long term successful bone marrow transplantation and HLA-A,B specificity matching is of undoubted benefit in platelet provision for HLA sensitised patients. However, future donor allocation and selection is likely to be regularly influenced by further immunogenetic considerations, including those of the cytokines, minor histocompatibility antigens, e.g. HA-1, and the human platelet antigen system (Haldar *et al.,* 1999; Kekomaki *et al.,* 1997; Rufer *et al.,* 1998).

Amongst the resources required for success in these areas are, jointly: energetic central government and professional body role in training, regulation, accreditation and audit; a robust clinical and laboratory foundation and superior liaison and communication between clinical and scientific, including informatics, professionals.

References

Haldar, NA, McLaren, A, Marshall, SE, Morris, PJ and Welsh, KI (1999) Is renal graft survival predetermined by the recipient's cytokine profile? *Transplant Proc* **31**: 289-290

Hektoen, L (1907) Iso-agglutination of human corpuscles *J Amer Med Assoc* **48**: 1739-1740

Kekomaki, S, Salmela, K, Partanen, J, Koskimies, S and Kekomaki, R (1997) Alloimmunization against platelet antigens in renal transplant patients with acute vascular rejection *Clin Transplant* **11**: 19-24

Rufer, N, Wolpert, E, Helg, C, Tiercy, J-M, Gratwohl, A *et al.* (1998) HA-1and the SMCY-derived peptide FIDSYICQV (H-Y) are immunodominant minor histocompatibility antigens after bone marrow transplantation *Transplantation* **66**: 910-916

CHAPTER 12

ALLOCATION OF SOLID ORGANS FOR TRANSPLANTATION

P. A. Dyer and S. Sheldon
Transplantation Laboratory
Manchester Royal Infirmary
Manchester M13 9WL, England

Introduction

Despite 30 years in the development of clinical human organ transplantation, without exception, suitable organs remain in short supply throughout the world. For example in the UK in 1996, 1780 new patients were entered to the renal transplant waiting list but only 1515 transplants were performed. At the end of 1996 this waiting list totalled 5421 patients in all. Clearly demand exceeds supply and unless a significant increase in the number of organs available is achieved, the allocation process of the organs available must be agreed and audited. Unfortunately in the situation of insufficient organ supply the decision process will usually identify those patients who shall not receive organs rather than those who shall.

The ethics of organ allocation are complex; Gutmann and Land (1997) see the need for ongoing debate to evolve "a systematic and rational decision procedure that could please patients, the public and the medical profession". These same reviewers state that organs for transplantation are a "social good" rather than "something morally owned by clinicians" and allocation is "not a medical question".

In Europe and North America nearly all countries have centralised organ allocation agencies:

- United Network for Organ Sharing (UNOS), USA
- UK Transplant Special Service Authority (UKTSSA), UK
- Eurotransplant (based in Leiden, Netherlands), Netherlands, Benelux, Germany and Austria
- Francetransplant, France
- Scandiatransplant, Denmark, Norway, Sweden and Finland
- North Italy Transplant Programme (NITP), Northern Italy
- Swisstransplant, Switzerland

In other countries there is usually a central government role in regulating organ supply since the origin of organs from dead persons is separate from the recipient unit and the transplant team. Unfortunately in some countries there remains no regulation leading to inefficient allocation and potential illicit use of cadaver donor organs.

The World Health Organisation has issued a statement on the availability of organs for transplant which aims to preserve the rights of donors, both cadaver and living, as well as ensuring efficient and fair use of the organs available. In addition at the international level, the Transplantation Society, which is the professional body for all persons actively involved in transplantation, has issued its own guidelines to which its members must adhere (Council of the Transplantation Society, 1985). Most countries also have national professional bodies which have adopted or endorsed guidelines.

Some countries have statutory legislation definition the condition of "brain death", protecting the rights of organ donors and regulating the supply and allocation of organs for transplantation. In the UK the Human Organ Transplants Act (1989) and its accompanying Regulations limit transplantation to the following instances:

(1) All cadaver donor organ transplants must be registered

(2) All living donor organ transplants are prohibited unless:

- the donor is established to be a close genetic relation of the recipent by an approved Tester
- the donor and recipient are not genetically related but approval for the transplant to proceed is endorsed by the Unrelated Live Transplant Regulatory Authority (ULTRA)

The regulation of organ transplantation has evolved because of the necessity to define brain death of cadaver organ donors, to prevent unethical use of organs donated, to protect living organ donors especially those of minority age and those unable to make informed decisions and to ensure transplantation takes place in units capable of achieving acceptable outcomes. These legal and organisational restrictions are probably unique to transplantation within medicine.

Principles of allocation

When cadaver donor organs are available, it is the responsibility of the transplant surgeon to ensure that allocation procedures are met. This does not mean the procedures are to be defined exclusively by the surgical team since legislation or formal agreement and professional body guidelines must be complied with.

Organs can be allocated on the basis of either of two broad factors: "equity" or "justice". In practice these conflicting issues are apparent in six categories:

- A. Clinical need or urgency - "who will die without a transplant"
- B. Waiting time - "first come, first served"
- C. Agreed rules based on outcomes - "evidence based"
- D. Random - "lottery"
- E. Bias - "most deserving case, in my opinion"
- F. Payment - "who has the most money"

Persons able to actively influence these options include patients, doctors, politicians and those "in possession" of the donated organs at any specific time. In developed countries agreed systems have been developed. For example, in the USA, UNOS committees regulate allocation rules which Organ Procurement Organisations (OPOs) operate. UNOS committees are constituted with representatives from all parties with an interest in transplantation. OPOs are independent non-profit groups which interact with donor centres. Once organs are available, the UNOS rules facilitate the OPOs to allocate organs to transplant centres and to specified recipients.

A. *Clinical need or urgency*

Clinical urgency is acceptable as the sole allocation rule in a restricted number of instances such as thoracic organ transplantation (see below) but should no longer apply in some areas such as renal transplantation where ill patients can be better treated with alternative, lower risk, therapies. In the early days of transplantation and in developing areas, then those recipients most likely to die without the opportunity of a transplant were primary candidates thus adding to the risk of transplant outcome. This approach limited transplant success rates leading to considerable criticism from informed but uninvolved persons. In low risk organ transplants, such as corneal transplantation, where the treatment may be for penetrating injury and the only reasonable treatment is transplantation then clinical urgency must be an acceptable form of allocation. Corneal transplantation has the advantage of organ banking and in consequence almost no waiting list.

B. *Waiting time*

Allocation of organs for transplantation on the basis of the time waited for an organ to become available at first appears to be the most fair but usually ignores important clinically considerations. Nearly all recipient groups place waiting time as a high priority. In the rare situations where there is an adequate supply of organs, such as corneas or possibly paediatric livers in the UK, then waiting time may become an important factor. In practice, organ transplantation is not a surgical event limited to a few hours in an operating theatre but must be considered a long term treatment involving:

- adequate recipient preparation
- careful donor management
- selection of the most suitable recipient

- quality transplant surgery
- post-transplant recipient care usually involving long-term immunosuppression and monitoring of rejection.

Waiting time can be included in allocation algorithms but its level of influence should be carefully determined.

C. *Evidence based*

The allocation system most acceptable to all concerned parties must be one based on the evidence available through efficient audit of transplant programmes. This necessitates efficient transplant registries which, without exception, record consecutive transplants from all units within a jurisdiction. These registries can be statutory or voluntary or units may contribute to both. Examples include:

Multiorgan registries:

- UNOS, USA
- UKTSSA, UK
- Eurotransplant
- Collaborative Transplant Study (CTS), Heidelberg

Single organ registries:

- European Dialysis and Transplant Association (EDTA)
- International Society for Heart and Lung Transplants (ISHLT)
- Corneal Transplant Follow-up Study (CTFS), UK
- International Pancreas Transplant Registry, Minnesota, USA

These registries, and others, publish regular audits from their databases and can make specific enquiries to ascertain the influences on transplant success rates. UNOS openly publishes the outcomes achieved by individual centres, together with an explanatory comment from each centre, but most registries anonymise their data. An example of deriving an allocation strategy based on review of registry data is that recently adopted within Eurotransplant (Wujciak and Opelz, 1993). Such outcome driven allocation policies are based on survival rates of a group of recipients who share a given characteristic; other outcome measures such as organ function or recipient quality of life are rarely used.

D. *Random lottery*

It is hard to accept that true random allocation of organs would ever occur; in practice there will always be some selection on clinical grounds, waiting time, need or even financial inducement. Any such system would demand close monitoring to ensure fairness and this would lead to a more logical process in a very short time.

E. *Biased allocation*

No doubt many allocation systems have been or are still biased. The observation of the occurrence of bias implies a degree of independence and thus a value judgement implying a less acceptable option. Most organ transplant programmes evolve away from bias in allocation as they mature but a strong influence of specific individuals in a position of power or of financial considerations may prevent change. Un-intentioned bias is an issue particularly for ethnic minorities since both ABO blood groups and HLA specificity frequencies vary between populations. If recipient and donor populations are composed of different ethnic groups then allocation will inevitably be biased.

F. *Financial profit*

Payment for profit in human organ transplantation is universally condemned and increasingly illegal. The practice has flourished in poorer countries where the survival of whole families can be ensured by one member donating a kidney for transplantation. No self respecting person active in organ transplantation should participate in "for profit" organ donation and must respect the sanctity of the human body. It is not always obvious that such events take place and anyone dealing with organ donors or recipients who originate from outside their normal area of practice must establish that no financial transactions will take place. When training others in any aspect of organ transplantation, those working in regulated countries must demand compliance with internationally recognised ethical practice. Periodically, the press have published claims that donor organs are obtained by murder of suitable persons. These claims have been investigated but never substantiated. Such "urban myths" ignore the need for expert surgeons to remove and implant the organs and for prolonged post-transplant care.

Organs for transplantation can only be allocated to those patients who have been identified as being in need of a transplant due to failure of an organ or organs. How are such patients identified? There is usually a list of such potential recipients referred to as the **waiting list**; this is an inappropriate term since it implies that all those on the list will receive an organ, given time. This will not happen for a proportion of those on the list due to the inadequate supply of organs for transplantation. Patients waiting for a kidney may be on a list for many years whilst those waiting for a heart, lung or liver are at a 30% risk of dying whilst waiting for an organ (UKTSSA, 1996). A more appropriate term would be a **transplant eligibility list** reflecting the true function of such lists. Access to the transplant eligibility list is itself a restriction and filters will exist dependent on the country and unit policy. Most units probably don't have a unified policy as to which patients may become eligible for a transplant and interesting theoretical case reviews by professional audiences are revealing. In the USA a complex algorithm to facilitate a decision making process leading to entry to the transplant eligibility list has been published by the American Society of Nephrologists

(Kasiske, 1995). To be fair to all patients the reasons for non-entry to eligibility lists must be recorded and must be open to review.

Histocompatibility in solid organ transplantation

The barrier to successful transplantation of organs would at first appear to be the surgical event but the technical challenges posed have been rapidly overcome by the ability of pioneering surgeons. Today many transplant operations are carried out routinely by trained surgeons and technical failure rates are very low and will often reflect the clinical condition of the recipient rather than the transplant procedure itself. The failure of most organs is the result of allogenic disparity between donor and recipient which drives antibody- and/or cell-mediated rejection mechanisms. To combat the influence of this disparity two strategies have evolved, firstly matching of donor genetic allotypes to those of the recipient and secondly, in vitro crossmatching between donor and recipient. These issues are detailed elsewhere is this volume.

To a degree, matching and crossmatching are linked but current understanding of each is different. For donor / recipient matching it is widely accepted that:

- ABO blood groups must be compatible to prevent thrombosis of the transplanted organ. This does not apply to cornea grafts.
- HLA specificity matching reduces transplant failure, acute rejection episodes and sensitisation to mismatched specificities in kidney, pancreas and heart transplant recipients
- Use of multi-drug, high dose immunosuppressive regimens can minimise the influence of HLA mismatching but with increased post-transplant morbidity.

Despite over thirty years of clinical transplantation some basic issues remain to be resolved: for example it is not known whether ABO blood group compatibility is relevant to corneal grafting. Some issues have been investigated but there are conflicting reports such as the role of HLA specificity matching and outcome in liver and multi-organ transplantation. With improving technology the role of matching for HLA alleles rather than specificities in kidney transplantation has to be established. Also evolving technology has identified many other genes which may influence transplant outcomes and the role of cytokines and chemokines needs to be examined.

The role of the pre-transplant crossmatch is central to successful immediate kidney transplant function and is important in some, but not all, thoracic organ transplant recipients. In contrast to HLA matching, the list of "unknowns" for crossmatching remains long including: crossmatching in non-renal transplantation; the clinical relevance of highly sensitive crossmatching techniques; the role of antibodies with specificity other than for HLA; and the isotype of antibodies (IgG, IgM, IgA) in combination with their specificity.

Allocation of kidneys

Cadaver donors

The existence of efficient artificial kidney dialysis places kidney allocation policies in a unique position. Potential recipients should be medically fit at the time of transplant to optimise success of the transplant event. Furthermore, apart from corneas, more kidneys are transplanted world-wide than any other organ. Data available for review is therefore substantial in both single-centre and multi-centre registries.

Without exception, all centres allocate donor kidneys solely to ABO blood group compatible recipients. In practice ABO identity is preferable to avoid the accumulation of ABO-O recipients on eligibility lists due to the allocation of ABO-O kidneys to ABO-A recipients.

Although allocation of kidneys on the basis of HLA specificity matching is still debated (Starzl *et al.,* 1997) the evidence from most studies is increasingly convincing that HLA mismatched transplants have poorer outcomes (Rosenberg *et al.,* 1997; Dyer *et al.,* 1998). In the USA it is mandatory to share kidneys when a donor has no HLA-A, -B or -DR ("000") mismatch with a recipient but beyond that kidneys are allocated locally using other criteria. In Eurotransplant, emphasis is placed on minimising HLA mismatches whenever possible by sharing kidneys between centres.

The UK has recently adopted a three-tier approach following a comprehensive review of the role of HLA and other factors on kidney transplant outcome:

- Both donor kidneys shared for "000" mismatched recipients
- One donor kidney shared for "100, 010 or 110" mismatched recipients
- Local allocation rules for other degrees of mismatch with a recommendation to minimise HLA mismatching when possible

When a "tie" exists non-HLA factors will be used including recipient sensitisation to HLA specificities, donor / recipient age disparity, ease with which a recipient could predictably receive a kidney and recipient waiting time. The geographical distance between donor and recipient centres will also be taken into account to minimise cold storage times. In all instances paediatric recipients will receive priority over adults.

No doubt there are other factors which play a role in determining outcome and which could therefore be used in allocation strategies but increasing complexity leads to conflict of opinion and logistical difficulties in operation. Some policies might consider the following candidates of lesser priority:

- Pre-dialysis patients
- Repeat transplants
- High-risk diagnoses: diabetes, vascular disease
- Co-morbidity: heart failure, hepatitis

Living donors

Live donor kidney transplantation poses special problems with allocation usually restricted to within close genetic relationships when the donor is over the age of consent and is capable of giving informed consent. The following relationship hierarchy is preferred:

- Monozygotic twins
- HLA-A, -B, -DR identical siblings
- "000" mismatched siblings or parents
- "111" mismatched siblings or parents
- other close genetic relations with no HLA-DR mismatch

The use of offspring as a donor for their parents is controversial and will depend on family circumstances but should probably only occur when the potential donor is over 30 years of age. With child-to-mother donation the issue of donor specific sensitisation because of in utero exposure must be carefully evaluated.

Live donors who are genetically unrelated to the recipient demand exceptionally careful consideration to comply with international guidelines and national legislation and consideration of motive to exclude coercion or payment. This practice will normally be limited to donation by partners, by strongly emotionally related friends or by distant genetic relations. The "altruistic unrelated donor" such as the life-long blood donor aged over 50 years who demands to make further contributions to society is a resource which is largely unused because of the huge potential problems which might be encountered after donation.

Allocation of livers

In the UK in 1996 639 liver transplants were performed and the waiting list at the end of that year was 195 patients. These figures reflect those throughout Europe and North America. The shortfall of liver donors is therefore less acute than that of kidney donors in part because of the absence of an effective artificial liver meaning that many patients with liver failure die or are not considered a suitable risk for transplantation. Liver transplantation is carried out in a restricted number of centres in contrast to kidney and heart transplantation because the surgery for removal of the liver from the donor and its transplantation into the recipient is challenging. Also although liver transplantation was attempted in the early 1960's its success did not reach acceptable levels until the early 1980's. As a result of these evolutionary differences and because the liver is apparently not susceptible to hyperacute rejection even in the presence of pre-formed donor-specific antibodies (Donaldson and Williams, 1997) histocompatibility issues are not usually considered in the allocation of livers. Compatibility for ABO blood groups is nearly always required although some ABO incompatible liver transplants have been performed with moderate success.

Sharing of livers between centres in the UK is therefore done on a rotational basis with availability of facilities and clinical urgency of the recipient taking priority. The size match of donor and recipient is taken into account. The allocation rules were agreed by all liver transplant centres through the auspices of the Royal College of Surgeons and activity is regularly audited. A facility for high-urgency recipients exists and again use of this option is carefully monitored.

A further advantage of liver transplantation is the possibility of splitting the lobes of a single donor liver so that more than one recipient can benefit. This is particularly relevant if the recipient is a child.

Use of liver lobes from living donors has commenced in the UK although this practice is more common in Japan where cadaver donation is limited due to religious and cultural objections to the definition of brain-death. Live liver lobe donation is most often between parent donors and their young children where emotional bonds are very strong. Since the liver is the only organ known to regenerate, the risks to the donor may appear to be less than in live kidney donation however the surgery is more complicated. One ethical issue in liver allocation is the consideration of the cirrhotic recipient who has liver failure because of abuse of alcohol. The approach differs between countries when sometimes the number of such recipients is low (Europe) and in others the incidence is higher (USA).

Allocation of thoracic organs

The allocation procedures for hearts, lungs or hearts and lungs as a combined transplant have also evolved in different circumstances. In the USA there are a large number of centres performing small numbers of thoracic organ transplants while in Europe the are fewer, busier centres. Allocation procedures are most similar to those agreed for livers in that clinical urgency of a recipient is prioritised. Again, mechanical support for heart and lung failure patients is still under development although a few centres do use “bridging” techniques of intra-thoracic mechanical pumps prior to a donor heart becoming available.

The role of histocompatibility in thoracic organ transplantation remains to be established perhaps because heart and lung recipients always receive comprehensive immunosuppression since failure of their transplant will be fatal. Furthermore the diagnosis of rejection in such recipients is effectively aided by invasive biopsy procedures which facilitate augmentation of drug treatments to overcome rejection precipitated by histoincompatibility.

A number of retrospective studies of HLA matching (Opelz and Wujciak, 1994, Smith *et al.,* 1995) and crossmatching (Smith *et al.,* 1993) have claimed an influence of HLA-DR mismatches on the incidence of acute rejections and reduced patient survival. In practice, the number of thoracic organ transplant candidates who are found to be sensitised to the majority of a cell-screening panel is small. It is difficult to ascertain the fate of such patients but it is probable that in most cases they do not receive a transplant. Repeat transplantation of thoracic organs is uncommon because of the poor success rates. As heart and lung transplants are “one off” opportunities it would seem reasonable that all possible is done to ensure the success of these transplants and therefore proving the case for prospective crossmatching and HLA matching remains a challenge to those active in the field. The evidence in favour of a role for HLA matching is accumulating, perhaps as other clinical issues are resolved. Unfortunately the use of high dose multi-drug immunosuppression in the face of histoincompatible donor organs means that heart and lung recipients are at high risk of associated morbidity such as post-transplant lymphoproliferative disease (Opelz and Henderson, 1993).

To avoid unnecessary travel of surgical teams the UK thoracic organ transplant community has agreed that local teams remove organs from cadaver donors and the organs are then allocated on a rotational basis through the UKTSSA. Prioritisation for clinical urgency is possible and ABO blood group compatibility is mandatory.

On first hearing, living donor heart transplantation seems an impossibility but it occurs when both heart and lungs from a cadaver donor are transplanted to a recipient with a specific diagnosis, usually cystic fibrosis. Such patients have a healthy heart but their own transplant surgery is more straightforward if both heart and lungs are transplanted (in turn their heart can be offered to a heart-only transplant candidate). Since the transplant team knows such living donors sometime before the donor organs are available, then consideration of recipients sensitised to HLA specificities is possible. Some centres consider use of both lungs and the heart from a donor for a single recipient to be wasteful and have pioneered both single and double lung transplantation leading to improvements in surgical technique. The incidence of combined heart and lung transplants is therefore in decline.

Living donor lung lobe donation is a rare but developing technique, which is pioneered in California. Usually one lobe from each parent is transplanted into a paediatric recipient. There are considerable ethical problems since the agreement of both donors is essential, putting pressure on both parents to agree to donate.

Allocation of corneas

The cornea has been transplanted for longer than any other human tissue reflecting the relative ease of the surgical procedure and the low degree of immunologically mediated rejection. Today corneas can be successfully banked with storage of up to 38 days possible. This has lead to a very small waiting list and a transplant procedure, which can be carried out electively. Allocation is therefore on the basis of the most suitable morphological matched cornea from the bank. UK cornea transplant units are currently studying the need for orientation of the transplanted cornea.

Despite these advantages which should allow prospective allocation studies, the role of ABO blood group compatibility in outcome of cornea transplants has yet to be agreed on (Borderie *et al.*, 1997). Also the role of HLA mismatching is debated (Gore *et al.*, 1995). In the main, cornea transplant recipients rarely receive immunosuppression although topical steroids may be applied. Studies of systemic immunosuppression are limited because of the considerable side effects.

A sub-group of cornea transplant patients are those who rapidly vascularise their transplanted cornea and go on to reject. They may receive multiple transplants over a period of time and these patients could benefit from receiving only HLA matched donor corneas. The incidence of antibodies in the serum of such patients is not well-documented (Roy *et al.*, 1992). The existence of cornea banks makes HLA matching for high-risk recipients quite feasible.

Corneas from living donors are obtained when normal eyes are removed incidental to facial surgery such as removal of a tumour. These will be banked to allow virological testing prior to issue from the bank.

Surrounding the eye is a region of stem cells, which can be transplanted from one or two living donors to recipients in need of such tissue. In time the stem cells grow over the recipient's cornea to resolve the clinical condition. In most instances the stem cell donors are close relatives of the recipient.

Organ allocation for multi-organ transplants

The number of multi organ transplants is small but increasing. Those documented include kidney and pancreas, liver and kidney, liver, heart and kidney, liver and small bowel and all the visceral organs. Allocation of organs to such recipients is on an individual basis with most agreed rules being suspended because of the nature of the transplant and the need for carefully planning and organisation. ABO blood group compatibility is usually required. Multi organ transplants should occur only in those centres with sufficient expertise to ensure a favourable outcome. Recipients of multi organ transplants will be acutely aware of the considerable resources needed for their treatment.

Problems of waiting times and clinical urgency

Surveys of potential organ transplant recipients usually highlight waiting time as the most emotive issue in deciding who should receive an organ. Unfortunately with insufficient supply of organs a “best use” policy is most acceptable. Whilst evidence based reviews of organ allocation strategies cannot easily assess the influence of waiting time on outcome it is usually considered fair to include a weighting for this factor, at least when two or more potential recipients compete for one organ. The precise waiting time of each recipient will be influenced by the clinical suitability of the patient over time and by the availability of the patient should an organ become available.

The type of organ needed will also influence the waiting time as heart, lung and liver failure patients cannot receive effective artificial organ support and might therefore be in a life-threatening situation prior to transplantation.

Clinical urgency of a patient is a factor which most would agree to be prioritised in an organ allocation strategy. Those who might die without a transplant were usually selected first in the early days of transplantation but it is now clear that such transplants are usually high risk because of the poor health of the patient and so might are not always the best option available. There can be no universally acceptable medical definition of "clinically urgent" and in cases where such transplants are an option a written statement of the patient's condition is usually required. Efficient audit of organs allocated to clinically urgent patients is essential if the continued goodwill of co-operating transplant teams is to be continued. In kidney transplantation there should not be a need to transplant a sick patient since there are preferred treatments to prevent death. In some cases there may be confounding co-morbid factors but they may beg the question whether a kidney transplant is the best option in a difficult case.

From the point of view of potential recipients and society as a whole, allocation of organs to ensure the longest survival of the rare resource, that of the donated organ, must be the first priority.

References

Borderie, VM, Lopez, M, Vedie, F and Laroche, L. (1997) ABO antigen blood group compatibility in corneal transplantation. *Cornea* **16**:1-6

Council of the Transplantation Society (1985) Commercialisation in transplantation: the problems and some guidelines for practice. *Lancet* **2**:715-716

Donaldson, PT and Williams, R. (1997) Cross-matching in liver transplantation. *Transplantation* **63**:789-794

Dyer, PA, Taylor, CJ and Martin, S (1998) HLA and clinical solid organ transplantation: recent publications and novel approaches. In: *HLA 1998* (Ed. Terasaki, PI and Gjertson, DW). UCLA Tissue Typing Laboratory, Los Angeles (in press)

Gore, SM, Vail, A, Bradley, BA, Rogers, CA, Easty, DL and Armitage, WJ. (1995) HLA-DR matching in corneal transplantation. *Transplantation* **60**:1033-1039

Gutmann, T, and Land, W. (1997). The ethics of organ allocation: the state of debate. *Transpl Rev* **11**:191-207

Kasiske, BL, Ramos, EL, Gaston, RS, Bia, MJ, Danovitch GM, *et al.* (1995) The evaluation of renal transplant candidates: clinical practice guidelines. *J Am Soc Nephrol* **6**:1-34

Opelz, G, and Henderson, R. (1993). Incidence of non-Hodgkins lymphoma in kidney and heart transplant recipients. *Lancet* **342**:1514

Opelz, G, and Wujciak, MS. (1994) The influence of HLA compatibility on graft survival after heart transplantation. *New Engl J Med* **330**:816-819

Rosenberg, JC, Kukuruga, D and Williams, T. (1997). HLA and clinical solid organ transplantation: A review of the literature of the 90s. In: *HLA 1997* (Ed. Terasaki, PI and Gjertson, DW), pp.7-38. UCLA Tissue Typing Laboratory, Los Angeles

Roy, R, Boisjoly, HM, Wagner, E, Langlois, A, Bernard, P-M, *et al.* (1992) Pretransplant and posttransplant antibodies in human corneal transplantation. *Transplantation* **54**:463-467

Smith, JD, Danskine, AJ, Laylor, RM, Rose, ML and Yacoub, MH. (1993) The effect of panel reactive antibodies and donor specific crossmatch on graft survival after heart and heart-lung transplantation. *Transpl Immunol* **1**:60-65

Smith, JD, Rose, ML, Pomerance, A, Burke, M and Yacoub, MH. (1995) Reduction of cellular rejection and increase in longer term survival after heart transplantation and HLA-DR matching. *Lancet* **346**:1318-1322

Starzl, TE, Eliasziw, M, Gjertson, DJ, Terasaki, PI, Fung, JJ, *et al.* (1997) HLA and cross-reactive group matching for cadaver kidney allocation. *Transplantation* **64**:983-991

UK Transplant Support Service Authority (1996) Cardiothoracic organ transplant audit 1985-1995. ISSN 1366-7939

Wujciak, T, and Opelz, G. (1993) A proposal for improved cadaver kidney allocation. *Transplantation* **56**:1513-1517

CHAPTER 13

SELECTION OF HAEMOPOIETIC STEM CELL DONORS FOR TRANSPLANTATION

A. Green
Histocompatibility and Immunogenetics Laboratory
National Blood Service Bristol Centre
Southmead Road
Bristol BS10 5ND, England

Introduction

Until recently bone marrow transplantation (BMT) has been indicated mostly for the treatment for acute lymphoblastic leukaemia (ALL) (reviewed by Kersey, 1997) and chronic myelogenous leukaemia (CML) (Savage and Goldman, 1997) but increasingly, BMT is now also being used to treat non-malignant diseases: examples include thalassaemia (Lucarelli, 1997), sickle cell disease (Vermylen and Corn, 1996), certain inherited metabolic diseases and more recently, autoimmune disease (Tyndall and Gratwohl, 1997). Furthermore, BMT is the treatment of choice for ALL in second complete remission, but it is now a matter of debate whether ALL in first complete remission with a good risk should be transplanted at all (Oakhill *et al.* 1996).

Haemopoietic stem cells may now be harvested from a number of sources including bone marrow, peripheral blood, and umbilical cord blood. Further, a stem cell collection may be made from a variety of donors, examples being:

- autologous
- an identical twin
- an HLA identical sibling
- a non-HLA-identical sibling
- a haploidentical parent
- an unrelated HLA-matched or HLA-mismatched donor

Both the source of stem cells and the way in which they are used in transplantation has become finely tailored to the individual patient. The classification and stage of disease, the age of the patient, the availability of a matched donor and the patient's response to previous therapy all contribute to a decision about what type of stem cells are most appropriate and how these might be best used. For example, patients with CML are routinely treated with stem cells from bone marrow, but are treated at a later stage if their disease returns with anti-leukaemic donor peripheral blood T cells. The stem cells infused may be unmanipulated or processed by a variety of techniques including T-cell depletion or CD34 selection. Infusions may consist of a combination of marrow with subsequent donor leucocytes, or may be purged of tumour cells using specific monoclonal antibodies or specific T cells.

Sources of stem cells

Apart from autologous stem cells, the principal sources are:

1. Bone marrow from related donors

A human leucocyte antigen (HLA) identical unaffected sibling is the ideal stem cell source. It has been estimated that the probability of finding an HLA-identical sibling donor is 1- (0.75n) where n represents the number of potential sibling donors (Armitage, 1994). This is the most common source of bone marrow for allogeneic transplants: in this situation, patients and siblings are genotypically matched. Example statistics for 1996 (Gratwohl and Passweg, 1998) show that bone marrow was the clinical source of only 10% of autologous transplants (n = 10,200) but of 74% of allogeneic transplants (n = 4,393). Where no HLA-identical sibling donor is available, HLA-haploidentical transplantation (from parent or sibling), or unrelated donor transplantation may be clinical options.

2. Bone marrow from unrelated donors (UD-BMT)

Worldwide, there are currently 41 registries of volunteer unrelated marrow donors, the largest of which is the National Marrow Donor Program (NMDP) based in the USA (Confer, 1997; Stroncek *et al.*, 1992). This has over 2.7 million registered donors of which just 35% are HLA-A, -B , -DR typed. In the UK there are two national registries: the Anthony Nolan Bone Marrow Trust (ANBMT) with 280,000 donors (156,000 of which are HLA-A,-B &-DR typed); and the British Bone Marrow Registry (BBMR) with 111,000 donors (75,000 of which are HLA-A,-B &-DR typed).

The extent and resolution of HLA typing on each volunteer registry is highly variable. As an example, donors recruited to the BBMR are now HLA typed by PCR-SSO/SSP DNA methods for HLA-A, -B and -DR: however when the BBMR was originally set up (as a source of HLA matched platelets) typing was for HLA Class I only and generally typing was performed using conventional serological methods. The consensus typing strategy for new donors worldwide, is that of high volume, low cost: and at level of HLA resolution which provides a reasonable chance of securing a number of potential donors for each patient depending on the frequency of their HLA type.

Searching for HLA-A,-B, -DR typed donors on NMDP normally reveals at least one full match for 75% of patients. For paediatric patients this figure can be extended further by the use of a single HLA-A or HLA-B mismatch (Anasetti *et al.* 1989). A study of consecutive searches for 1012 patients (Ottinger *et al.* 1994) demonstrated that searching a series of co-operative registries reduced the mean search-to-transplant time from 7.2 to 4.8 months and increased the final number donors found from 13.8% to 50%.

Together, the UK registries have contributed over 2500 bone marrow donors who have donated bone marrow stem cells actually used in transplantation (though not all were used for UK patients). These registries form a sophisticated network of donor databases and can be simultaneously accessed in the search for an unrelated donor. Despite the availability of international registries, it is still not possible to find a suitably matched donor for some patients. It has recently been suggested that this situation may be improved through better international communication, a better understanding of the HLA system and the significance of HLA matching, use of improved HLA databases, and through the use of alternative stem cell sources (Confer, 1997).

3. Peripheral blood stem cells (PBSC)

Until recently, the biological source of donor stem cells has been confined to bone marrow: however, a pilot joint clinical trial has now been given ethical approval to investigate the use of granulocyte colony stimulating factor (G-CSF) to promote the use of peripheral blood stem cells from unrelated volunteer donors. PBSC mobilised by haemopoietic growth factors such as G-CSF are rapidly replacing bone marrow as the preferred source of autologous haemopoietic stem cells for engraftment after myeloablative therapy (Haynes and Russell, 1995). The advantages include:

- ease of collection
- more rapid platelet and neutrophil engraftment
- reduced stay in hospital
- no requirement for anaesthesia
- less expense incurred

The use of PBSC, primarily for autologous transplants, has now led to its adoption in allogenic transplants (Haynes and Russell, 1995).

Early studies on stem cell expansion highlighted difficulties in achieving a significant ex-vivo increase in numbers of stem cells. High numbers of stem cells in donations are advantageous since animal experiments have shown that an increase in bone marrow stem cell dose by four to fivefold can lead to full donor chimerism, to the extent of overcoming MHC barriers when mice are sublethally irradiated prior to transplantation. In human clinical trials it has been demonstrated that by using a combined megadose (i.e. $>10^7$ nucleated cells per kg body weight) with an increased immunosuppressive and myeloablative conditioning regime, 75% of HLA-A, -B, -DR mismatched patients were able to sustain engraftment (Bachar-Lustig *et al.* 1995).

This method has recently been applied to the very high risk acute leukaemia patients and CML patients who do not respond to α-interferon, are in relapse after an autologous transplant, and have no HLA-matched donor available (Aversa *et al.* 1994). It has been suggested that there is potential for this treatment in nonneoplastic diseases e.g. aplastic anaemia and severe combined immunodeficiency (SCID), where engraftment problems may be overcome.

4. Cord blood stem cells

The clinical use of umbilical cord blood (UCB) cells has recently been reviewed (Cairo and Wagner, 1997). There are a number of centres world-wide, set up to collect and store cord blood on a large scale under good manufacturing conditions (GMP). These include the New York Blood Centre and the UK Cord Blood Banks.

Several groups are currently expanding umbilical cord stem cells in vitro and it is becoming clear that if such cells are capable of giving rise to sustained engraftment and immunological recovery, the use of this stem cell source may have a role in adult transplantation (Fietz *et al.* 1997; Denning Kendall *et al.* 1998).

Currently the majority of clinical results are from paediatric transplants: two recent preliminary studies indicated that where unmanipulated cord blood was transplanted from unrelated donors (n = 337) there was an incidence of severe acute graft-versus-host disease (GVHD) of 21-23%. These studies also showed delayed platelet engraftment compared to UD-BMT (Wagner and Kurtzberg, 1997).

There are a number of reported advantages of using UCB as a source of stem cells. Possibly the most important of these is the potential for increasing the ethnic mix of the donor pool. Other advantages include:

- the immediate availability of stored UCB where patients with a high probability of relapse do not have to wait
- the low risk of transmissible disease
- the apparently lower risk of acute and chronic GVHD
- the absence of donor risk
- the reduction in time between the search and transplant (although here, one group reported the time between search request and donor confirmation ranged from 12-291 days (Cairo and Wagner, 1997).

Clinical effect of HLA matching in stem cell transplantation

There have now been a large number of large single-centre based studies which have attempted to dissect the role of HLA matching in clinical transplant outcome. A number of important factors need to be considered when reviewing such studies. Thus, the patient disease group is particularly important since this tends to reflect the patient age: some published studies have included a mixture of paediatric and adult cases. In other studies, the marrow has been T cell depleted and in yet others, the marrow is T cell replete. An important aspect of the analysis of the clinical effects of HLA matching is the variability of methods employed: which range from serology to DNA sequencing.

1. ID-BMT versus MUD-BMT

A number of early studies compared the clinical results of HLA-identical sibling bone marrow transplants (ID-BMT) with HLA-matched unrelated transplants (MUD-BMT) (Bearman *et al.*, 1994; Davies *et al.*, 1994) and with transplants using haploidentical donors (Beatty *et al.*, 1985). These studies provided the first indications that HLA matching in BMT was clinically important. In one study (Bearman *et al.*, 1994), while there was no significant increase in either toxicity or transplant related mortality (TRM), there was an increase in the incidence of acute GVHD, from 21% for ID-BMT to 31% for MUD-BMT, with a concomitant further 3 day stay in hospital.

A second study of ID-BMT versus MUD-BMT (Davies *et al.*, 1994) revealed that CML patients who received non-T cell depleted grafts showed a significant increase in both primary & secondary graft failure in the MUD-BMT group: and it was clear at this time, that even serologically matched pairs were much more antigenically disparate than previously recognised. In particular it was reported that HLA Class I disparities were associated with increased graft failure.

There have been a number of other reports linking HLA disparity with graft failure (see Anasetti *et al.*, 1989). We have since confirmed this in a study of ALL patients during the period 1988-1997, in which we analysed 137 paediatric patients who received T cell depleted grafts. Our results showed a significant increase in primary graft failure in the HLA-mismatched group ($p=0.026$) compared with the matched group. However, these results also revealed that the severity of acute GVHD, the relapse rate and overall survival were not statistically different in the two groups (Green *et al.*, 1999).

Three studies have indicated that younger age is associated with better overall survival and transplant related mortality. One study of young adults, who were mismatched for HLA-A or -B or DRB1 subtype, showed no difference in survival when compared with fully HLA-matched children, but in adults the HLA-matched group showed significantly increased survival comparted with the HLA-mismatched group (Davies *et al.*, 1995). In a second study it was demonstrated that HLA disparity at one HLA Class I locus within the same cross reactive group (CREG) can be tolerated in young children: here, the incidence of acute GVHD is lower than in the adult group (Beatty *et al.*, 1985). A more recent study has suggested that the reason for the clinical success in children may be that they receive a higher stem cell dose per kg of body weight than adults, and that this might overcome the possible effect of HLA disparities (Sierra *et al.*, 1997).

2. HLA Class I mismatch

A recent analysis of the role of HLA Class I has shown that HLA-C disparity is associated with graft failure in unrelated donors. HLA-A and HLA-B were also implicated independently in this study (Petersdorf *et al.*, 1997). In another study,

TRM and and GVHD were also shown to be a consequence of HLA-C mismatching, in a patient group with a variety of diseases and in whom T cell depleted or T cell replete marrow was transplanted (Nagler *et al.*, 1996).

3. HLA Class II mismatch

The impact of HLA Class II mismatches has also been investigated in a number of studies. In a study of 360 T cell replete transplants, the probability of severe acute GVHD was greater with an HLA-DRB1-mismatched graft (0.48 versus 0.70, n = 59). Further, HLA-DRB1 matching to the allelic level decreased the risk of TRM and suggested that HLA-DRB1 allelic typing was important in both children and adults (Petersdorf *et al.*, 1995).

A further multicentre study of 366 CML patients confirmed that HLA-DRB1 matching was the most significant factor affecting survival (p = 0.04), leukaemia-free survival (p = 0.013), and TRM (p = 0.0049) (Devergie *et al.* 1997).

A study of the potential role of HLA-DPB1 mismatch in MUD-BMT (Petersdorf *et al.*, 1993) indicated that matching patients and donors for HLA-A, -B, DRB and DQB does not predict matching for DPB1. This is to be expected, since it has been proposed that there might be a recombination hotspot between the HLA-DQ and HLA-DP genes. This study also failed to provide evidence of an effect of HLA-DPB1 mismatching on acute GVHD, and it was suggested that HLA-DPB1 incompatibility should not therefore be used as an exclusion criterion for donor selection.

Several molecular studies have shown that significant numbers of patient-donor pairs, thought to be matched on the basis of HLA serology, were in fact HLA-DR-incompatible. Further, this observation is likely to be repeated by the recent adoption of molecular methods for HLA Class I allelic typing. It is thus now clear that high resolution HLA typing by molecular methods (see Chapters 5, 6, 7 and 8) can reveal incompatibilities not previously detected by conventional serological typing. Such incompatibilities are associated with an increase in severe acute GVHD, TRM and actuarial survival (Speiser *et al.*, 1996)

Donor Selection Procedures

Although the donor selection procedure differs between centres, the following procedural notes and criteria are relevant to most schemes.

A. Potential family donors

1. On referral from a transplant centre to the histocompatibility laboratory, a 20ml blood sample suitable for DNA extraction is required for use in PCR based HLA typing methods. The blood should be obtained from the patient using a suitable anticoagulant (3.3% trisodium citrate; or acid-citrate/dextrose, ACD). A further

5ml clotted blood sample should be taken for cytomegalovirus antibody screening, since this may be useful in donor selection.

2. Samples for HLA typing should be requested from both parents wherever possible. Parental HLA types should be used for family pedigree analysis and parental HLA typing may be required if a one-haplotype-mismatched transplant is being considered.

3. Information should be recorded concerning the family relationships and dates of birth of individuals from family members who have given samples, together with disease diagnosis for the patient. This information may help to indicate a potential donor if an HLA-matched sibling cannot be obtained.

4. One or more molecular methods may be used to determine the HLA type of the patient (see Chapters 5, 6, 7 and 8). Initially, high resolution HLA-A, -B, -C, -DR and -DQ typing is often performed since a high-resolution HLA type can facilitate an unrelated donor search, should a matched related donor be unavailable.

5. Siblings may be HLA typed using low-resolution molecular methods or by serological techniques, to select a matched sibling donor. In some centres low-resolution HLA typing is used to select a sibling family donor.

6. Where there is a single sibling for a patient and where no parental HLA typing has been performed, and the sibling inherits maternal and paternal haplotypes not inherited by the patient, a further blood sample should be requested to rule out human error and to confirm the result.

7. When there is more than one HLA-A, -B, -C, -DR, DQ-matched sibling donor available, the decision may be purely a clinical one. Factors such as body weight, social circumstances, CMV antibody status or gender may need to be considered. In the case of patients transplanted for autosomal recessive genetic diseases carrier status in a potential donor may need to be considered.

8. A number of additional laboratory tests can been performed to distinguish between apparently fully matched sibling donors. The one-way mixed lymphocyte culture (MLC) assay (see Chapter 11) has been widely performed to confirm HLA Class II incompatibilities between two serologically typed sibling donors. More recently, high resolution class II matching performed by molecular methods has arguably made the MLC redundant for the selection of related donors.

9. The helper T-lymphocyte precursor (HTLp) assay is used by some centres to quantify the frequency of donor helper T-lymphocyte precursors capable of responding to mismatches with patient cells. This frequency has been shown in some groups to correlate with acute GVHD (Schwarer *et al.* 1993). The impact of the HTLp assay may require validation using the local patient group. In paediatric transplants, it has been difficult to relate the results of these assays with clinical results because T cell depletion and less severe acute GVHD in children have made this hypothesis difficult to test. Patients with ALL may need to be

transplanted within 4 to 8 weeks due to a high probability of leukaemic relapse. Samples from these mainly paediatric patients may not contain sufficient lymphocytes to perform routine cellular assays and also there may not be sufficient time for the assays. A contrasting situation occurs for adult CML patients: here, there is more time available for donor selection and normally in this disease, there is sufficient material available to do further cellular investigations.

10. If an HLA-identical sibling is not found, the family study could be extended to a search of relatives who have inherited the same HLA haplotype as the patient; or by chance be phenotypically matched for a second haplotype with the patient. If an unrelated donor search is considered, this should be carried out simultaneously with the family search since the likelihood of finding a donor by extended family HLA typing is small unless the patient has inherited a haplotype that is common in the population.

Where the above strategies are unsuccessful the next option is to search for an unrelated HLA-matched or mismatched donor. However, the use of such donors may not be clinically appropriate or desirable: in this case, the use of other stem cell sources or other treatments may be eventually indicated.

B. HLA-matched unrelated donors

1. *Donor search.* High resolution HLA typing results from the patient, obtained by molecular methods, should be submitted to either of the registries using the appropriate forms. The search request will then be automatically faxed to other panels. Figure 13.1 shows the details required by the registries in order that a search can be instigated. Results of the searches should be available the same day and there should be no delay at this stage. A search report provides the following details:

- patient reference number
- local donor number
- donor panel number
- donor age and sex
- blood group
- donor CMV antibody status (if available)
- subpanels (donor centres)
- HLA match status:
  - A, B and DR matched
  - A and B matched, DR mismatched
  - A and B matched, DR not tested
  - one A mismatch, B and DR matched
  - A matched, one B mismatch, DR matched
- readout from Bone Marrow Donors Worldwide (BMDWW) of donors that have been listed on international panels

Unrelated Marrow & Cord Blood Donor Search Request Form

PATIENT DETAILS

Cord Blood Search Required Yes/No (delete as appropriate)

If Yes indicate the weight of the recipient (see 8 below)

1. **Family name** ____________
2. **Forename** ____________
3. **Country of Residence** ____________
4. Country of Birth ____________

5. **Sex (M male; F female)** [ ]

6. Race [ ]
   1 Caucasian; 2 Black; 3 Oriental; 4 Hispanic; 5 Asian; 6 other; 7 Mixed Race; 8 Arab;

7. **Date of birth (day / month / year)** [ ]
8. Recipient Weight ____________
9. **Diagnosis** ____________
10. **Date of diagnosis (day / month / year)** [ ]
11. Risk category: (Please code using table overleaf) [ ]
12. **If leukaemia please give**
    current status (1 remission; 2 relapse) [ ]
    number of remissions achieved [ ]
13. **Patient hospital number** [ ]
14. Intended transplant centre ____________
15. Intended time to transplant (if known) ____________
16. Transplant physician ____________

PERSON REQUESTING SEARCH
(to whom initial registry report will be sent)

Name ____________
Address ____________
Tel. ____________
Fax. ____________
Signed ____________
Date signed (day / month / year) [ ][ ][ ][ ][ ][ ]

INVOICEE

Name ____________
Address ____________
Tel. ____________
Fax. ____________
Signed ____________
Date signed (day / month / year) [ ][ ][ ][ ][ ][ ]

TESTING CENTRE

17. Tissue Typing Laboratory ____________

TISSUE TYPING DETAILS
Please attach family tree if available

18. PATIENT

HLA -A ______ ______
B ______ ______
Cw ______ ______
DRB1* ______ ______
DRB3* ______ ______
DRB4* ______ ______
DRB5* ______ ______
DQA1* ______ ______
DQB1* ______ ______
DPA1* ______ ______
DPB1* ______ ______

Patient CMV Status ____________
Blood Group ____________

19. FATHER — Trace code [ ]
1 tissue typed; 2 not typed; 3 no siblings; 4 dead or unavailable

Family name ____________
Forename ____________
Race (see question 6) [ ]
HLA - A ______ ______
B ______ ______
DRB1* ______ ______
DQB1* ______ ______

20. MOTHER — Trace code (see question 18) [ ]

Family name ____________
Forename ____________
Race (see question 6) [ ]
HLA - A ______ ______
B ______ ______
DRB1* ______ ______
DQB1* ______ ______

21. FULL SIBLING — Trace code (see question 18) [ ]

Family name ____________
Forename ____________
HLA - A ______ ______
B ______ ______
DRB1* ______ ______
DQB1* ______ ______

22. FULL SIBLING — Trace code (see question 18) [ ]

Family name ____________
Forename ____________
HLA - A ______ ______
B ______ ______
DRB1* ______ ______
DQB1* ______ ______

Fig 13.1. Example of a donor search request form.

It does not provide:

- details of donor availability
- high resolution DNA typing of the majority of donors

2. *High resolution confirmatory typing (CT).*

Donor samples need to be requested from registries for CT, which should include HLA-A, -B, -C, -DR and -DQ, using high resolution PCR-SSP or PCR-SSO based methods. Requesting centres need to allow a minimum of two weeks for donors to be contacted by the local registries and for arrangements for samples collection to be made.

At this stage there is a 20-30% attrition rate on some local panels where donors are either temporarily or permanently withdrawn from panels for a variety of medical and social reasons.

3. *Initial donor selection criteria*

Age of the patient

- for paediatric patients, samples should be requested from donors who are potential full matches or in their absence one antigen mismatched.
- for adult patients, samples from potential fully matched donors may be requested: at the same time, it is advisable to request a formal international search based on the printout from Bone Marrow Donors Worldwide (BMDWW).

Disease of the patient

- Patients with ALL are usually children: consequently, the search to transplant time should be minimised. Cord blood searches should also be considered.
- Adult CML patients generally show a longer time from remission to relapse: therefore international searches may be appropriate where there are no potential full matches available.

Sex of donors

There is evidence to suggest that young male donors may have a better transplant outcome, presumably because they will not have been sensitised to HLA, which may occur in females during pregnancy.

CMV antibody status of donors

CMV antibody-negative patients should be transplanted with stem cells from CMV-negative donors, in order to prevent the potential for primary CMV infection or CMV reactivation from the donor stem cells. Where cord blood donors are selected, other criteria such as total nucleated cell count, volume of the collection, and sometimes CD34+ cell content, are also considered.

4. *HLA typing of donors*

- Preferentially select donors that have been typed to the highest resolution: i.e. those that have been typed using molecular methods and those that have been HLA-C and DQ typed.
- If there are only a few donors matched to the patient, all donors should be selected regardless of typing level on the search report, since it is possible that the HLA typing results, if performed some years ago, are imprecise in the face of current technology.
- The majority of DNA samples are stored by donor centres and thus high resolution allelic typing can be performed on site to speed up selection. However, the disadvantage of this approach is that donors may no longer be active, ultimately delaying the procedure.

5. *HLA matching*

When HLA-DR and -DQ typing was performed using restriction fragment length polymorphism (RFLP) analysis, the time taken was a cause of considerable delay to the selection of a suitable donor. Hence it became advantageous to use one of a number of rapid DNA conformational methods: these include heteroduplex analysis and single stranded conformational polymorphism (SSCP) analysis. For example, heteroduplex techniques have been applied to HLA Class I matching (Pursall *et al*., 1996.) to effectively rule out mismatched donors rapidly, and to select donors suitable for further testing in cellular assays. Although these methods are technically easy to perform easy and relatively inexpensive, some HLA differences may not be easily detected. The use of high resolution PCR-SSP has largely replaced the need for DNA conformational analysis matching methods, with certain exceptions, e.g. heteroduplex matching for HLA-Class I in the absence of routine Class I allelic typing. A further disadvantage of conformational analyses is that HLA types of panel donors are not increased in resolution by the use of such techniques. DNA conformational analysis methods have subsequently been developed to the stage where HLA allelic typing is now possible: this is described in detail in Chapter 8.

6. *HLA-typing methods*

In recent years HLA typing has concentrated on the molecular analysis of genes which encode the HLA molecules. The two main methods currently used in routine laboratories for stem cell donor selection are PCR using sequence-specific primers (PCR-SSP: Chapter 5) and PCR using sequence-specific oligonucleotides (PCR-SSOP: Chapter 6). The introduction of sequencing-based typing (Chapter 7) has been slower but is likely to impact greatly on the routine service in the near future.

Currently in many laboratories, donors are selected using high resolution HLA-DRB1, -DRB3, -DRB4, -DRB5, -DQB1, -Cw typing and low resolution HLA-A and -B typing by molecular methods. Serological typing for HLA has been completely superceded by these methods in many laboratories: however, serology may provide a a useful role in confirming whether certain HLA alleles are expressed (*cf* "null" alleles) and in confirming inter-relationships between alleles. (See Hurley *et al.*, 1997).

7. *Additional selection methods: cellular assays*

HLA-DRB1 allelic typing by PCR-SSP, PCR-SSO and other high resolution molecular analyses is considered by many investigators to be superior to the mixed lymphocyte culture (MLC) in terms of speed, cost and precision for predicting clinical outcome following haemopoietic cell transplantation (Mickelson *et al.*, 1996). It has also been demonstrated that the MLC is not predictive of acute GVHD or survival (Segall *et al.*, 1996). Consequently, many laboratories have now ceased using this assay for donor selection.

Cytotoxic T-lymphocyte precusor (CTL-p) frequency assays are described in detail in Chapter 11. The relevance of the assay in the selection of HLA compatible unrelated donors is still a matter of debate. It has been suggested by a number of groups that the CTL-p frequency assay is predictive for acute GVHD (Kaminski *et al.,* 1989). This conclusion, however, has not been universally accepted (Fussell *et al*, 1994). The assay detects mainly HLA Class I differences and thus is useful where this has not been performed to allelic level. It is therefore a matter of current contention that, as with the MLC assay, CTL-p frequency assays may be superseded by HLA typing at the allelic level by molecular techniques.

A problem with the validation of these cellular assays is that most studies are of adult CML patients where lymphocytes counts are generally high. The fact that it takes 10 days to carry out a CTL-p assay has also made it impracticable to use for donor selection in paediatric patients, because cell counts in these patients are lower and transplants must be carried out more urgently. Such transplants are also normally T cell depleted, making it difficult to establish a causal relationship between graft outcome & CTL-p frequency. In cases of HLA-Class I mismatched transplants, the fact that CTL-p frequencies are usually high is thus predictable.

8. *HLA and non-HLA factors*

It is important that HLA typing is performed on patient-donor pairs to the allelic level in order to select best matched donor. At present, the question of which level of resolution and which HLA loci are important is only just beginning to be answered. It is also clear that we should consider typing/matching for other non-

HLA loci including minor histocompatibility antigens. It is important that the influence of HLA and non-HLA factors in haemopoietic cell transplantation continues to be analysed in large multicentre studies and that conclusions are supported by clear statistical evidence.

Summary

The current donor selection policy depends upon a number of interacting factors and upon the local transplant activity. Thus, the strategy for haemopoietic cell donor selection depends upon patient disease category, availability of an HLA identical sibling donor, age, genotype, number of available donors, patient CMV status and donor gender. It is also clear that good communications between the transplant centre, the histocompatibility laboratory, and the bone marrow donor registries, are essential for the rapid selection of the best matched donor. The final decision is simple when the selection process reveals a single donor but it is likely that where there a number of donors further selection procedures may be required.

References

Anasetti, C, Amos, D, Beatty, PG, Appelbaum, FR, Bensinger, W, *et al.* (1989) Effect of HLA compatibility on engraftment of bone marrow transplants in patients with leukaemia or lymphoma. *N Engl J Med* **320:** 197-204

Armitage, JO (1994). Bone Marrow Transplantation. *N Engl J Med* **330:** 827-838

Aversa, F, Tabilio, A, Terenzi, A, Velardi A, Falzetti F, *et al.*(1994). Successful engraftment of T cell depleted haploidentical ‘three loci’ incompatible transplants in leukaemia patients by addition of recombinant human granulocyte colony-stimulating factor-mobilised peripheral blood progenitor cells to bone marrow inoculum. *Blood* **84:** 3948-3955

Bachar-Lustig, E, Rachamin, N, Hong-wei, L, Lan, F and Reisener, Y (1995). Megadose of T-cell depleted bone marrow overcomes MHC barriers in sub lethally irradiated mice. *Nature Medicine* **12:** 1268-1273

Bearman, SI, Mori, M, Beatty, PG, Meyer, WG, Buckner, CD, *et al.* (1994). Comparison of morbidity and mortality after marrow transplantation from HLA-genotypically identical siblings and HLA-phenotypically identical unrelated donors. *Bone Marrow Transpl* **13:** 31-35

Beatty, PG, Clift, RA, Mickelson, EM, Nisperos, BB, Flournoy, N, *et al.* (1985) Marrow Transplantation from related donors other than HLA-identical siblings. *N Engl J Med* **313**: 765-771

Beatty, PG, Anasetti, C, Hansen, JA, Longton, GM, Sanders, JE, *et al.* (1993) Marrow transplantation from unrelated donors for treatment of hematologic malignancies: effect of mismatching for one HLA locus. *Blood* **81:** 249-253

Cairo, MS and Wagner J.E. (1997). Placental and/or umbilical cord blood: An alternative source of hematopoietic stem cells for transplantation. *Blood* **90:** 4665-4678

Confer DL (1997). Unrelated marrow donor registries. *Curr Opin Hematol* **4:** 408-412

Davies, SM, Ramsay, NKC, Haake, RJ, Kersey, JH, Weisdorf, DJ, *et al.* (1994). Comparison of engraftment in recipients of matched sibling or unrelated donor marrow allografts. *Bone Marrow Transpl* **13**: 51-57

Davies, SM, Shu, XO, Blazar, BR, Filipovich, AH, Kersey, JH, *et al.* (1995) Unrelated donor bone marrow transplantation: influence of HLA A and B incompatibility on outcome. *Blood* **86:** 1636-1642

Denning-Kendall, PA, Nicol, A, Horsley, H, Donaldson, C, Bradley, B, *et al.* (1998). Is in vitro expansion of human cord blood cells clinically relevant? *Bone Marrow Transpl* **21:** 225-232

Devergie, A, Apperley, JF, Labopin, M, Madrigal, A, Jacobsen, N, *et al.* (1997). European results of matched unrelated donor bone marrow transplantation for chronic myeloid leukaemia. Impact of HLA class II matching. *Bone Marrow Transpl* **20:** 11-19

Fietz, T, Hilgenfeld, E, Berdel, WE, Hopp, H, Wenzel U, *et al.* (1997) Ex vivo expansion of human umbilical cord blood does not lead to co-expansion of contaminating maternal mononuclear cells. *Bone Marrow Transpl* **20:** 1019-1026

Fussell, ST, Donnellan, M, Cooley, MA and Furrel, C. (1994) Cytotoxic T lymphocyte precursor frequency does not correlate with either incidence or severity of graft-versus-host disease after matched unrelated donor bone marrow transplantation. *Transplantation* **57**: 675-676

Goldman, MJ (1997). Chronic myeloid leukaemia. *Curr Opin Hematol* **4:** 277-285

Gratwohl, A, Passweg, J, Baldomero, H and Hermens, J (1998) Blood and marrow transplantation activity in Europe 1996. *Bone Marrow Transpl* **22**: 227-240

Green, A, Clarke, E, Hunt, L, Canterbury, A, Lankester, A, *et al.* (1999) Children with acute lymphoblastic leukaemia who receive HLA mismatched allografts from unrelated donors have increased incidence of primary graft failure but overall outcome is not adversely affected. *Blood* (in press)

Haynes A P and Russell, N (1995). Blood stem cell allografting. *Curr Opin Hematol* **2:** 431-435

Hurley, CK, Schreuder, GMT, Marsh, SGE, Lau, M, Middleton, D, *et al.* (1997) The search for HLA-matched donors: a summary of HLA-A*, -B*, DRB1/3/4/5* alleles and their association with serologically defined HLA-A, -B, -DR antigens. *Tissue Antigens* **50:** 401-418

Kaminski, E, Hows, J, Man, S, Brookes, P, Mackinnon, S, *et al.* (1989) Prediction of graft-versus-host disease by frequency analysis of cytotoxic T cells after unrelated donor bone marrow transplantation. *Transplantation* **48**: 608-613

Kersey, JH. (1997). Fifty years of study of the biology and therapy of childhood leukaemia. *Blood* **90:** 4243-4251

Lucarelli, G (1997). Bone marrow transplantation for thalassaemia. *J Int Med Suppl* **740:** 49-52

Mickelson, EM, Longton, G, Anasetti, C, Martin, PJ, Guthrie, LA, *et al.* (1996). Evaluation of the mixed kymphocyte culture (MLC) assay as a method for selecting unrelated donors for marrow transplantation. *Tissue Antigens* **47**: 27-36.

Nagler, A, Brautbar, C, Slavin, sincerely and Bishara, A. (1996). Bone marrow transplantation using unrelated and family related donors: the impact of HLA-C disparity. *Bone Marrow Transpl* **18:** 891-897

Oakhill, A, Pamphilon, DH, Potter, MN, Steward, CG, Goodman, S. *et al.* (1996). Unrelated donor bone marrow transplantation for children with relapsed acute lymphoblastic leukaemia in second complete remission. *Brit J Haem* **94**:574-578

O'Shea, J, Madrigal, A, Davey, N, Brookes, P, Scott, I, *et al.* (1997). Measurement of cytotoxic T lymphocyte precursor frequencies reveals cryptic HLA class I mismatches in the context of unrelated donor bone marrow transplantation. *Transplantation* **64:** 1353-1356

Ottinger, H, Grosse-Wilde, M, Schmitz, A and Grosse-Wilde, H (1994). Immunogenetic marrow donor search for 1012 patients: a retrospective analysis of strategies, outcome and costs. *Bone Marrow Transpl* **14 (Suppl. 4):** 34-38

Petersdorf, EW, Smith, AG, Mickelson, WEM, Longton, GM. Anasetti, C, *et al.* (1993). The role of HLA-DPB1 disparity in the development of acute graft versus host disease following unrelated donor marrow transplantation. *Blood* **81:** 1923-1932

Petersdorf, EW, Longton, GM, Anasetti, C, Martin, PJ, Mickelson, WEM, *et al.* (1995). The significance of HLA-DRB1 matching on clinical outcome after HLA-A, B,DR identical unrelated donor marrow transplantation. *Blood* **86:** 1606-1613

Petersdorf, EW, Longton, GM, Anasetti, C, Mickelson, WEM, McKinney, S, *et al*. (1997) Association of HLA-C disparity with graft failure after marrow transplantation from unrelated donors. *Blood* **89:** 1818-1823

Pursall, MC, Clay, TM and Bidwell, JL. (1996) Combined PCR-heteroduplex and PCR-SSCP analysis for matching of HLA-A,-B,-C allotypes in marrow transplantation. *Eur J Immunogenet* **26:** 41-53

Savage, DG and Goldman, DM (1997). Allografting for chronic myeloid leukaemia. *Curr Opin Hematol* **4:** 369-376

Schwarer, AP, Jiang, YZ, Brooks, PA, Barret, AJ, Batchelor, JR, *et al.* (1993) *Lancet* **341**: 203-205

Segall, M, Harriet, N, Edwins, L, Haake, R, Shu, XO, *et al*. (1996) Lack of correlation of MLC reactivity with acute graft-versus-host-disease and mortality in unrelated bone marrow transplantation. *Hum Immunol* **49:** 49-55

Sierra, J, Storer, B, Hansen, JA, Bjerke, JW, Martin, PJ, *et al*. (1997). Transplantation of marrow cells from unrelated donors for treatment of high-risk acute leukaemia: the effect of leukaemic burden, donor HLA- matching, and marrow cell dose. *Blood* **89:** 4226-4235

Speiser, DE, Tiercy, J-M, Rufer, N, Grundshober, C, Gratwohl, A, *et al*. (1996). High resolution matching associated with decreased mortality after bone marrow transplantation. *Blood* **87:** 4455-4462

Stoncek, D, Bartsch, G, Perkins, BL, Randall, BL, Hansen, JA, *et al.* (1992) The National Marrow Donor Program. *Transfusion* **33**: 567-577.

Tyndall, A and Gratwohl, A (1997). Hemopoeitic blood and marrow transplants in the treatment of severe autoimmune disease. *Curr Opin Hematol* **4:** 390-394.

Vermylen, C and Corn, G (1996). Bone marrow transplantation for sickle cell anaemia. *Curr Opin Hematol* **3:** 163-166

Wagner, JE and Kurtzberg, J. (1997) Cord blood stem cells. *Curr Opin Hematol* **4:** 413-418

CHAPTER 14

SELECTION OF PLATELET DONORS AND PROVISION OF HLA-MATCHED PLATELETS

J. Harrison and C. Navarrete
NBS - London & The South East
North London Centre
Colindale Avenue
London NW9 5BG, England

Introduction

Platelet refractoriness, which is characterised by the failure to gain adequate increments (less than 10 x 10^9/l, one hour post-transfusion), following at least two platelet transfusions from random donors, is a serious clinical complication in transfusion-dependent patients. Approximately 30-70% of these patients become refractory to platelet transfusions (Murphy and Waters, 1990).

The effectiveness of the platelet transfusion is normally assessed by the platelet count obtained 15 minutes, 1 or 24 hours following the transfusion. This can be measured as the corrected count increment (CCI) or as percentage (%) of post transfusion recovery of platelets:

Corrected count increment (CCI)

This is the value calculated from the formula below but it requires the knowledge of the patient's body surface area (BSA):

$$\text{CCI} = \frac{\text{Platelet increment } (10^9/\text{L}) \times \text{BSA}}{\text{No of platelets transfused} \times 10^{11}}$$

In general, a CCI greater than 7.5x10^9/L within an hour post transfusion and greater than 4.5x10^9/L if measured after 18-24 is considered to be successful. In reality, in the majority of cases a pre and a post platelet transfusion count is performed and a good response is considered to be either a post-transfusion increment of greater than or equal to 10x10^9/L after one hour or a decrease/arrest of clinical bleeding.

If the response to a dose of random platelets is poor on two consecutive occasions, it is then advisable to use fresh (<48 h old), random, ABO identical platelets. If this approach also fails, laboratory investigation of the possible causes of platelet refractoriness should commence. The causes of platelet refractoriness may be immunological or non-immunological, although in the majority of patients both immunological and non- immunological factors are present.

Non-immunological refractoriness

There are a number of factors which can contribute to the non-immunological destruction of transfused platelets. These include the use of old and/or badly stored platelets, products containing small platelet doses, other clinically related conditions such as splenomegaly, hepatomegaly, disseminated intravascular coagulation (DIC), septicaemia, fever, infections, (e.g. CMV) and malignancies. In addition, drugs used as part of the treatment including antibiotics, e.g. amphotericin B, vancomycin and ciprofloxacin can contribute to refractoriness.

If no non-immunological causes are identified, investigation into possible immunological causes should commence.

Immunological refractoriness to random donor platelet transfusions

HLA and to a lesser extent HPA and high titre ABO alloantibodies present in the patient reacting with donor platelets are the main cause of immune destruction of transfused platelets. Platelet destruction is thought to occur via the monocyte/macrophage system. The Fab terminus of the antibody will recognise and bind to the incompatible platelet and the Fc receptor (FcR) of monocytes will bind to the exposed Fc leading to the phagocytosis and destruction of the opsonised platelets. Since the FcR expressed on monocytes preferentially binds IgG3 and IgG1, the main type of antibodies involved are IgG.

HLA antibodies are found in approximately 50% of multitransfused patients but only approximately 30% of these patients are immunologically refractory. The titre and specificity of the antibodies present is important since patients with HLA-specific antibodies and with a low percentage panel reactivity (PRA) may not necessarily be immunologically refractory. Furthermore, a number of patients never develop HLA antibodies nor do they become refractory, despite receiving multiple platelet transfusions. The production of antibodies may be influenced by a number of factors including the level of mismatch between patient and donor, previous sensitisation, the immune status of the patient and the original disease. In addition to HLA, both HPA and high titre ABO antibodies have also been identified in these patients. The reported frequency of HPA antibodies varies from 3-30% but in most cases these are found in highly HLA immunised patients (Schnaidt *et al.,* 1996).

Refractoriness due to high titre ABO has been reported in two patients receiving HLA-matched platelets. Furthermore, the transfusion of HLA-matched but ABO mismatched platelets into alloimmunised patients results in a 20% reduction in the platelet increments post transfusion (Carr *et al.,* 1990). On the other hand, circulating immune complexes involving the ABO system have also been shown to affect the survival of transfused platelets (Heal *et al.,* 1993)

Other antibodies such as drug induced have also been implicated in platelet refractoriness but their occurrence is rare. Finally, although secondary thrombocytopenia due to the presence of platelet autoantibodies (PAIg) has been observed, these have not been shown to affect allogeneic platelet survival (Godeau *et al.,* 1992).

Management of immunological platelet refractoriness

Patients refractory to random platelet transfusions should first be tested for the presence of HLA antibodies and, if positive, they should be HLA typed in case HLA-matched platelets are required. The management of these patients involves the following 4 steps:

1. *HLA antibody screening*

The lymphocytotoxicity test (LCT) has been the standard technique used for the detection of HLA antibodies. When tests are performed for cytotoxic antibodies, the presence of non-HLA lymphocyte reactive autoantibodies should be excluded since these are common in thrombocytopenic patients, particularly in post bone marrow transplant patients who have a dysfunctional immune system. Furthermore, the clinical relevance of these antibodies in immunological platelet refractoriness is not clear. The detection of these autoantibodies is normally carried out using DTT (see Chapter 2). In our laboratory, 104 serum samples from patients receiving platelet transfusions were tested and 50% of sera were positive by LCT but only 40% were positive when screened with DTT illustrating the importance of using DTT to remove the reactivity due to IgM, non-HLA lymphocytotoxic antibodies (10%). One of the main disadvantages of the LCT test is that it only detects cytotoxic antibodies, therefore the detection of non-cytotoxic HLA-specific antibodies is performed using flow cytometry or ELISA assays as described in Chapter 2.

Furthermore, one of the main advantages of the ELISA technique is that not only can it detect non-cytotoxic but more importantly it detects HLA-specific antibodies since it relies on the binding of the antibodies to wells coated with pools of solubilized HLA antigens. It is also more sensitive and in our laboratory the ELISA test achieves a 7% increase in sensitivity over the LCT test (49 versus 42%). The precise identification of the type, specificity and titre of antibodies is not only important for the diagnosis but also to establish the best course of treatment since the majority of these patients can benefit from the provision of HLA-matched or crossmatch negative platelets (see below) (Contreras and Navarrete, 1997).

2. *HLA class I (A & B) typing*

The HLA class I (A & B) typing of patients should be performed as soon as HLA-specific antibodies are detected in order to identify the most suitable HLA-matched platelet unit. Platelets express all classical HLA class I (HLA-A, -B) and to a lesser degree -Cw antigens. At present, and since most laboratories only perform HLA-A & -B typing on these patients and on platelet donors, the clinical significance of HLA-Cw antibodies to immunological refractoriness has not been established. The main reason for this is that until recently the serological detection of Cw antigens was limited but with the availability of molecular DNA based techniques to define these antigens, the precise contribution of both the HLA-Cw antigens and -Cw antibodies to immunological platelet refractoriness may be elucidated.

Furthermore, by using DNA based techniques it is now possible to perform HLA typing on patients with such low cell counts who could not be typed by previous methods (these are the majority of patients requiring platelet support). Similarly, the use of PCR-based techniques can provide a higher level of resolution of the HLA-A, -B and -Cw alleles which may result in the identification of immuno-dominant serological epitopes involved in the process of alloimmunisation.

3. *Provision of HLA-matched or crossmatch-negative platelets*

For refractory patients in whom non-immune causes have been excluded, and HLA-specific antibodies are detected, HLA-matched platelets should be provided. However this is only possible if large panels of HLA-typed platelet donors are available. Alternatively, crossmatch negative platelets could be used but this approach also relies on the availability of large numbers of platelets to be crossmatched for each individual patient. The relative benefits of each of these two approaches is still controversial and is generally determined by the infrastructure available to support each type of treatment rather than by sound clinical and scientific evidence.

3.1. *Provision of HLA-matched platelets.*

Due to the high degree of polymorphism of the HLA system, large panels of HLA-typed platelet donors are required to provide HLA-matched platelets. In most laboratories the matching is carried out based on the serological definition of the HLA antigens at the specificity levels including serological splits. However, with the introduction of DNA based techniques to type patients and platelet donors at the high resolution allele level, it will soon be possible to assess the clinical relevance of HLA matching at the allele level in these patients.

The provision of HLA-matched platelets is also carried out on the basis of the known serological crossreactivity that exists between different antigens of the HLA-A and -B loci as described by Duquesnoy *et al.,* (1977). Although this is a useful alternative approach to overcome the difficulties arising from the lack of large HLA typed platelet panels and patients with rare HLA types, patients with antibodies to antigens within the CREG groups have been described.

The degree of matching used in the UK are defined as follows:

A grade matching. This involves serological compatibility for the four HLA-A and -B locus antigens including the use of HLA homozygous donors, e.g.

- Patient = HLA-A1,A2/B8,B44
- Donor = HLA-A1,A2/B8,B44 or
- Homozygous Donor = HLA-A1,A1/B8, B8 or HLA-A2, A2/B44, B44

B grade matching (B1-B4). In this case the patient and donor are mismatched for 1 to 4 serologically crossreactive* antigens, e.g. a B1 match would be:

- Patient = HLA-A1, A2*/B8,B44
- Donor = HLA-A1,A28*/B8,B44

C grade matching (C1-C4). In this grade the patient and donor are mismatched for a serologically non-crossreactive* antigen, e.g. a C1 match would be:

- Patient = HLA-A1, A2*/B8,B44
- Donor = HLA-A1, A30*/B8,B44

A similar matching criteria is used in most countries, although the nomenclature varies slightly in that B (B1-B4) grade matching distinguishes between the cross-reactive donor antigen mismatch as either unknown (B1U) or crossreactive (B1X). Similar criteria is used for the C grade matching (Duquesnoy *et al.,* 1977)

3.2. *Use of HLA- A and -B homozygous platelet donors*

The provision of HLA-matched platelets for people with relatively common HLA types can be facilitated by the use of donors homozygous for common HLA haplotypes. In a study of the French Bone Marrow Panel published in 1995 (Lonjou *et al.,* 1995), 65,700 donors from all parts of France were typed for HLA class I antigens. The frequency of the HLA-A1, B8 haplotype was 5.6%, and that of the HLA-A2, B44 haplotype was also 5.6%. On this basis, it can be calculated that HLA-A1, B8 homozygotes and A2, B44 homozygotes would have a frequency of 0.3% in the population and would be found in approximately 1/300 people.

In 1997, HLA-matched platelets were provided for 78 patients by the North London Centre. Of these, the number of patients for whom HLA-A1, B8 homozygotes would have provided an A grade match was 10 (12.8%) patients. The number of patients for whom HLA-A2, B44 homozygotes would have provided an A grade HLA match was 12 (15.4%) patients. Overall, 22 (28.2%) of the 78 patients could have been managed using platelets from donors homozygous for HLA-A1, B8 or HLA-A2, B44.

In another study of North London patients transfused in 1997, it was shown that over a three month period (January to March 1997) 424 doses of HLA-matched platelets were provided. Of these, the number of doses of platelets where an HLA-A1, B8 homozygote would have provided an A grade HLA match was 54 (12.7%) doses. The number of doses where an HLA-A2, B44 homozygote would have provided an A grade HLA match was 111 (26.2%) doses. Thus, during this period using HLA-A1, B8 or HLA-A2, B44 homozygotes, 165 of the 424 doses of platelets could have been provided as an A grade HLA match (38.9% of doses). It should be noted that platelets donated by HLA-A2, B44 homozygotes would have provided an A grade match more than twice as often as those donated by HLA-A1, B8 homozygotes. This is because the HLA-A2, B44 haplotype is more commonly found in people of several different ethnic groups, whereas the HLA-A1, B8 haplotype is common only in people of Northern European origin. Patients in the UK, and particularly in London, come from various ethnic backgrounds, but the majority of platelet panel donors are ethnically Northern European. Current platelet donor recruitment strategies are designed to try to address this problem.

3.3. Provision of crossmatched platelets.

If no HLA-A, -B or -C matches are available and the specificity of the antibody is known, single donor (SD) platelets negative for the relevant antigen are provided. If this is not possible, available apheresis platelets are crossmatched with the patient's serum. A number of platelet crossmatch techniques have been described (Kakaiya *et al.,* 1984) but most laboratories use a commercially available solid phase technique (CAPTURE-P®, Immucor Inc., Norcross, GA 30071, USA). The limitation of this technique is that it detects all antibodies reacting with platelets and therefore does not distinguish HLA from non-HLA antibodies. Crossmatch-negative platelets are also the only alternative for patients with low cell counts and in whom no HLA typing is available.

In our laboratory, preference is given to HLA-matched over cross-matched platelets because of the need to avoid further HLA alloimmunisation via the indirect allorecognition of the transfused HLA antigens, a complication of significance in women of child bearing age and younger patients. Ideally both HLA-matched and crossmatch-negative platelets should be provided depending on patient requirements. However, the clinical benefits or cost effectiveness of this approach needs to be determined, particularly in view of the recent introduction of universal leucodepletion in the UK.

More recently, a method to eliminate the HLA class I antigens from the membrane of platelets using acid treatment has been described (Shanwell *et al.,* 1991). After transfusion of the acid treated platelets it was possible to obtain increments in an alloimmunised thrombocytopeneic patient.

4. *Correlation between platelet support with increments following platelet transfusion*

Following the issue of HLA-matched or crossmatched platelets, clinicians are requested to perform a pre-transfusion platelet count and a one hour post-transfusion platelet count. If the response to a grade A matched or solid phase crossmatch negative platelets is poor, the possible additional effect of HPA or high titre (HT) ABO alloantibodies should be considered. If HT ABO antibodies are present, both ABO and HLA compatible platelets are provided whenever possible. Although the provision of HLA and HPA compatible platelets is not impossible, it requires a large panel of HLA and HPA typed platelet donors. In the London & South East Zone of the National Blood Service, approximately 2,200 platelet donors are fully HLA-A and -B typed and of these 800 are active donors, i.e. donate regularly. Approximately 30% of these donors are also fully HPA typed.

Recruitment and selection of platelet donors

In the London & South East Zone, recruitment of plateletpheresis donors is from existing panels of volunteer whole blood donors. Since 90% of people in the UK are either Group O or Group A, regular whole blood donors of these groups are targeted. Platelet donor recruiters use a computer program to select donors from those called to donor sessions in the vicinity of the apheresis clinic, who may be suitable to donate platelets. Donors of groups O and A under the age of 55 who have donated blood at least twice previously and at least once in the past year are listed. The donor recruiters attend the donor sessions and as donors who have been selected as potentially suitable to donate platelets are registered at the whole blood donor session, they are handed a leaflet about platelet donation. Whilst they are waiting to donate their blood they are approached by the platelet donor recruiter who gives further information about what is involved in donating platelets. Donors are informed that they will be selected only if they have platelet counts in the upper range of normal and that only about 20% of people have high platelet counts. They are also informed that donating platelets involves attending an apheresis clinic by appointment. The donor can expect to allow two hours for the attendance at the apheresis clinic as the plateletpheresis donation procedure takes about 90 minutes. Donors may attend as often as every two weeks although many donors attend on a monthly basis. For donors who are interested in becoming platelet donors, details are taken of the donor's weight and the veins of both antecubital fossae are examined to ensure that the veins are large enough to permit a flow of 80 ml per minute during the apheresis procedure. A blood sample is taken from the potential volunteer (it is usually at the end of the whole blood donation) so that the platelet count and haematocrit can be measured.

In order to try and recruit donors from ethnic minority groups to the HLA panel, particular attention is paid by the platelet recruiters to any donor who is from a Black, Asian, Oriental or Jewish ethnic background. Donors of these ethnic types and of groups B and AB will be approached as potential volunteers in addition to those of groups O and A. At the end of the blood donor session, the completed recruitment forms and samples are returned to the transfusion centre for analysis.

Apheresis medical staff review the results of the full blood counts and volunteers are divided into three categories:

1. Donors who weigh more than 10 stones - 64kg (blood volume > 4 litres) with haematocrit (Hct) > 40 and platelet count > 250 x 10^9/l or donors who weigh between 8 to 10 stones - 51-64kg (blood volume < 4 litres) with platelet counts > 265 x 10^9/l. These donors are suitable to enrol as high yield platelet donors and are sent a letter inviting them to make an appointment for their first donation. At the end of the first donation, if the donor has not experienced untoward effects and wishes to continue as a platelet donor, a blood sample is collected for class I HLA typing.

2. Volunteers who do not fulfil the criteria in (1) and are not from an ethnic minority group, are sent a letter thanking them for volunteering, but informing them that they are not suitable as high yield platelet donors. They are invited to continue as regular whole blood donors and the value of this is stressed.

3. Donors from ethnic minority groups who do not fulfil the criteria outlined in (1), but have a platelet count ≥200 x 10^9/l are sent a letter telling them that they are not suitable to act as high yield platelet donors, but that they would be valuable tissue typed platelet donors. Such donors are given an appointment to donate a single dose of platelets, to ensure that the donor can undergo an apheresis procedure without untoward effects. At the end of this donation, a blood sample is taken for class I HLA typing and the donor is enrolled on the 'HLA only' panel. He or she will be called to donate a single dose of platelets if HLA-matched for a particular patient. The donor is asked to continue as a whole blood donor until required as an HLA-matched platelet donor.

The result of this type of platelet recruitment is that there are a group of high yield platelet donors who attend regularly to donate two or three doses of platelets at each attendance. All these donors are HLA class I typed and, when HLA-matched platelets are required for a patient, a search will first be made of the panel of high yield regular platelet donors to see whether suitable HLA-matched platelets can be provided by these donors. There is a second, larger panel of donors who are HLA class I typed and have indicated that they would be prepared to attend to donate a single dose of platelets (as their platelet count would not allow the collection of a double or triple dose) if they are HLA-matched for a particular patient. If, on a search of the panel of regularly attending high yield platelet donors, sufficient matched donors are not found to support a particular patient, then a search will be undertaken of the 'HLA only' panel. 'HLA only' donors are then contacted and invited to donate or asked to 'stand-by' and not to donate whole blood for a period so that they can be available to donate platelets if required.

Patients who require HLA-matched platelets fall broadly into two groups. The first group is of patients whose HLA class I types are relatively common in the UK and for whom HLA-matched platelets are readily found from the panel of high yield platelet donors. The second group of patients have HLA types which are not common, particularly amongst the panel of platelet donors in SE England, largely composed of people of Northern European ethnic type. To provide HLA-matched platelets for patients with less common HLA types, a search is undertaken of both the pool of high yield donors and the 'HLA only' donors. A small panel of suitable donors is created for each patient and both regular and 'HLA only' donors can be notified that they will be needed over a period of time to support a particular patient.

For both patients who have common HLA types and those who have less common types and require the creation of a special panel, the provision of well-matched HLA typed platelets is greatly assisted where the patient requires long term support and the laboratory can be informed in advance of the dates when the patient will be attending hospital. In this case the HLA-matched donors who are to supply platelets for the patient can be booked well in advance to attend apheresis clinics. For patients with disorders such as Myelodysplasic Syndrome (MDS) who require long term regular HLA-matched platelet support, the relevant donors can be given appointments at least a month in advance. In such cases, if donors can be informed of the fact that they are supporting a particular patient with a particular type of disease, then those donors become extremely motivated to help 'their' patient and are likely to make every effort to keep their appointments to donate platelets. Donors are even willing to reorganise their work schedules and travel long distances to donate their platelets because they feel committed to helping a particular patient.

Prevention of platelet refractoriness and HLA alloimmunisation

The production of HLA antibodies is initiated by the direct allorecognition of HLA class II antigens on donor antigen presenting cells (APC), present in the platelet transfusion, by the patient's CD4+ T helper lymphocytes (Lechler and Batchelor, 1982). The most important APCs are dendritic cells and these cells express high levels of HLA class I and II and are capable of delivering the co-stimulatory signals to activate patient lymphocytes. Donor APCs migrate to the secondary lymphoid organs and initiate a primary immune response via direct allorecognition of the foreign MHC molecules (Rodey, 1993).

1. *Leucodepletion*

Although it has been shown that platelet transfusions filtered to remove the leucocytes can reduce the alloimmunisation rate (Kickler *et al.,* 1989), this does not prevent the induction of HLA antibodies in an already sensitised patient since platelet alloantigens can still be recognised by the indirect pathway of allo-recognition (Semple *et al.,* 1995). This also includes women who have been sensitised by pregnancy. Shed antigen or soluble HLA molecules can thus be taken up, processed and presented to the recipient's T lymphocytes by the recipient's own (Rodey, 1993). Once allorecognition has occurred activated CD4 T-cells can stimulate allospecific B cells to produce antibody.

With the recent introduction of universal leucodepletion in the UK, primary alloimunisation following the transfusion of blood or platelets should decrease in the coming years.

2. *Ultraviolet irradiation*

An alternative approach to the removal of leucocytes from the transfused product is the use of UV light to reduce the immunogenicity of the transfused leucocytes.

It has been shown that UVR renders lymphocytes unable to either stimulate or respond to alloantigens in the *in vitro* mixed lymphocyte culture (MLC). Furthermore, animal data have shown that 92% of recipients of UV irradiated platelets did not become platelet refractory following 8 transfusions of single donor platelets in contrast to only 14% recipients receiving unmodified platelets (Slichter, 1990).

3. *Reduced donor exposure*

Reduction in the number of donors used in each platelet concentrate by using platelets from single apheresis donors should contribute to decreased alloimmunisation.

If none of the above mentioned alternatives overcome the platelet refractoriness, the following procedures have been used but with less success:- massive transfusions of ABO identical platelets, intravenous immunoglobulin (IVIG), plasma exchange, acid treatment of platelets to restrict the HLA antigens or treatment of platelets using epsilon amino caproic acid (EACA). Of all of these the massive platelet transfusion seems to be the most successful.

Summary

Platelet refractoriness characterised by the failure to achieve adequate increments following platelet transfusions from random donors can be a serious clinical condition in transfusion dependent patients. This failure can be caused by immunological or non-immunological factors although in most patients both causes are present simultaneously. Various types of antibodies including high titre ABO, platelet-specific (HPA) and HLA have been shown to be involved in the immune destruction of platelets. However, of all these, HLA antibodies play a predominant role. Patients known to be immunologically refractory to platelet transfusion can be supported with HLA-matched or crossmatched platelets. The former type of treatment requires the existence of large panels of HLA typed platelet donors, carefully selected and regularly attending the apheresis clinics. The latter can be a suitable alternative providing there are sufficient numbers of platelet doses to be crossmatched but in the long term it may lead to further alloimmunisation particularly in already sensitised patients.

Thus, the establishment of selected, and sufficiently large HLA and HPA typed panels are essential for the management of patients who are immunologically refractory to random platelet transfusions.

References

Carr, R, Hutton, JL, Jenkins, JA, Lucas, GF and Amphlett, NW. (1990) Transfusion of ABO-mismatched platelets leads to early platelet refractoriness. *Brit J Haem* **75**: 408-413

Contreras, M and Navarrete, C. (1997) The management of alloimmunised patients in need of platelet transfusions. *Vox Sanguinis* **73:** 194-195

Duquesnoy, RJ, Filip, DJ. Rodey, GE, Rimm, AE, Aster, RH, *et al.* (1977) Successful transfusion of platelets "mismatched" for HLA antigens to alloimmunized thrombocytopenic patients. *Am J Hematol* **2**: 219-226

Godeau, B, Fromont, P, Seror, T, Duedari, N and Bierling, P. (1992) Platelet alloimmunization after multiple transfusions: a prospective study in 50 patients. *Brit J Haem* **81**: 395-400

Heal, JM, Masel, D, Rowe, JM and Blumberg, N. (1993) Circulating immune complexes involving the ABO system after platelet transfusion. *Brit J Haem* **85**: 566-572

Kakaiya, RM, Gudino, MD, Miller, WV, Sherman, LA, Katz, AJ, *et al.* (1984) Four crossmatch methods to select platelet donors. *Transfusion* **24**: 35-41

Kickler, TS, Bell, W, Drew, H and Pall, D. (1989) Depletion of white cells from platelet concentrates with a new adsorption filter. *Transfusion* **29**: 411-414

Lechler, R and Batchelor, J. (1982) Restoration of immunogenicity to passenger cell depleted kidney allografts by the addition of donor strain dendritic cells. *J Exp Med* **155**: 31-41

Lonjou, C, Clayton, J, Cambon-Thomsen, A and Raffoux, C. (1995) HLA-A, -B, -DR haplotype frequencies in France - Implications for recruitment of potential bone marrow donors. *Transplantation* **60**: 375-383

Murphy, MF and Waters, AH. (1990) Platelet transfusions: The problem of refractoriness. *Blood Rev* **4**: 16-24

Rodey, GE. (1993) Cellular immune responses to alloimmunisation. In: *Alloimmunity: 1993 and Beyond* (Ed. Nance, SJ), pp.1-23. American Association of Blood Banks, Arlington, VA

Schnaidt, M, Northoff, H and Wernet, D. (1996) Frequency and specificity of platelet-specific alloantibodies in HLA-immunized haematologic-oncologic patients. *Transfusion Med* **6**: 111-114

Semple, JW, Speck, ER, Milev, YP, Blanchette, V and Freedman, J. (1995) Indirect allorecognition of platelets by T helper cells during platelet transfusions correlates with anti-major histocompatibility complex antibody and cytotoxic T lymphocyte formation. *Blood* **86**: 805-12

Shanwell, A, Sallander, S, Olsson, I, Gulliksson, H, Pedajas, I, *et al.* (1991) An alloimmunized, thrombocytopenic patient successfully transfused with acid-treated, random-donor platelets. *Brit J Haem* **79**: 462-465

Slichter, SJ. (1990) Mechanisms and management of platelet refractoriness. In: *Transfusion Medicine in the 1990's* (Ed. Nance, SJ), pp.95-179. American Association of Blood Banks, Arlington, VA

PART 5

STATISTICAL METHODS

PART 5 OVERVIEW

STATISTICAL METHODS

J. D'Amaro and R. F. Schipper
Department of Immunohematology & Blood Transfusion
Leiden University Medical Center
The Netherlands

The extensive polymorphism of HLA makes it an excellent marker system. Some of the most common analytical aspects of HLA typing results are set out in Chapters 15 to 18. Paternity testing and genetic counselling are two additional areas, outside the scope of the present volume.

Since its first use by Van Rood in 1963 to define the first leukocyte group system, data analysis has been an integral activity of Histocompatibility Testing laboratories. The Histocompatibility Testing series published after the periodic international Histocompatibility Workshops and Conferences since 1965, reveals the methodology and results of numerous population and immunogenetic analyses. The comprehensive report by Mattiuz *et al.* in the 1970 volume is a particularly good methodology reference. Two sources of background information on the HLA system with extensive analytical examples have been published by Cavalli-Sforza and Bodmer in 1971 and Cavalli-Sforza *et al.* in 1994.

Tests for goodness of fit of HLA typing results involve the following three stages:

- a statement of the null hypothesis, which is usually that the distribution of observations in a population under study agrees with the theoretical distribution
- the choice of the level of significance which defines the risk of Type I errors (erroneously rejecting the null hypothesis), usually 5 percent
- calculation of the Chi-square

Rejection or acceptance of the null hypothesis depends upon the probability of obtaining such an agreement between observations and theoretical expectations, which, in turn, is related to the number of degrees of freedom in the calculations.

Mather (1967) suggested that "the level of probability chosen as indicating significant departure from the null hypothesis is simply the level at which the worker is willing to be misled." In the same publication he reminded the reader that "a hypothesis can never be proven or disproved by a test of significance", but "they only make it a more or less unlikely one."

Mather also clearly defined the limitations that one should bear in mind when dealing with either single or multiple hypotheses. Significant departure from the hypothesis at the 5 percent level of probability could be justification for rejection of the hypothesis in single trials but not in multiple trials, since such departures are expected to occur once by chance more often with increasing numbers of trials.

He also emphasized that "the probability taken as setting the level of significance is a matter of personal decision, that the choice of level must be in fact determined by what is at issue and that the stringency of the test should match the importance of the consequences of rejection." For example, significance levels should be much more stringent for bone marrow transplantation studies, where the consequences of rejection may be fatal, than for renal transplantation where they are infrequently so.

Mather also suggested the rule that "in setting out the results of a comparison between observations and hypothesis, the probability corresponding to observation actually made should be stated. Any other person can then assess the agreement between them for himself using any level of significance that he may feel the circumstances of the experiment and the consequences of rejection to warrant."

Many analyses of HLA determinants produce large numbers of comparisons because of the polymorphism within HLA loci. Consequently, the probability of observing random deviations may be large. The practice of correcting p values by multiplying them by the number of comparisons should be avoided since, especially when the number of comparisons is large, it may yield corrected p values which are greater that 1. The exact method of Edwards should be used (Edwards, 1974) by preference and in particular when the number of comparisons is greater than 1/significance level. In n independent tests of significance, the chance of finding no significance, in the absence of interaction, at the pth level is $(1 - p)^n$. The chance of asserting that at least one test is significant, also in the absence of interaction, is $1 - (1 - p)^n$ which is always less than $n \times p$ which it approximates when p is considerably smaller than $1 / n$.

P value correction techniques are best used when there is only one deviation among a number of comparisons. When the number of comparisons is large, both methods will certainly reduce the number of Type I errors, but they will just as certainly increase the chance of Type II errors.

Significant associations should be considered as tentative, subject to confirmation by other investigators. An effective alternative to that procedure is to carry out a self-confirming study. When large amounts of data are available, it should be partitioned into two subsets. 'True significances' should be observed in both subsets. See D'Amaro *et al.* (1984) for a practical example.

Finally, since population and immunogenetic analyses of HLA data are complex applications, expert advice should be sought at the design phase of studies.

References

Cavalli-Sforza, LL and Bodmer, WF (1974) *The Genetics of Human Populations.* Freeman, San Francisco

Cavalli-Sforza, LL, Menazzi, P and Piazza, A (1994) *The History and Geography of Human Genes*. Princeton University Press, Princeton

D'Amaro, J, Bach, FH, van Rood, JJ, Rimm, AA and Bortin, MM (1984) HLA-C associations with acute leukaemia. *Lancet* **2**: 1176-1178

Edwards, JH (1974) HL-A and disease. The detection of associations. *J Immunogenet* **1**: 249-50

Mather, K (1967) *The Elements of Biometry*. Chapman and Hall, London

Mattiuz, PL, Ihde, D, Piazza, A, Ceppellini, R and Bodmer, WF (1970) New approaches to the population, genetic and segregation analysis of the HL-A system. In: *Histocompatibility Testing 1970* (Ed. Terasaki, PI), pp.193-205. Munksgaard, Copenhagen

Svejgaard, A, Jerslid, C, Nielsen, LS and Bodmer, WF (1974) HL-A antigens and disease. Statistical and genetical considerations. *Tissue Antigens* **4**: 95-105

Van Rood, JJ and van Leeuwen, A (1963) Leukocyte grouping. A method and its application. *J Clin Invest* **42**: 1382-1390

CHAPTER 15

POPULATION GENETICS OF THE HUMAN MAJOR HISTOCOMPATIBILITY COMPLEX

R. F. Schipper and J. D'Amaro
Department of Immunohematology & Blood Transfusion
Leiden University Medical Center
The Netherlands

Introduction

This chapter deals with the question of population genetic analyses of HLA, the most complex genetic system known thus far. We begin with a brief review of the history and genetic structure of that system and then proceed on to an overview of a few applications of population genetics relating to the study of HLA.

History

The history of modern genetics and population genetics is closely linked to the discovery of the genetic markers that are expressed on red and white blood cells. It is also closely linked to the names of a number of famous scientists, who worked in the field of genetics, statistics and population genetics. The views of Hardy (1908) and Weinberg (1963) could be integrated into a law of genetic equilibrium in populations. The theoretical fact that a population, in the absence of migration and admixture, will reach an equilibrium state (Hardy-Weinberg equilibrium) in the course of just one generation is of prime importance to the methods of population genetics. Fisher (1918) resolved the controversies between the Mendelians and the followers of Galton (who claimed that genetic traits of the parents were blended in their offspring), clearing the way for the development of population genetics theory.

This book focuses on the human HLA system. HLA genes are principally expressed on white blood cells (leukocytes) but can be found on the membranes of many other cells. The system is generically called a Major Histocompatibility Complex (MHC) (Frelinger and Shreffler, 1975) and similar ones can be found in all vertebrates. For an extensive introduction and historical overview of MHCs, see Klein (1986).

Definition of populations

A general usable definition of the term "population" is difficult to establish. See Cavalli-Sforza and Bodmer (1971) for a definition of Mendelian populations, and Cavalli-Sforza *et al.,* (1994) for an extensive discussion of population definitions. A "Mendelian population" is one in which *random mating* occurs and that is not the subject of strong selection (Cavalli-Sforza and Bodmer, 1971). Such populations are ideal and defined by the existence of Hardy-Weinberg (HW) equilibrium.

Much anthropological research has been done based on ethnic definitions of populations (Baur and Danilovs, 1980a,b; Baur *et al.,* 1984a,b,c; Ohayon and Cambon-Thomsen, 1986; Dupont, 1989a,b; Tsuji *et al.,* 1992; Cavalli-Sforza *et al.,* 1994). Of course many populations still exist that can be ethnically defined because of their geographically and/or sociologically relative isolation. However, many other populations, especially those in the industrialized parts of the world, consist of mixtures of other populations. Consequently, when we perform genetic analyses on the HLA antigens of populations in order to use the results for disease studies and for match prognosis in transplantation, ethnic definitions of populations are far from suitable. It is more sensible to use operational definitions of populations for such purposes (Schipper *et al.,* 1997; Gjertson and Terasaki, 1998). In the case of bone marrow transplantation, for example, it is possible to define populations on the basis of local registration of volunteer donors, because there is a practical difference between the use of local donors and of donors from other registries.

Irrespective of the criteria which have been used to define a population, prior to performing population genetic analyses on a sample of that population, one should establish that the population is in HW equilibrium. Also see the discussion of HW equilibrium in the 'Summary of population genetic parameters' below.

The genetics of the HLA system

The genes of the HLA system are located on the short arm of chromosome 6 (see Campbell and Trowsdale, 1993, and the Introduction to this volume). They form not only a cluster (a region of closely located genes) but also a complex of genes that are functionally related, which is quite rare. A number of HLA loci are of prime importance in transplantation and have been studied extensively.

A striking feature of many of these genetic loci is that they are highly polymorphic, i.e. a single locus may have numerous alleles. Because of the short distances between the HLA loci on the chromosome, recombination between them is rare: in the order of less than 1% for HLA-A and -B (Svejgaard *et al.* 1971).

Although much is still to be discovered about the function of the HLA gene products, it is clear that they are all involved in the immune response against bacterial and viral pathogens. Their discovery was particularly accelerated by three factors:

- the recognition that the immune system is an important barrier in transplantation
- the acceptance of kidney transplantation as the treatment of choice for end stage renal failure
- the numerous International Histocompatibility Workshops and Conferences held since 1964 which represent a level of collaboration within a single scientific discipline which is unique in the annals of science

The number of HLA genes and alleles discovered by this combined effort has made it clear that the human MHC, HLA, is the most polymorphic genetic system known.

In the context of transplantation, HLA phenotypes are often called "tissue types". When the tissue types of donor and recipient are completely identical, the immune system of the patient does not "recognise" any foreign, non-self, antigens and graft survival is optimal. In the case of bone marrow transplantation patient and donor can be mismatched for Minor Histocompatibility Antigens (Beatty and Hervé 1990; Bortin *et al.,* 1991; Martin, 1991; Goulmy *et al.,* 1991; see Chapter 19) which can induce Graft-versus-Host disease even in the absence of HLA mismatches (Goulmy *et al.,* 1996). Population genetic analysis of these minor antigens will not be possible until many individuals have been tested for these factors. When patient and donor differ for one or more of the HLA genes, graft survival is sub-optimal. Consequently, histocompatibility testing laboratories (or "tissue typing" laboratories) have been set up all over the world and millions of individuals have been "HLA typed" for various reasons.

The HLA gene products are often called antigens. The term 'antigen' originates from the fact that the protein products of the alleles of the HLA genes can induce immunization after transfusion or transplantation. The terms antigen and allele are often used interchangeably. However, when the HLA phenotype is determined by the use of antisera it is not proper to use the term allele, since serologic techniques detect gene products. One should try to reserve the term allele for HLA specificities that are determined by the analysis of the DNA of the HLA genes.

Tissue typing laboratories use many different techniques to determine the HLA phenotypes of individuals. These techniques are the subject of this volume, and can be divided into classes according to the reagents that they require. The oldest typing techniques rely on the use of antisera against one or more HLA antigens present on leukocytes. These techniques are called "serological" (Chapters 1 to 4, this volume). In the mid 1980s, the HLA phenotype of individuals began to be determined using their DNA. A wide variety of DNA typing techniques have been developed (Chapters 5 to 9, this volume). Initially, DNA techniques were used to confirm the results of serologic typing. The number of recognized alleles at the HLA loci, revealed by DNA typing, exceeds the number of gene products recognized by serology. Since these fine specificities may also be important in transplantation, especially of bone marrow, DNA typing to determine HLA phenotypes may eventually replace serologic typing. Moreover, DNA typing techniques offer practical advantages over serologic techniques.

An HLA genotype consists of two HLA alleles per locus. The alleles of HLA genes are expressed as "co-dominant" entities, which means that both alleles of a locus (one from the father and one from the mother) are equally expressed on the cell membrane. Therefore, if the phenotype of an individual appears to have only one allele at a particular locus, that individual could be homozygous. There are, however, three complicating factors that must be considered. A second allele at that locus might have been missed because the typing technique could or did not reveal it. Also, the two alleles might seem similar phenotypically using a certain typing technique, when they in fact differ. This second factor can often be resolved by expanding the typing technique, in the case of serology with more sera, or by typing family members. Thirdly, some genes are only present on certain haplotypes, e.g.: the DRB3, DRB4 and DRB5 genes expressing DR52, DR53 and DR51 respectively.

Historically, HLA antigens are assigned numbers which reflect the sequence of their discovery. Some antigens may be partitioned into two or more so-called 'split' antigens by serologic techniques, e.g. HLA-B5 contains the splits HLA-B51 and HLA-B52. Some antisera react only against one or more of these split specificities, like B51 and B52, while others are directed against the so-called 'broad' specificity, B5, and therefore appear to react against cells which carry any of its split specificities.

When DNA typing and sequencing became commonplace, the nomenclature for the system was expanded with a numeric system that allows for a maximum of 99 variants of each serologically defined specificity by adding two digits to the allele name. An asterisk after the locus name signifies that an allele is defined by DNA typing. We will try to illustrate this complex nomenclature with an example. The first level of the nomenclature are the serologically defined broad and split specificities. For instance, HLA-B21 has two splits, B49 and B50. The most detailed level of the nomenclature is defined by DNA typing techniques. For example HLA-B49 and B50 are called HLA-B*4901 and HLA-B*5001 respectively when typed by DNA technology. The third and fourth digit indicate the subtypes of the serologic specificity. B49 has only one subtype, but HLA-DRB1*04 has at least thirty-two. A fifth digit is available for so-called 'silent mutations', but these are irrelevant to the contents of this chapter.

A complicating factor in HLA typing is the existence of 'serological masking'. This happens when the antisera in a typing set can not distinguish one antigen in the presence of another antigen. For example, if a serum set contains sera that can detect both HLA-A2 and HLA-A28 together on the same cell and HLA-A2 alone, while no sera can detect HLA-A28 monospecifically, then it is not possible to identify HLA-A28 in the presence of HLA-A2.

Such masking can have a serious disturbing effect on results of tests for the goodness of fit for Hardy-Weinberg equilibrium. Phenotypes that appear to be homozygous may be in fact heterozygous with one antigen masked. Two additional reasons why an antigen might be missed are:

- antisera that fail to react
- the absence of any sera in the typing set that react against the antigen

These problems must be recognised and dealt with in population genetic analyses.

Phenotypes should not be simple listings of 'positive' antigens since all of the remaining antigens are then 'negative' by default. They should be constructed so that there is a clear distinction between 'negative' scores and 'untested' or 'uninterpretable' antigens. Untested loci should also be clearly marked. These unambiguous phenotypes avoid the danger of underestimating phenotype and gene frequencies due to 'false' negative scores.

One of the earliest discovered groups of HLA antigens were the Bw4 and Bw6 specificities (van Rood, 1962; van Rood *et al.*, 1970). All the alleles of the HLA-B locus (and surprisingly, some HLA-A antigens) are 'included' in either of those two groups. They were originally thought to be a bi-allelic system, but it has been shown recently that the Bw4 and Bw6 antibodies recognize two different epitopes on HLA class I molecules. Many problems of masking or weak serologic reactions against antigens of the HLA-B locus can be resolved by using the extra information that Bw4 and Bw6 offer. In addition, their scores may be predictive of as yet undetected ('new') antigenic specificities. For example, if a phenotype contains a single HLA-B locus antigen which is included in Bw4, and Bw4 and Bw6 are both positive, then the positivity of Bw6 indicates presence of a new or untested HLA-B locus specificity which is included in Bw6.

The genetic term *haplotype*, was introduced by Ceppellini *et al.,* (1967). A haplotype can be defined as 'half of a genotype', the genotype being the genetic composition at two or more loci. The genes in one haplotype are located on the same chromosome and are all inherited from one parent. Because of tight 'linkage' between the HLA loci and the effect of selective forces, many haplotypic combinations (alleles of two ore more loci in one haplotype) have frequencies that are higher (sometimes much higher) than the frequency that would be theoretically expected from the frequencies of their composing alleles. This phenomenon, *linkage disequilibrium*, was first communicated to Race by Fisher in 1943 (Race, 1944). We will illustrate it with an example. The frequencies of HLA-A1 and HLA-B8 in the Dutch population are estimated at 0.173 and 0.128 respectively. If recombination between HLA-A and -B was not low and no selection for or against the A1, B8 haplotype existed, one would expect that the equilibrium frequency of the A1, B8 haplotype would be equal to the product of their allele frequencies (0.022). However, the frequency of the A1, B8 haplotype in the Dutch population is estimated at 0.097. Consequently, the two antigens are said to be in strong linkage disequilibrium. Linkage disequilibrium is an important subject for population genetic studies, since it has many biological and clinical implications.

The haplotypes of an individual can only be determined by studying the genetic composition of that individual's pedigree, especially his/her parents and siblings. In population genetics, we usually study samples of unrelated individuals. If we estimate the frequencies of the haplotypes in such samples, we are not dealing with haplotypes as defined in pedigrees. The difference is that in families we know, again under the assumption of no recombination, that the haplotypes of an individual are copies of one haplotype from each parent. All the alleles of genes that were not tested but that are located between the genes we did test, will also be identical between parents and child. If, however, we could compare the haplotypes of two unrelated individuals as determined by studying their respective pedigrees, they may seem to have similar haplotypes, while in fact they could differ for the genes that were not tested. To distinguish between these two uses of the term haplotypes, Yunis (Awdeh *et al.,* 1985) introduced the term "extended haplotype" which is defined as "a specific combination of alleles from different loci that are in significant linkage disequilibrium in chromosomes of unrelated individuals". Therefore, when we study unrelated individuals, their estimated haplotype frequencies are in fact (implicitly) the frequencies of extended haplotypes in their population.

Students may be puzzled by the paradox between Hardy-Weinberg (HW) equilibrium and linkage disequilibrium. It is important to understand the difference between these equilibria. HW equilibrium exists at the *phenotype* level. The genetic composition of a generation of diploid individuals (individuals with two copies of each chromosome, one from their father, one from their mother) can be considered a pool of alleles from which, by mating, combinations are formed in their offspring. Those combinations are said to be in HW equilibrium when all of them have a likelihood of occurring equal to twice the product of the frequencies of the composing alleles. When mating is random, this equilibrium is established in the course of one generation. Since each phenotype can be seen as a combination of two haplotypes, HW equilibrium still exists when considering more than one locus. Linkage disequilibrium, however, exists at the *haplotype* level. This simply means that not all combinations (haplotypes) of the alleles of the composing loci occur with frequencies equal to the product of their allele frequencies.

Summary of population genetic parameters

Not all known population genetic parameters are the subject of, or relevant to, this chapter. Most of the parameters described here are routinely denoted by one or more symbols.

One very useful parameter in HLA population genetics is the *phenotype frequency* (PF) (see also section 1 of the Appendix to this chapter), which for the HLA system is simply how often an antigen has been found in the phenotypes of the sample of tested individuals, i.e. the proportion of individuals tested positive for an antigen. In the HLA system, phenotypes can be a complex of antigens from a variable number of loci, for example: A2, B18, B40, B60, Bw6, Cw3, Cw10, Cw5, DR3, DR17, DR6, DR13, DR52, DQ1, DQ6, DQ2. This phenotype is composed of antigens from the HLA-A, -B, -C, -DR and -DQ loci. More than two antigens per locus may be listed since both broad specificities and their splits can be part of the phenotype. Actually, it is not possible to speak of *the* phenotype of a person, since information of any locus can be left out or added arbitrarily. For analytical purposes the phenotype should also contain codes indicating untested antigens or loci.

The *gene frequency* (GF) (see also section 2 of the Appendix to this chapter), or more appropriately, the *allele frequency* of an HLA antigen is defined as the number of times that the allele occurs divided by the total number of alleles (twice the number of individuals). It is more difficult to determine because of uncertainty about homozygosity. Because of that fact and differences in the ease of typing between antigens, which may lead to 'undecided' scores, the sum of the GFs does not always add up to one. The difference is usually assigned to the theoretical *null gene frequency* (GF_{null}). This theoretical allele includes all of the alleles that were not typeable. The *observed homozygosity* of the alleles of a locus is simply derived by counting how many times an allele was the only one observed in a single locus. The *probability of homozygosity* for the alleles can be calculated from their GFs and the GF_{null}. The combined homozygosity of the locus can be compared to the *expected homozygosity* (also called the homozygosity statistic F) using a goodness of fit test. The *heterozygosity* of the locus is the complement of the homozygosity of the locus.

The *haplotype frequency* (HF) (see also section 3 of the Appendix to this chapter) (Ceppellini *et al.,* 1955) is analogous to the gene frequency but extended to combinations of single alleles from multiple loci instead of single alleles. For gene frequencies it is not relevant on which chromosome (the father's or the mother's) an allele is located. For haplotypes, that is essential information. Therefore the only exact method to determine haplotypes and their frequencies is by examining the genetic information of individuals in families (pedigrees).

A very important concept in population genetics is the goodness-of-fit for Hardy-Weinberg (HW) equilibrium (Hardy, 1908; Weinberg, 1963). Most of the other parameters depend on this equilibrium as a premise. The estimation of gene and haplotype frequencies and the analysis of disease associations all require that the population under investigation is in HW equilibrium. If that is not the case, the laws of Mendelian segregation cannot safely be applied and genetic analyses will yield invalid results.

Delta (Δ) (Fisher, 1958; Cavalli-Sforza and Bodmer, 1971) is the absolute measure of linkage disequilibrium, (see also section 4 of the Appendix to this chapter), and is defined by the difference between the observed HF and the HF that would be expected from the GFs of the alleles in the haplotype, in the absence of linkage disequilibrium. If we consider haplotypes consisting of the alleles of 2 hypothetical bi-allelic loci (A and B), then Table 15.1 gives the relation between the HF and the GFs at perfect equilibrium, while Table 15.2 gives the same relation when disequilibrium exists (Lewontin, 1988). This can easily be expanded to multi-allelic loci, if we say that the letter 'A' denotes allele A positive, while 'a' denotes any non-A and similarly for locus B.

	A	a	
B	HF_{AB}	HF_{aB}	GF_B
b	HF_{Ab}	HF_{ab}	$1\text{-}GF_B$
	GF_A	$1\text{-}GF_A$	

Table 15.1. Relationship between HF and GF at perfect equilibrium.

	A	a	
B	$HF_{AB} + \Delta$	$HF_{aB} - \Delta$	GF_B
b	$HF_{Ab} - \Delta$	$HF_{ab} + \Delta$	$1\text{-}GF_B$
	GF_A	$1\text{-}GF_A$	

Table 15.2. Relationship between HF and GF when linkage disequilibrium exists

Because Δ is an absolute measure of linkage disequilibrium, it is difficult to compare Δs of haplotypes with different frequencies. The relative measure of linkage disequilibrium, *Relative Delta* (Lewontin, 1964) (RD), makes such comparisons possible. It is defined as Δ divided by the theoretically possible maximum Δ. See Hedrick (1987) for an overview of parameters of linkage disequilibrium. The significance of Δ can simply be calculated using Chi-square for goodness of fit. The resulting P-value then has to be corrected for the number of comparisons made, being the number of different haplotypes potentially present in the sample (which have an estimated HF> 0). The method for correction of P-values as described by Edwards (1974) is preferred over the widely used Bonferroni method, because the former calculates exact corrected probabilities through a simple probabilistic algorithm, while the latter does not.

The *genetic distance* (f) (Cavalli-Sforza and Bodmer, 1971) between populations is a parameter that quantifies the overall genetic diversity between populations. Its results may be used to draw phylogenetic trees of populations. Such trees illustrate the degree of relationship between different populations.

Because of the complexity and polymorphism of the HLA, tissue typing techniques usually cannot detect all antigens that may exist in a population. Some alleles may be difficult to detect in the presence of other alleles (masking), resulting in false homozygotes. Other alleles may still be undiscovered, which means that the typing technique used can never detect them. A theoretical allele, called the *null-gene* (or null-allele) is used in the analysis of HLA loci in order to accommodate for this incompleteness of the data. The frequency of this allele is the combined frequency of all alleles that are undetected by the typing technique.

By definition, the GFs of the alleles of one locus add up to one. Therefore, the estimated GF_{null} is simply one minus the sum of all estimated GFs of the detectable alleles. The definition of the null-gene enables estimation of maximum likelihood HFs. Such HF estimates are mathematically correct in the sense that they also add up to one.

Establishing reliable population genetics parameters

The precision of population genetic parameters is crucial when they are used to compute prognostic factors or used directly as factors in clinical investigations. The precision of GFs and HFs can be expressed in terms of their standard error (SE), which, however, often is an estimation just as the frequencies are. Therefore it is necessary to investigate the behaviour of different estimation methods. One such investigation is described in Schipper (1998).

Population genetics and its applications

Population genetics is the branch of genetics that deals with the distribution of genes in groups of individuals, i.e. populations. There are several reasons to study such distributions. They can help us to understand the history of mankind. By comparing the distributions of many genes in many populations, it has been possible to draw extensive conclusions about the origins of human populations and their spread over the different continents (Mourant, 1954; Mourant *et al.,* 1976; Roychoudhury and Nei, 1988; Bodmer and Cavalli-Sforza, 1976; Cavalli-Sforza *et al.,* 1994; Bontrop *et al.,* 1990).

Another application of the analytical techniques of population genetics is the identification of genetic factors which may be involved in the pathogenesis of diseases (Svejgaard *et al.,* 1983). Those techniques reveal, for example, which alleles have significantly different, higher or lower, frequencies in diseased than in healthy members of a population.

A third useful application of the analytical techniques of population genetics is to provide assistance in the estimation of the likelihood of finding suitably matched donors for patients in need of a graft. Since HLA matching has been shown to provide a significant beneficial effect on graft and patient survival (Ceppellini *et al.,* 1966; van Rood *et al.,* 1966; Amos *et al.,* 1969; Persijn *et al.,* 1977; Persijn *et al.,* 1978; Thorogood *et al.,* 1990) the likelihood of finding well matched donors is vital information.

In many studies the HLA haplotypes are of prime importance. Without pedigree data, however, genotypes cannot be deduced from phenotypes with complete certainty. Using reliable haplotype frequencies, it is in most cases possible to assign haplotypes for unrelated individuals with a high degree of certainty (Hanifi Moghaddam *et al.,* 1998).

Finally, the results of population genetic analyses can be used for tissue typing quality control. This application is discussed in detail in the next section.

Population genetics for data validation

Assessment of the quality of HLA typing is partly inherent in the practice of population genetic analysis and HLA and disease association studies, but also a useful tool that can help improving the performance of laboratories.

When immediate feed-back exist between population genetic analysis and laboratory practice, the quality of the data and the quality of the estimated population genetic parameters improve simultaneously.

The techniques that are used for tissue typing are not perfect (Schipper *et al.*, 1996a). The serum sets used are frequently not standardized and the identification *per se* of some antigens is difficult or impossible, while other antigens may be masked by the presence of other antigens. The incompleteness of typing results introduces 'false homozygotes' in the phenotypes which has an adverse effect on the goodness of fit for HW equilibrium. Moreover, typing serum sets should be appropriate for the population being tested. Some HLA antigens are unique to certain populations, therefore typing sera which are defined in one population may not necessarily perform the same when they are used to type individuals in other populations. Quality assessment should be carried out prior to all further population genetic analyses in order to establish the suitability of loci, broad specificities and split specificities in the analyses (Schipper *et al.,* 1996a).

Presuming that the population under study is in HW equilibrium, analysis of the HW equilibrium can be used to assess the quality of the phenotypes of the individuals typed by a certain laboratory. Ideally, all antigens known should be used in the analysis of GFs and HFs. However, for each locus, the goodness of fit for HW equilibrium must be acceptable.

The evaluation of split antigens is particularly sensitive to the problems mentioned above. Evaluation of split antigens should be limited to broad antigens of which all splits are well-defined serologically. For the practical use of the analytical results, however, as many split antigens should be included in the analyses as possible. The procedure of stepwise HW analyses (Schipper *et al.,* 1996b) effectively deals with this problem.

A useful indicator of the completeness of typing results is the magnitude of the hypothetical 'null-gene' frequency, as calculated by the Maximum Likelihood (MXLK) GF estimation method. In the ideal situation the sum of the gene frequencies is one and the frequency of the null-gene is zero. A low null-gene frequency is an indication that the typing technique (in the case of serology, particularly the composition of the serum set) used is adequate for the sample under study and that all of the possible alleles at the locus have probably been detected. When many antigens are difficult or impossible to determine in the laboratory, the GF_{null} will be high. Therefore, a high GF_{null} may be an indication of bad phenotype data quality.

Concluding remarks

The field of population genetics is specialistic. It requires knowledge of statistics, genetics and of the biological function of the genes under study. Some computer software for population genetics analyses is available in the public domain. Most of this software is complex, rather user-unfriendly and usage should be discouraged by others than trained specialists. To stimulate the use of population genetics, national or, preferably, international organisations could consider setting up a central population genetic data analysis working group. Such a working group could cover international collaboration, training and teaching, centralisation of data acquisition, legal aspects, ethical aspects and other relevant issues.

References

Amos, DB, Seigler, HF, Southworth, JG and Ward, FE (1969) Skin graft rejection between subjects genotyped for HL-A. *Transpl Proc* **1**: 342-346

Awdeh, ZL, Alper, CA, Eynon, E, Alosco, SM, Stein, R, *et al.* (1985) Unrelated individuals matched for MHC extended haplotypes and HLA-identical siblings show comparable responses in mixed lymphocyte culture. *Lancet* 2: 853-856

Baur, MP and Danilovs, JA (1980) Reference tables of two and three-locus haplotype frequencies for HLA-A, B, C, DR, Bf, and GLO. In: *Histocompatibilty Testing 1980* (Ed. Terasaki, PI), pp.994-1210. UCLA Tissue Typing Laboratory, Los Angeles

Baur, MP and Danilovs, JA (1980) Population analysis of HLA-A, B, C, DR, and other genetic markers. In: *Histocompatibility Testing 1980* (Ed. Terasaki, PI), pp.955-993. UCLA tissue Typing Laboratory, Los Angeles

Baur MP, Neugebauer, M, Deppe, H, Sigmund, M, Luton, T, *et al.* (1984) Population analysis on the basis of deduced haplotypes from random families. In: *Histocompatibility Testing 1984* (Ed. Albert, ED, Baur, MP and Mayr, WR), pp.333-341. Springer-Verlag, Berlin

Baur, MP, Neugebauer, M and Albert, ED (1984) Reference tables of two-locus haplotype frequencies for all MHC marker loci. In: *Histocompatibility testing 1984* (Ed. Albert, ED), pp.677-678. Springer-Verlag, Berlin

Baur, MP, Neugebauer, M, Albert ED (1984) Reference tables of three-locus haplotype frequencies and delta values in Caucasians, Orientals, and Negroids. In: *Histocompatibility Testing 1984* (Ed. Albert, ED, Baur, MP and Mayr, WR), pp.756-760. Springer Verlag, Berlin

Beatty, PG and Hervé, P (1990) Immunogenetic factors relevant to acute graft-versus-host disease. In: *Graft-versus-host disease: immunology, pathophysiology and treatment* (Ed. Burakoff, SJ, Deeg, HJ, Ferrara, S and Atkinson, K), pp.415-423. Marcel Dekker, New York

Bodmer, WF and Cavalli-Sforza, LL (1976) *Genetics, Evolution, and Man.* Freeman, San Francisco

Bontrop, RE, Elferink, DG, Otting, N, Jonker, M and de Vries, RRP (1990) Major histocompatibility complex class II-restricted antigen presentation across a species barrier: conservation of restriction determinants in evolution. *J Exp Med* **172**: 53-59

Bortin, MM, Horowitz, MM, Mrsic, M, Rimm, AA and Sobocinski, KA (1991) Progress in bone marrow transplantation for leukemia: a preliminary report from the Advisory Committee of the International Bone Marrow Transplant Registry. *Transpl Proc* **23**: 61-62

Campbell, RD and Trowsdale, J (1993) Map of the human MHC. *Immunol Today* **14**: 349-352

Cavalli-Sforza, LL and Bodmer, WF (1971) In: *The Genetics of Human Populations* (Ed. Kennedy, D and Park, RB). Freeman, San Francisco

Cavalli-Sforza, LL, Menozzi, P and Piazza, A (1994) *The history and geography of human genes*. Princeton University Press, Princeton

Ceppellini, R, Siniscalco, M and Smith, CAB (1955) The estimation of gene frequencies in a random-mating population. *Ann Hum Genet* **20**: 97-115

Ceppellini, R, Curtoni, ES, Mattiuz, PL, Leigheb, G, Visetti, M, *et al.* (1966) Survival of test skin grafts in man. Effect of genetic relationship and of blood group incompatibility. *Ann N Y Acad Sci* **129**: 421-421

Ceppellini, R, Curtoni, ES, Mattiuz, PL, Miggiano, V, Scudeller, G, *et al.* (1967) Genetics of leukocyte antigens: a family study of seggragation and linkage. In: *Histocompatibility testing 1967* (Ed. Curtoni, ES, Mattiuz, PL and Tosi, RM), pp.149-187. Munksgaard, Copenhagen

Dupont B (1989) *Immunobiology of HLA - Histocompatibilty Testing 1987*. Springer Verlag, Berlin

Edwards, JH (1974) HL-A and disease. The detection of associations. *J Immunogenet* **1**: 249-257

Fisher, RA (1918) The correlation between Relatives on the Supposition of Mendelian Inheritance. *Trans Roy Soc Edinb* **52**: 399-433

Fisher, RA (1958) *The Genetical Theory of Natural Selection*. Dover, New York

Frelinger, JA and Shreffler, DC (1975) The major histocompatibility complexes. In: *Immunogenetics and Immunodeficiency* (Ed. Benacerraf, B). MTP: Lancaster

Gjertson, DW and Terasaki, PI (1998) *HLA 1998*. American Society for Histocompatibility and Immunogenetics, Lenexa

Goulmy, E, Voogt, P, *et al.* (1991). The role of minor histocompatibility antigens in GVHD and rejection: a mini-review. *Bone Marrow Transpl* **7 (Suppl. 1):** 49-51

Goulmy, E, Schipper, RF, Pool, J, Blokland, E, Falkenburg, F, *et al.* (1996). Minor histocompatibility antigen mismatches influence the development of GvHD after HLA identical related bone marrow transplant. *N Engl J Med* **334**: 281-285

Hanifi Moghaddam, P, de Knijff, P, Roep, BO, van den Auwera, B, Naipal, A, *et al.* (1998) Genetic structure of IDDM1: two separate regions in the major histocompatibility complex contribute to susceptibility or protection. *Diabetes* **47**: 263-269

Hardy, GH (1908) Mendelian proportions in a mixed population. *Science* **28**: 49-50

Hedrick, PW (1987) Gametic disequilibrium measures: proceed with caution. *Genetics* **117**: 331-341

Klein, J (1986) *Natural History of the Major Histocompatibility Complex*. Wiley, New York

Lewontin, RC (1964) The interaction of selection and linkage. I. General considerations; Heterotic models. *Genetics* **49**: 49-67

Lewontin, RC (1988) On measures of gametic disequilibrium. *Genetics* **120**: 849-852

Martin, PJ (1991) Increased disparity for minor histocompatibility antigens as a potential cause of increased GVHD risk in marrow transplantations from unrelated donors compared with related donors. *Bone Marrow Transpl* **8**: 217-223

Mourant, AE (1954) *The Distribution of the Human Blood Groups*. Blackwell Scientific, Oxford

Mourant, AE, Kopec, AC and Domaniewska-Sobczak, K (1976) *The Distribution of the Human Blood Groups and Other Polymorphisms*. Oxford University Press, London

Ohayon, E and Cambon-Thomsen, A (1986) *Human Population Genetics*. Les Editions INSERM, Paris

Persijn, GG, Hooff, JP, Kalff, MW, Lansbergen, Q and van Rood, JJ (1977) Effect of blood transfusions and HLA matching on renal transplantation in The Netherlands. *Transpl Proc* **9**: 503-505

Persijn, GG, van Leeuwen, A, Hoogeboom, J, Gabb, BW, Nagtegaal, A, *et al.* (1978) Matching for HLA antigens of A, B, and DR loci in renal transplantation by Eurotransplant. *Lancet* **1**: 1278-1281

Race, RR (1944) An 'incomplete' antibody in human serum. *Nature* 153: 771-772

Roychoudhury, AK and Nei, M (1988) *Human Polymorphic Genes: World Distribution.* Oxford University Press, New York

Schipper, RF, Oudshoorn, M, D'Amaro, J, van Zanden, HGM, de Lange, P, *et al.* (1996a) Validation of large data sets, an essential prerequisite for data analysis: an analytical survey of the Bone Marrow Donors Worldwide. *Tissue Antigens* **47**: 169-178

Schipper, RF, Schreuder, GMTh, D'Amaro, J and Oudshoorn, M (1996b) HLA gene and haplotype frequencies in Dutch caucasoids. *Tissue Antigens* **48**: 562-574

Schipper, RF, D'Amaro, J, Bakker, JT, Bakker J, van Rood, JJ and Oudshoorn, M (1997) HLA gene and haplotype frequencies in Bone Marrow Donors Worldwide registries. *Hum Immunol* **52**: 54-71

Schipper, RF, D'Amaro, J, de Lange, P, Schreuder, GMTh, van Rood, JJ, *et al.* (1998). Validation of haplotype frequency estimation methods. *Hum Immunol* **59**: 518-523

Svejgaard, A, Bratlie, A, Hedin, PJ, Högman, C, Jersild, C, *et al.* (1971) The Recombination Fraction of the HL-A System. *Tissue Antigens* **1**: 81-88

Svejgaard, A, Platz, P and Ryder, LP (1983) HLA and disease 1982 - a survey. *Immunol Rev* **70**: 193-218

Thorogood, J, Persijn, GG, Schreuder, GMTh, D'Amaro, J, Zantvoort, FA, *et al.* (1990) The effect of HLA matching on kidney graft survival in separate post-transplantation intervals. *Transplantation* **50**: 146-150

Tsuji K, Aizawa, M and Sasazuki, T (1992) *HLA 1991*. Oxford University Press, Oxford

Van Rood, JJ (1962) Leukocyte grouping: A method and its application (Thesis). University of Leiden

Van Rood, JJ, van Leeuwen, A, Schippers, AMJ, Ceppellini, R, Mattiuz, PL, *et al.* (1966) Leucocyte groups and their relation to homotransplantation. *Ann N Y Acad Sci* **129**: 467-472

Van Rood, JJ, van Leeuwen, A and Zweerus, R (1970) The 4a and 4b antigens. Do they or don't they? In: *Histocompatibility testing 1970* (Ed. Terasaki, PI), pp.93. Munksgaard, Copenhagen

Weinberg, W (1963) On the demonstration of heredity in man (1908). In: *Papers on Human Genetics* (Ed. Boyer, SH). Prentice-Hall: Englewood Cliffs

Appendix

Frequency analysis: Further notes and examples

E. Albert
Labor für Immungenetik
Kinderpoliklinik der LMU
Pettenkoferstr. 8a
80336 München, Germany

1. Phenotype Frequencies

The *phenotype frequency* (PF) describes how frequently one particular allele is found in a theoretical sample of 100 individuals, regardless of whether this allele is found in heterozygous (i.e., inherited from only one parent) or homozygous (i.e., inherited from both parents) state. Thus, if the HLA allele A*0101 is found in 20 out of 100 individuals in a given population, then the phenotype frequency is 20 out of 100 = 0.2. This frequency simply describes the probability under which in a given population an individual will be found positive for A*0101. It should be stressed here, that it is important to clearly distinguish between frequency per 100 individuals which is the phenotype frequency and frequency per 100 genes, which is the gene frequency. When HLA alleles were tested exclusively using serological methods, we spoke about *antigen frequencies*, because the HLA molecules were recognised by means of antibodies. Since nowadays, the majority of the HLA polymorphism is detected by DNA methodology at the level of the gene, we cannot possibly speak about antigen frequencies anymore, because the detected structures are genes and not antigens. In the age of DNA typing, we are defining HLA alleles and if we describe the frequency of such alleles in the population, the term *allele frequency* is used, however it remains frequently unclear whether this is frequency per 100 individuals (phenotype frequency, PF) or frequency per 100 genes (gene frequency, GF). The development towards DNA typing has led many authors of investigations on HLA disease associations to perform analyses exclusively at the level of the gene frequencies. This is not entirely appropriate, since HLA-disease association studies are frequently based on the working hypothesis that HLA molecules have a functional relationship to the disease studied, and that the function of a gene product is mainly dependent on the presence or absence of the gene product and not so much on the gene dose (homozygous *versus* heterozygous). For this reason, we recommend the use of phenotype analyses before complicated genotype analyses are performed.

2. Gene Frequencies

The *gene frequency* (GF) describes the frequency of a particular allele among a sample of 100 genes. In the days of serology, when there was still a considerable gene frequency not covered by serologically detected antigens, one could use the simple formula:

$$GF = 1 - \sqrt{1 - PF}$$

where GF is the gene frequency and PF is the phenotype frequency expressed as a fraction of 1. This formula is based on the assumption of a Hardy-Weinberg equilibrium in the population tested. It follows that, in the given population, the selection of partners for reproduction is not influenced by the markers under study, i.e., the HLA alleles. This means, that there is random mating with respect to HLA alleles. Random mating, for populations, can be assumed if there has been no HLA-related selection in the sample to be tested and if there has been no deliberate inbreeding. If, however, a sample was for example selected for a disease such as ankylosing spondylitis, which is associated with HLA-B27, then it is clear that such a patient population cannot be in Hardy-Weinberg (HW) equilibrium. The HW equilibrium is described in the most simple case of a bi-allelic system by the formula $p^2 + 2pq + q^2$, where p is the gene frequency of allele 1 and q is the gene frequency of allele 2. It can be derived from this formula, that the frequency of homozygotes is p^2 or q^2, and the frequency of heterozygotes is $2pq$ (for more details see Cavalli-Sforza and Bodmer, 1971). The HW equilibrium as given by the above formula is a very convenient method to investigate whether in the testing procedures for defining the alleles, there might have been a systematic error discriminating against homozygotes or heterozygotes of any kind. For example, in HLA serology, it is difficult to distinguish between an individual who is homozygous for HLA-A2 and an individual who is HLA-A2, A28 heterozygous. This is because many antibodies directed against A28 have sublytic reactivity against HLA-A2. This is relevant particularly in HLA-A2 homozygous individuals, because there is a higher quantity of expressed HLA-A2 molecules on the cell surface, causing truly A2 homozygotes to be falsely typed as A2, A28, which will lead to a perceived excess of A2, A28 and a lack of A2 homozygotes. For this reason, one could use the HWequilibrium and postulate that the number of A2 homozygotes should correspond to the square of the gene frequency for HLA-A2 and the number of A2, A28 heterozygotes would be equal to 2 x GF(A2) x GF(A28). If we assume that the GF of A2 is 0.3 and the GF of A28 is 0.05, then we expect in a sample of 1000 individuals which have not been selected for any MHC related factors, the number of A2 homozygotes to be $0.3^2 \times 1000 = 90$ individuals, and that the number of A2, A28 heterzygotes would be expected to be 2 x 0.3 x 0.05 = 0.03 x 1000 = 30 individuals. These expected numbers of homozygotes and heterozygotes in a given sample are then compared to the observed numbers and a simple Chi-square test is performed, for example:

A2/A2 expected: 90, observed 70
A2/A28 expected: 30, observed 50

X^2 A2/A2 = $(70 - 90)^2/90 = 4.4$, $p = 0.05$
X^2 A2/A28 = $(50 - 30)^2/30 = 13.3$, $p = 0.0005$

with one degree of freedom.

Thus, in the above given example, we have shown, that there has been a significant deviation from the HW expectations for A2/A2 and A2/A28 which indicates a systematic error in the assignment of A28 in the presence of A2. Such observations are the basis for the correction of assigning policies.

In the age of the DNA typing for HLA alleles, the determination of gene frequencies has become much simpler in that simple gene counting can be applied, using the assumption that any individual for which there is only one allele at a given locus recognisable, is homozygous for the allele in question. The number of new alleles which cannot be recognised with the DNA typing methods is very small indeed. For this reason, one can say that for all practical purposes, the gene counting method is appropriate for all DNA typed markers of the HLA system. The gene counting procedure simply determines the number of genes in a population which carry the information for example for HLA-A*0201. Individuals with only A*0201 and no other allele of the HLA-A locus account for two HLA-A*0201 genes and individuals with for example A*0201, *0301 will be counted as one allele for A*0201 and one allele for A*0301. In a sample of 1000 individuals, therefore, the number of genes counted must be 2000 and the number of A*0201 genes determined is divided by 2000 to arrive at the gene frequency by gene counting.

Listings of phenotype and gene frequencies for HLA alleles can be found in standard publications, such as Gjertson and Terasaki (1998).

3. Haplotype Frequencies

The term *haplotype* describes the unit of inheritance of a group of closely linked loci. Thus, a haplotype is the combination of all alleles coded for by closely linked loci in the cis-position, that is on the same parental chromosome in a family. Haplotypes and haplotype frequencies can also be determined by statistical methods from data of unrelated populations (Mattiuz *et al.,* 1970). A family-deduced haplotype in the HLA system could for example be HLA-A*0101, B*0801, DRB1*0301. The family-deduced second haplotype of a family member could then be HLA-A*0301, B*0702, DRB1*1501. The combination of these two haplotypes identified in one individual would then be the *genotype* of this individual. If the same individual is HLA typed without family analysis, one obtains the phenotype which is for this individual HLA-A*0101, *0301, B*0801, *0702, DRB1*0301, *1501.

Haplotype frequencies (HF) can be determined by simple haplotype counting, if a large enough sample is available in which by family analysis the genotype (i.e., the two haplotypes) have been deduced by family analysis. Family data of large sample sizes are difficult to obtain. Also in family analyses, the deduced haplotypes are sometimes ambiguous, i.e., for a given individual there may be two or more possible genotypes. Therefore, methods have been developed which can estimate HFs from phenotype data. The first formula by Mattiuz *et al.* (1970) estimates haplotype frequencies on the basis of a two-by-two table from the phenotype data for 2-point-haplotypes. For 3- and more-point-haplotypes, an alternative estimation procedure has been developed by Arnold *et al.* (1978) and by Baur *et al.* (1980), in which for each given phenotype the possible genotypes are deduced and divided according to their *a priori* probability, such that then fractions of haplotypes can be counted. For example, an individual with the above given phenotype of HLA-A*0101, *0301, B*0801, *0702 could have the following two genotypes with an *a priori* probability of 50%: A*0101, B*0801 and A*0301, B*0702 or A*0101, B*0702 and A*0301, B*0801. These four haplotypes are now counted according to their *a priori* probability of 0.5, such that for this individual a total of 4 x 0.5 = 2 haplotypes are counted. This procedure is performed for all individuals of the population sample to be analysed and a first table of HFs is obtained. In the second cycle, the genotypes of all individuals are analysed again and the counting is performed using the probabilities (frequencies) determined in the first preliminary frequency table. The third cycle uses probabilities of the second frequency table and so on. The procedure is iterated 30 times, after which stability usually results, i.e., the frequency changes from one cycle to the next become negligibly small. This procedure has the great advantage, that haplotypes with three and more loci can also be easily counted. One of the first observations which were made when HFs were determined in different populations, was that each population has a set of relatively characteristic HFs which are more distinctive than the set of GFs, which of course are also variable from population to population. The second observation was, that there are some haplotypes which occur relatively frequently and others which occur very rarely or are not found in a given sample (it should be stressed, that a haplotype which is not found in a given sample, is not necessarily non-existent, the only statement that can be made is, that this haplotype is present in a frequency smaller than 1 in *n*, where *n* is the size of the sample). Considering one particularly frequent haplotype, namely A*0101, B*0801, one can observe that this in the Caucasoid population most frequent haplotype is not formed by the most frequent alleles and conversely, one can observe that certain haplotypes involving quite frequent alleles as for example A*0301 and B*44 occur relatively rarely. The phenomenon, which is the basis of these observations is called linkage disequilibrium.

4. Linkage Disequilibrium

Very soon after the 3rd International Histocompatibility Workshop in Torino, where it had been recognised that the HLA system consists at least of two separate but closely linked loci, it became evident, that certain alleles of one locus exhibit an association with other alleles of the closely linked locus, such as the relationship between HLA-A1 and HLA-B8 mentioned above. It was observed, that the two markers A1 and B8 coded for at two closely linked loci, were found together more frequently than one would expect by chance alone. In an unrelated population, one expects the frequency of the A1, B8 haplotype (i.e., the joint occurrence of A1 and B8 on one haplotype) to correspond to the product of the GFs of the alleles involved. In the European caucasoid population, these frequencies are approximately 0.1 for HLA-B8 and approximately 0.14 for HLA-A1. Thus, the expected HF of HLA-A1-B8 is 0.1 x 0.14 = 0.014. The observed HF for A1-B8 in the European caucasoid population is, however, almost five times as great, namely 0.07. The difference between the observed HF and the expected HF has been called the *linkage disequilibrium parameter,* Δ. From these calculations, it can be immediately seen, that the Δ value is dependent on the frequencies of the alleles involved. Therefore, the *relative* Δ was defined, which measures the Δ value in relation to the maximal possible Δ value, which corresponds to the smaller of the two involved gene frequencies. In the above cited example of A1-B8, a maximum Δ value would be obtained if all haplotypes which carry HLA-B8 also carried HLA-A1. In the case of a negative association between two alleles, the lower limit for the HF is 0.

Significance testing for two-locus associations as an expression of the linkage disequilibrium can be performed from the two-by-two table of the phenotype data using the Chi-square or Fisher's Exact test.

The estimation of linkage disequilibrium can of course also be extended to three-point-haplotypes (Piazza, 1975). In such calculations, one has to take into account not only the GF of the three alleles of three closely linked loci, but also the two-way interactions which are included.Thus, the Δ value for an ABC haplotype is:

$$\Delta(a,b,c) = p(a,b,c) - p(a) \times p(b) \times p(c) - p(a) \times \Delta(b,c) - p(b) \times \Delta(a,c) - p(c) \times \Delta(a,b)$$

Again, the best measure of linkage disequilibrium is the *relative* Δ, which is the representation of the absolute Δ value defined by the formula given above, divided by the maximum Δ. Significance testing for the deviation from zero of the Δ value must use the second order interaction Chi-square test (Bartlett, 1935). It must be stressed, that due to the very large number of alleles at the various HLA loci, there is an extremely large number of theoretically possible three-point-haplotypes. Since the number of possible haplotypes must be taken into account if significance testing for three-point-haplotypes is performed, the tested panel sizes are rarely large enough for Chi-square values to remain significant after Bonferroni correction for the number of haplotypes possible.

Finally, one word of nomenclature and proper usage of genetic terms in the field of linkage association and linkage disequilibrium. The term *linkage* must remain restricted to the presence of at least two gene loci on the same chromosome. Two alleles of closely linked loci as for example HLA-A1 and HLA-B8 are associated in the random population, however they are not linked. The term haplotype does *per se* not imply linkage disequilibrium, the haplotype is simply describing the presence of at least two alleles of two closely linked loci on the same chromosome

When considering linkage disequilibrium, it is important to recognise that this phenomenon is a dynamic one which changes over time and which is defined by a given population tested. There has been a great deal of speculation about the origin of linkage disequilibrium and it is clear now, that linkage disequilibrium is a phenomenon found regularly for alleles of closely linked loci. It must be assumed that selection, as well as genetic drift, and the mixture of distant populations will produce linkage disequilibrium, and that the rate of recombination, a physiological process in genetics, determines the rate of decay of a once established linkage disequilibrium. Thus, if we observe today in a defined population a linkage disequilibrium, this means that since the establishment of this linkage disequilibrium, there has not been enough time for recombination to separate the two loci in question, in a way which would result in linkage equilibrium. Since the frequency of recombination depends largely, although not completely, on the physical distance between two loci, it is clear that very closely linked loci will in general have many pairs of alleles in linkage disequilibrium. However, it is conceivable that there are two very closely linked loci with a certain degree of polymorphism for which there will be no linkage disequilibrium measurable.

References

Arnold, A and Albert, ED (1976) Computer Programm zur Berechnung von Haplotypfrequenzen des HLA-Systems. In: *Proceedings of the 7th ISBN, Z Immun Forsch* **152**: 407-415

Bartlett, MS (1935) Contingency table interactions. *J R Stat Soc Suppl* **2**: 248

Baur, MP, Bertrams, J and Hintzen, U (1979) HLA-A, B, Bf Assoziationen bei 1972 Haplotypen. 10. Deutsche HLA Tagung, Tübingen

Baur, MP and Danilovs, JA (1980) Reference tables of two and three-locus haplotype frequencies for HLA-A, B, C, DR, Bf and GLO. In: *Histocompatibility Testing 1980* (Ed.Terasaki, PI), pp.994. UCLA Tissue Typing Laboratory, Los Angeles

Cavalli-Sforza, LL and Bodmer, WF (1971) *The Genetics of Human Populations*. Freeman, San Francisco

Gjertson, D and Terasaki, PI (1998) *HLA 1998*. ASHI Lenexa, Kansas

Mattiuz, PL, Ihde, D, Piazza, A, *et al.* (1970) New approaches to the population genetics and segregation analysis of the HLA system. In: *Histocompatibility Testing 1970* (Ed. Terasaki, PI), pp.193. Munksgaard, Copenhagen

Piazza, A (1975) Haplotypes and linkage disequilibrium from the three-locus phenotypes. In: *Histocompatibility Testing 1975* (Ed. Kissmeyer-Nielsen, F), pp.923. Munksgaard, Copenhagen

CHAPTER 16

SURVIVAL ANALYSIS IN SOLID ORGAN TRANSPLANTATION

P. A. Dyer
Transplantation Laboratory
Manchester Royal Infirmary
Manchester M13 9WL, England

Introduction

Audit of the clinical efficacy of solid organ transplantation is dependent on measuring outcome, usually the survival of the recipients or of their transplants, as a group. A survival study will have a start time point, which is usually the date the transplant was performed, a survival interval and an end point. The start time and survival interval are precise measurements in time but the end point or points, will vary within a group of recipients depending whether the transplant is judged to have failed or not and what the failure criteria are.

Survival data are usually presented in the form of a survival curve with the calculated proportion of the group surviving plotted on the vertical axis and the time interval after transplantation plotted on the horizontal axis (Figure 16.1). As the survival rate falls over time the line of the curve falls toward the horizontal axis. In general, survival curves of organ transplants show three rates of decline (Table 16.1).

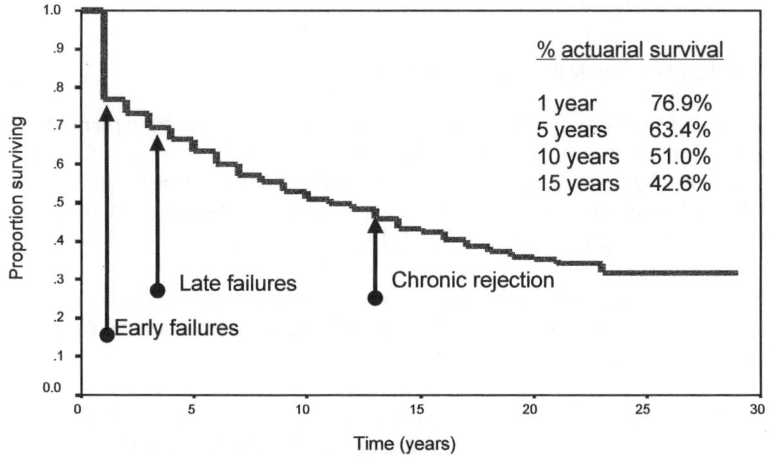

Figure 16.1. Kaplan-Meier survival curve of 2,146 Manchester cadaver donor kidney transplants 1968 to 1997. Three time periods of failure patterns are indicated.

Epoch	Post-transplant time	Clinical processes
Early	0-3 months	Technical complications Hyperacute rejection Irreversible acute rejection
Late	3-12 months	Ongoing acute rejection
Long-term	More than 12 months	Chronic rejection Non-adherence to anti-rejection drug treatment Recipient death.

Table 16.1. Periods of transplant failure

Survival curves must be clearly annotated to show the number of recipients entering the survival study and if more than one survival curve is plotted on a graph for purpose of contrast the statistical significance of any difference between survivals must be indicated. It can also be useful to indicate the specific survival rate at fixed time points such as 3, 12 and 60 months after transplantation.

Measuring outcomes

The outcome of a solid organ transplant evaluated, at any time after transplant must fall into one of three categories:

- ongoing function of the transplanted organ
- recipient has died
- transplant has failed but recipient is alive

It is possible to set other criteria based on the function of the transplanted organ, such as serum creatinine level for kidney transplant recipients, or quality of life measurements but such studies are often subjective and are not frequent. In such cases the end point will occur when the chosen factor reaches a specified level, *e.g.* serum creatinine is greater than 500 μmol/l.

If all transplants in a group of recipients were performed on the same day and all were followed for the same time after transplantation then survival calculations could be easily calculated as:

$$\% \text{ transplants surviving} = \frac{\text{number of functioning transplants} \times 100}{\text{total number transplants performed}}$$

The survival of the recipients would be:

$$\% \text{ recipients surviving} = \frac{\text{number of recipients alive} \times 100}{\text{total number of patients transplanted}}$$

For some types of organ transplants, such as hearts, the survival of the transplants and that of the recipients will usually be the same since failure of the organ means death of the recipient. Repeat transplantation of hearts has a poor outcome due to the high risk state of health of the recipient of a failing first transplant. In kidney transplantation, where repeat transplantation is common or alternative treatment is available, then these outcome measures will be different.

In reality, a group of transplant recipients will receive their individual organs over a period of time, most probably several years. This means that changes in recipient selection, organ allocation and post-transplant treatments must be evaluated and recognised as being variable (Figure 16.2).

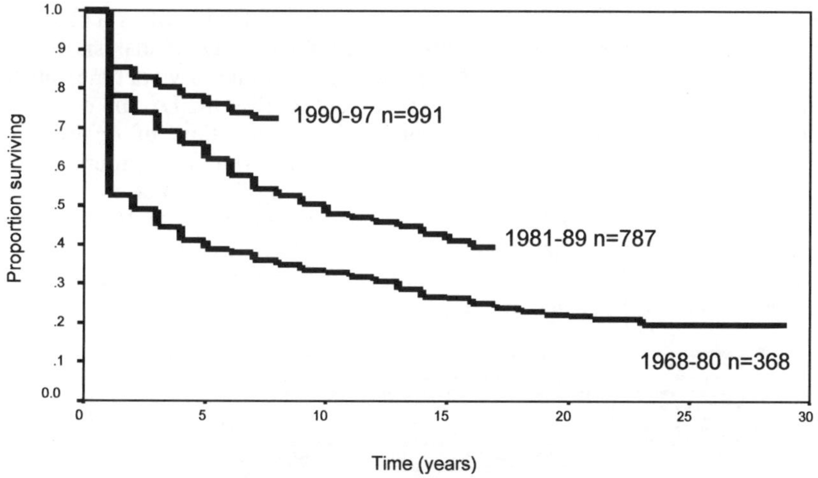

Figure 16.2. Survival of Manchester cadaver donor kidney transplants 1968 to 1997 according to anti-rejection immunosuppression treatment protocols. (a) 1968 to 1980, azathioprine with prednisolone; (b) 1981 to 1989, cyclosporin alone or with azathioprine and prednisolone; (c) 1990 to 1997, as (b) or various trials of new drugs including tacrolimus.

Within a specific time period there may also be variability such as the use of kidneys from cadaver or living donors or the use of whole or liver lobes for transplantation.

Within a group of recipients, several may have the same survival time but with different end points. For example:

- patient A received a kidney transplant on 1 January 1990 and has a functioning transplant 300 days later
- patient B received a kidney transplant on 30 April 1991 which was removed due to rejection 300 days later
- patient C received a kidney transplant on 15 August 1992 which remained in place 300 days later, but its function was insufficient and the patient was receiving haemodialysis
- patient D received a kidney transplant on 21 September 1992 and died 300 days later

Each recipient had the same transplant and patient survival of 300 days, but to accommodate these different outcomes the use of actuarial survival calculation methods has been widely adopted. Actuarial methods are both complicated and time consuming and have been encoded in computer programmes, which are now easily available (see below).

The main principle of actuarial calculations is that patients with functioning transplants at the time end point of follow-up, usually the date of analysis or last date of review, are not considered to have contributed a finite survival time, rather their ongoing transplant function is said to be "CENSORED". In contrast, recipients whose transplants are not functioning at the time of review are considered as "FAILED". A representation of follow-up in a group of 25 transplant recipients is shown in Figure 16.3. On-going function at one year of follow-up was observed in 15 cases as indicated by an arrow. In 10 cases the transplant event had taken place a year ago whilst in the remaining 5 cases follow-up varied from 3 to 300 days. In 10 other cases the transplant was judged to have failed at times between 10 and 360 days.

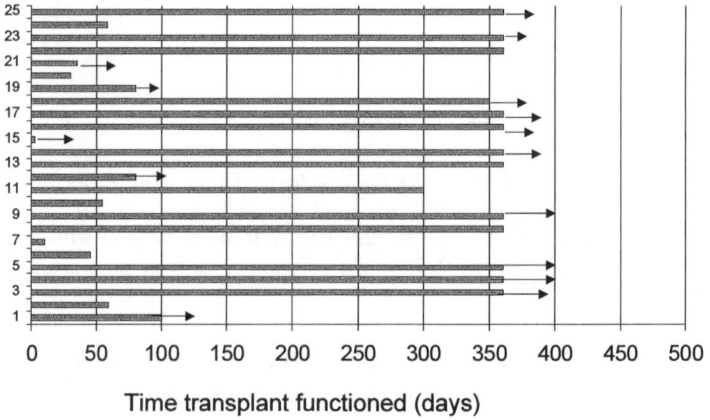

Figure 16.3. Survival intervals of a consecutive series of transplants up to one year of follow-up. Cases with continued function are indicated by horizontal arrows.

At each time point after transplant the number of cases from the initial group of recipients still contributing to the survival analysis will be reducing as transplants fail and as follow-up times are censored. The number of cases "AT RISK" can be indicated on the survival curve to reflect the relative strength of the study at lengthy time intervals after transplantation.

A group of transplant recipients must be continually reviewed to determine functioning and failed cases or the time of the last review should be recorded in each case. Recipients who are "lost to follow-up", such as those recipients living elsewhere, can be considered as functioning transplants only up to the time of last review. Inaccurate follow-up will result in incorrect survival calculations and inappropriate interpretation of the data. In practice, solid organ transplant recipients are usually followed-up with accuracy because of their need to attend clinics regularly for review of their anti-rejection therapy.

There is debate as to the relationship of the end point of follow-up with the transplant itself. The end point for **patient survival** is death of the recipient irrespective of cause since it is usually difficult to determine whether or not the transplant event influenced the patient's death. The resulting survival estimation will be the "worst case" but will be most acceptable to review. For **graft survival** the end point will be failure of the transplanted organ to alleviate other forms of treatment or death of the recipient for any reason. **Transplant survival** end point is taken as failure of the transplanted organ to alleviate other forms of treatment with the exclusion of recipients who died with a functioning transplanted organ.

Data collection and storage

Accurate collection of events relevant to survival analysis is essential. This is best done as a paper record initially but with rapid transfer to a computer database. The choice of database used is no longer critical since most database software is compatible with other applications such as the statistical package which will be used to perform the survival analysis itself. Some statistical software packages have database functions within their structure and can be used directly for data storage.

At the time of the transplant event all relevant data should be collected and noted. It is often far more difficult to collect data weeks or months after the transplant since clinical notes will have expanded and if the transplant has failed, the notes may have been re-located from the transplant centre. There is always the possibility of unintentionally introducing bias when collating data and this is more likely when some time has passed after an event.

The outcome measurements of the transplanted organ and the recipient must be pre-defined by establishing outcome categories. At each post-transplant clinic visit the category of outcome should be recorded. The value of survival calculations increases with the number of transplants available for analysis and with greater follow-up times. Both of these factors influence the statistical power of the survival analysis. With time, a consecutive series of transplants, accurately recorded and with accurate follow-up can become a valuable asset to the transplant programme.

As with all computerised records it is essential to make several copies of the database using different media. A useful additional function of the database will be the ability to generate reports of patients groups for audit and other management purposes. Most statistical packages have this function often with an associated graphical output.

Life table analysis.

All actuarial survival calculations are derived from a LIFE TABLE which sets out the history of a group of patients over time (see Table 16.2). The life table is structured according to the time intervals selected for each point of analysis; in Table 16.2 this is each year after transplantation as shown in the first column. The number of cases entered to the study at the start of each time is shown in the second column. During the study cases will be withdrawn, or censored, since the time during which they have been treated is limited by the day of review but they will continue in the study as further follow-up time accrues; these cases are shown in the third column. The calculated number of cases at risk in each time interval is shown in the fourth column. As cases are judged to have failed they are accumulated within a time interval and are totalled in the fifth column. Finally, in column six, the proportion of cases surviving based on an actuarial calculation taking into account failures and censored cases is shown in a cumulative manner for each time interval; this is displayed as a fraction but can readily be converted to a percentage. Table 16.2 shows that at the end of the first year of follow-up of 2146 transplants there were 104 cases censored and 483 failed transplants giving an actuarial survival of 77%. After five years of follow-up, which occurs at the end of the start time of the fourth year, the actuarial survival had fallen to 63%.

Time interval Start time in years	Number entering interval	Number withdrawn during interval	Number at risk	Number failing	Proportion surviving
0	2146	104	2094	483	0.77
1	1559	107	1505	69	0.73
2	1383	122	1322	70	0.69
3	1191	89	1146	50	0.66
4	1052	100	1002	47	0.63
5	905	88	861	44	0.6
6	773	77	734	37	0.57
7	659	99	609	18	0.55
8	542	90	497	21	0.53
9	431	79	391	15	0.51
10	337	37	318	8	0.49

Table 16.2. Life table using data from Figure 16.1. Manchester cadaver donor kidney transplants 1968 to 1997. Data output using SPSS computer application.

Further detailed explanation of using and interpreting life tables, as well as the calculations involved, can be obtained from the many medical statistics publications available, for example Bland (1995) or Campbell and Machin (1993).

Statistical packages

Actuarial survival calculations are only realistically achievable with a large number of cases by using a commercially available computer application. There are several good packages available with relevant programmes for survival analysis. Data storage, manipulation and analysis shown here was performed using the SPSS (SPSS Inc.) package but other commonly used applications are SAS and BMDP (Dixon, 1983).

Contemporary computer applications are relatively easy to use, which can also be their downfall. It is essential that the operator fully understands the nature of data input required and the meaning of the output. An apparently valid output can be meaningless if the user has not provided the correct instructions. Before embarking on survival analysis using a computer package it is essential to receive adequate training and instruction.

Survival curves

Survival data from a life table calculation is usually presented in the form of a survival curve and this form of output is usually automated when using a computer application. The most commonly used plot is the Kaplan-Meier survival curve, which illustrates the decline in survival of a group of cases over time. The interval between survival points can usually be varied within the computer application but for long follow-up times of several years, data points every six months are sufficient. In organ transplantation the most rapid period of decline in survival is usually within the first six months following transplantation.

Plotting two or more survival curves on the same axes is useful when comparing and contrasting the survivals of different groups of transplant recipients. The significance of the difference in outcomes between two or more groups is usually calculated by the Log Rank test (Peto *et al*, 1977) which gives a significance of difference value (p) derived from a chi-square calculation. Computer applications most often use the Log Rank test as a default although there are other methods available as set out in statistical texts.

Half life calculations

Although a group of transplant recipients may have an acceptable survival rate at one year of follow-up, or over even longer periods, the ongoing rate of decay is important. Some studies have used half-life calculations to measure decay rates and hence to predict total survival times. At its simplest, the half-life of a group of recipients is the point in time at which 50% of the transplants have failed or are predicted to fail. In the USA, for cadaver donor kidney transplants the half life is 9.2 years but for related living donor transplants it is 15.8 years (Cecka, 1997).

Post-transplant survival interval (months)	Percent of all 205 failures occurring
0-3	52.2
3-6	6.3
6-9	5.4
9-12	2.4
12-24	10.7
24-36	8.3
36-48	5.9
48-60	4.4
>60	4.4

Table 16.3. Rate of failure in 205 of 991 cadaver kidneys transplanted in Manchester between 1990 and 1997. All causes of failure, including death with function, are included.

Half-life calculations are useful in illustrating decay rates but there is a potential pitfall in that these calculations assume that the decay rate is constant over time. For organ transplant recipients the initial (three month) post-transplant period carries the highest risk of rejection, technical failure and infection. Thereafter transplant failures are less frequent (see Table 16.3). To overcome this problem some half-life studies include only those recipients with transplants functioning at six or 12 months after which the failure rate is approximately constant.

Multi-variate analyses

Generating survival curves for a group of transplant recipients depends on identifying a single factor which unifies the group, for example, the survival of a all male recipients of a heart transplant between the years 1990 and 1997. Following such an analysis a second survival calculation, perhaps of all female recipients transplanted during the same time period, could be warranted. These two survival experiences could then be compared using the log rank test. Such an approach is termed uni-variate analysis since a single variable, that of recipient gender, is examined for its influence on survival. When faced with the need to identify which variable or variables have a significant influence on survival in a group of transplant recipients uni-variate analysis is inappropriate and time consuming so a multi-variate method of analysis is essential.

The most widely used multi-variate analysis method is the Cox proportional hazards model. This is included in most statistical packages available as computer applications and is described in medical statistics texts. This model describes hazard functions (h) for each variable entered to the model: the hazard is the probability of transplant failure or death of the recipient occurring at a time point. It is assumed that any affect on the hazard occurs by the same ratio at all times. The calculated hazard rate is a relative risk of an end point occurring at any given time and so the confidence intervals of the relative risk can also be calculated. A computed hazard rate exceeding a value of unity indicates an increased risk associated with the factor analysed. An example of a multi-variate analysis using the Cox model is shown in Table 16.4. This analysis of the relative influences of HLA-A, -B and –DR mismatches in a recent large number of cadaver donor kidney transplants in a single centre reflects a well established hierarchy of influences.

Mismatched HLA specificity	Hazard rate	Confidence interval	Statistical Significance
A	0.9	0.7-1.1	0.5
B	1.1	0.9-1.3	0.5
DR	1.3	1.0-1.7	0.04

Table 16.4. Multi-variate analysis using Cox proportional hazards model. The relative effect of mismatching for HLA-A, -B and -DR specificities in Manchester cadaver donor kidney transplants 1990 to 1997.

Interpretation and pitfalls

As with any statistical test it is essential to interpret the results of a survival analysis with care. Since survival analysis is the result of a series of steps from data collection to computer based calculations the adage "garbage in, garbage out" is particularly relevant. Having established and checked the database, in particular for accuracy of the outcome data, it is always worthwhile performing a standard survival analysis, the outcome of which is well-known, as an expected predictor of results. This will not identify minor errors but will give confidence that in general no major error has been unintentionally introduced.

The most common pitfalls can be summarised as:

- Inaccurate collection of data
- Errors in entering data to database
- Inappropriate selection of cases for analysis
- Incorrect selection of parameters within a computer application
- Biased selection of groups of cases
- Ignoring significant statistical analyses

The final test of accuracy and analysis of data is to ask a colleague to repeat the entire process, but this can test the strongest of professional relationships!

References

Bland, M (1995) *An Introduction to Medical Statistics.* Oxford Medical Publications, Oxford

Campbell, MJ and Machin, D (1993) *Medical Statistics, a Commonsense Approach.* Wiley, Chichester

Cecka, JM (1997) The UNOS scientific renal transplant registry. In: *Clinical Transplants 1996*. (Ed. Cecka, JM and Terasaki, PI), pp.1-14. UCLA Tissue Typing Laboratory, Los Angeles

Dixon, WJ (1983) *BMDP Statistical Software.* University of California Press, California

Peto, R, Pike, MC, Armitage, P, *et al.* (1977) Design and analysis of randomized clinical trials requiring prolonged observation of each patient. *Br J Cancer* **35**:1-39

Supplier

SPSS Inc. 444 North Michigan Ave. Chicago IL 60611, USA.

CHAPTER 17

SURVIVAL ANALYSIS IN BONE MARROW TRANSPLANTATION

S. Richards
University of Oxford CTSU
Harkness Building, Radcliffe Infirmary
Oxford OX2 6HE, England

Introduction

There are standard techniques for analysing survival, calculating survival curves and comparing the survival of two or more groups of patients. These have mostly been described in Chapter 16, so only a few additional points are covered here. The standard methods can be applied satisfactorily to patients who have received a transplant, analysing from the time of the transplant. For comparisons of transplants versus other treatments, there are problems of bias which are often ignored. These are discussed in detail, with suggestions of ways of trying to minimise the effects due to bias, so that true treatment differences can be estimated.

Basic methods of survival analysis

Kaplan-Meier calculations give survival curves for a group of patients and survival curves for two groups of patients can be compared by the logrank method (Peto *et al.,* 1977; Altman, 1992). As well as giving a p value for the statistical significance of the difference between the groups, the ratio of the odds of death in one group to the odds in the other group, together with 95% confidence intervals, can also be calculated.

Allowance for other factors can be made by doing the analyses within strata defined by the factors, and summing certain statistics over strata to obtain overall values which can be used to obtain an adjusted p-value, odds ratio and its 95% confidence interval (see Appendix). For example, if gender and age are believed to be important prognostic factors, and we are comparing two treatment groups with different proportions of males and young patients in them, the analyses can be done for males and females separately within several age groups. This means that similar types of patients are compared only with each other, with the hope that the main difference between them is the treatment.

An alternative way of allowing for several variables at once is to use Cox's method of survival analysis (Cox, 1972; Altman, 1992). This is widely used and is available in many of the popular statistical packages such as SAS and SPSS. Baseline variables, including treatment group, can be included in the function which is fitted to the data. It has the benefit that continuous variables, such as age, do not have to be grouped. However, it is more difficult to understand and is less robust than the logrank method. That is, it is more likely to give misleading results if assumptions about proportional hazards (i.e. that the relative risk between the groups is similar at different times) and the linear effect of the variables used are wrong. This is particularly important in the case of bone marrow transplants, where the risk of treatment related mortality may be greater early on, with relapses becoming more important later, so that proportional hazards assumptions about variables which may affect one endpoint more than the other must be tested.

Comparison of transplants with other treatment

The most reliable way of assessing the difference between any two treatments is the large prospective randomised trial, which minimises the effects of both chance and bias. Within the area of transplants there have been randomised trials comparing different transplant methods, and these are generally analysed using the standard methods described above. When comparing bone marrow transplant with chemotherapy however, there have been very few completed randomised trials published so far.

Autologous transplants

Clearly, for autologous transplants, HLA matching is not a concern. In this case, the transplant is really a means of enabling very intensive treatment to be given, with the transplant used to rescue their bone marrow. Such treatment is best assessed in a randomised trial against the best current standard treatment. However, only a handful have randomised even as many as 200 patients in such comparisons: in acute lymphoblastic leukaemia (ALL) (Fiere *et al.,* 1993) in acute myeloid leukaemia (AML) (Zittoun *et al.,* 1995; Ravrindranath *et al.,* 1996; Burnett *et al.,* 1998), in myeloma (Harousseau and Attal,1997), and in non-Hodgkin's lymphoma (NHL) (Haioun *et al.,* 1997). In these diseases, as well as in breast cancer, there are randomised trials either ongoing or recently closed which will provide further information, but almost all are small compared with trials comparing other types of treatment.

Allogeneic transplants from a related donor

Where a matched related donor is available, it is even more difficult to achieve randomisation, but a comparison can be done, among those for whom a donor has been sought, of those with an HLA-matched relative versus those without one (Gray and Wheatley, 1991). This is sometimes called 'genetic' or 'Mendelian' randomisation, and provides unbiased comparison groups. Attempts have been made to use this method, for example in AML (Burnett *et al.,* 1996), adult ALL Bernasconi *et al.,* 1992; Sebban *et al.,* 1994), in childhood relapsed ALL (Chessells *et al.*, 1986) and high-risk childhood ALL (Chessells *et al.*, 1992). At present the numbers in such studies are small. Comparisons are weakened by the number of patients who have a donor but do not have a transplant. In a standard randomised trial this would be referred to as non-compliance, and it would be accepted that an 'intention-to-treat' analysis was the only way of obtaining an unbiased comparison. Although a non-compliance at the level found in these studies (sometimes as much as 30%) may be a cause of concern in interpreting the results, it should be born in mind that many of the so-called 'non-compliers' may be so because they relapsed or were in some other way not fit enough to receive the transplant, and hence the comparison is valid as a comparison of two treatment policies. Exclusion of such patients would produce serious bias.

Unrelated donor transplants

The evaluation of unrelated donor transplants is even more difficult. There is almost no evidence from randomised trials and the possible benefit generally has to be inferred from comparison with related donor transplants (Gordon-Smith, 1997). There is a great reluctance among both patients and clinicians to randomise between unrelated donor transplant and chemotherapy. The MRC attempts in the UKALLR2 trial to randomise between chemotherapy and unrelated donor bone marrow transplant in relapsed childhood ALL have failed, with only 5 patients randomised.

Non-randomised comparisons

As it has been extremely difficult to perform randomised trials comparing even autologous transplant and standard therapy, there is a vast amount of literature which attempts to evaluate transplants by comparing those who have received a transplant with those receiving chemotherapy. This is prone to all the caveats which apply to the comparison of any two treatments in a non-randomised way, and even has additional problems. Attempts have been made to overcome some of the problems, but there is no means of allowing for the many unknown factors involved in the selection of patients for a particular treatment group.

Time-to-transplant bias

A problem particular to transplants is the difference between the treatment groups in terms of initiation time of treatment. For patients who receive a transplant there is an inevitable delay before the procedure is done. This means that those patients who relapse or die early are automatically assigned to the chemotherapy group. Those who are transplanted have survived for a certain length of time before they receive their transplant and so are often better prognosis than those who are newly diagnosed (Gray and Wheatley, 1991).

Statistical methods can be used to adjust treatment comparisons for this bias. The most reliable, and yet easiest to understand, is a modified version of the logrank method known as Mantel-Byar analysis (Mantel and Byar, 1974). This method uses the number of patients at risk and the number of events in each treatment group in each time period in the same way as the logrank method, but patients are initially regarded as belonging to the chemotherapy group. They only count towards the transplanted group from the time at which they receive their transplant. The effect of this is that transplant patients are only directly compared with patients who have survived for at least as long as the time-to-transplant interval. Unfortunately, this method is not readily available in the software packages most frequently used for survival analyses, and so has rarely been used. It can, however, be combined with adjustment for known prognostic factors and used to provide a graphical display of the relative effects of transplant and chemotherapy (Early Breast Cancer Trialists' Collaborative Group, 1992; Wheeler *et al.,* 1998).

An example of how the apparent relative effects of treatments change when adjustments are done is given in figures 17.1 to 17.3. Figure 17.1 shows event free survival from the time of relapse for the 432 patients in the MRC UKALLX trial who relapsed before October 1993, and were in second remission 6 weeks after relapse. Figure 17.2 shows the results of using the Mantel-Byar method to compare either allogeneic or autologous transplant with chemotherapy, allowing for the delay to transplant. Figure 17.3 shows these comparisons after additionally adjusting for the most important known prognostic factors: site of relapse, duration of first remission and age. For allogeneic transplant, a difference of 16% at 5 years is reduced to 7% after allowance for time to transplant, but increased back to 14% when adjusted for prognostic factors. For autologous transplant, an apparent improvement of 2% at 5 years becomes a decrease of 1% after allowance for transplant delay, and an improvement of 7% after adjustment for prognostic factors.

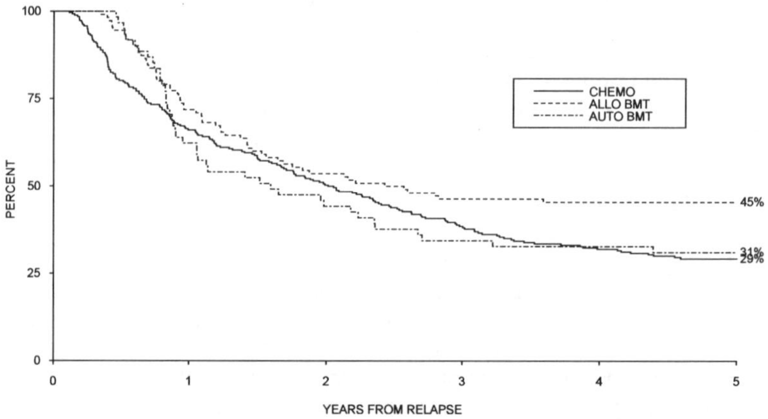

Figure 17.1. UKALLX outcome after relapse by treatment group. Unadjusted event-free survival of patients who received chemotherapy, allogeneic BMT or autologous BMT after relapse.

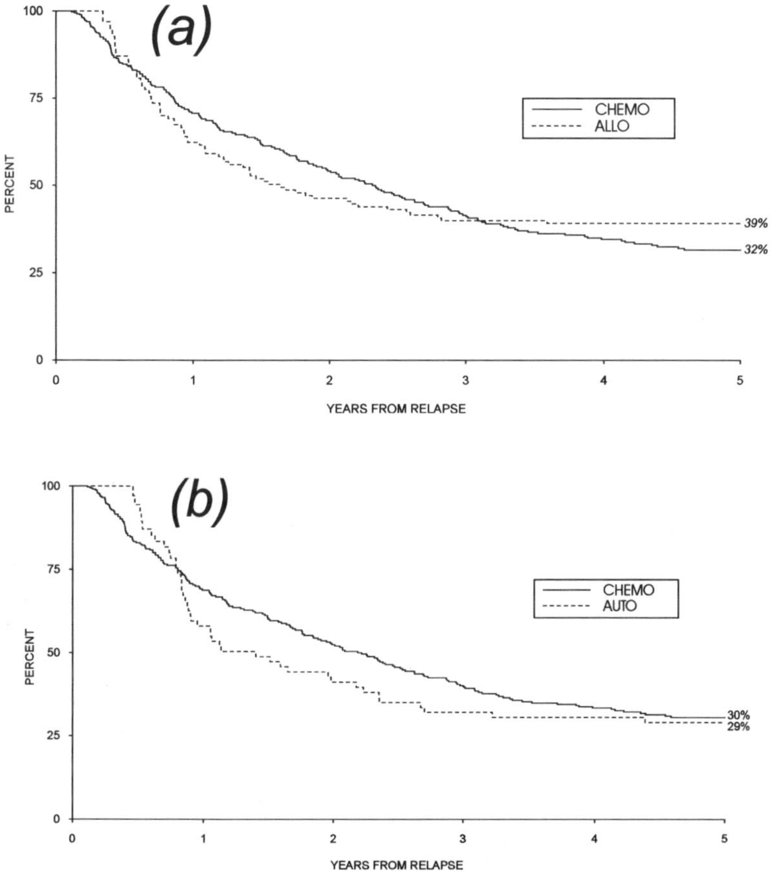

Figure 17.2. UKALLX comparison of (a) allogeneic BMT and (b) autologous BMT with chemotherapy-treated patients following relapse. Event-free survival comparisons after adjustment for time-to-transplant by Mantel-Byar method.

One alternative method is to apply Cox regression analysis with a time-dependent variable which indicates transplant status (i.e. done or not done yet) (Cox, 1972). This is available in the PHREG procedure of the SAS computer package. The allowance for time-to-transplant is analogous to the Mantel-Byar method of adjusting Log Rank analyses. Examples of results obtained by this method include comparisons of allogeneic BMT with chemotherapy in second remission childhood ALL (Uderzo *et al.,* 1995) and in firs remission adult ALL (Zhang *et al.,* 1995). There is no obvious way of displaying the comparative survival of the two groups of patients using this method, although one suggestion is to derive a time-to-transplant function for the transplant cohort and to use this to derive a survival distribution for the chemotherapy group conditional on the assumption that patients survive long enough to receive a transplant (Begg *et al.,* 1984). This

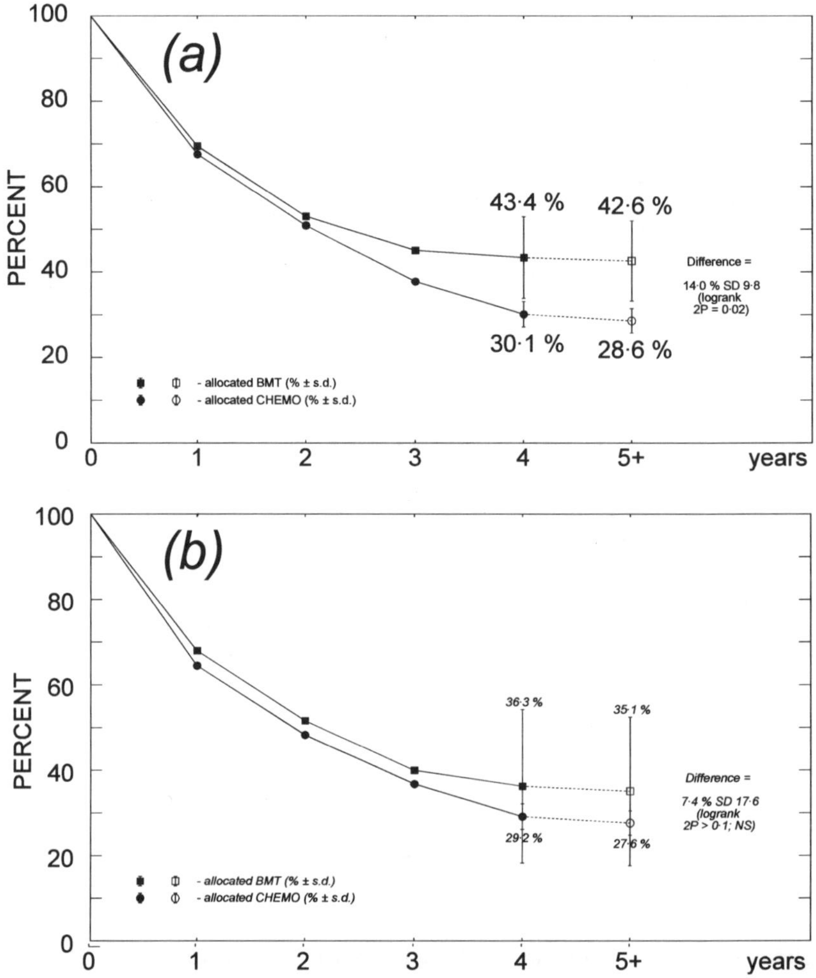

Figure 17.3. Adjusted UKALLX comparison of (a) allogeneic BMT and (b) autologous BMT with chemotherapy-treated patients following relapse. Event-free survival comparisons allowing for relapse type, duration of first remission and age, as well as time-to-transplant.

method is difficult to understand and it is not clear how an overall adjusted statistical comparison of survival can be obtained, rather than a comparison at a single time point (Horowitz *et al.,* 1991).

Another possible method is to use some sort of matching or case-control analysis. Thus transplanted patients can be matched with chemotherapy patients whose event-free survival is at least as long as the time to transplant (Barrett *et al.,* 1994, Borgmann *et al.,* 1995; Hoogerbrugge *et al.,*1995). Although this goes some way towards dealing with the time-to-transplant bias, it is not the most robust method since it will usually mean that either matching has to be done inexactly (in the case of a small cohort of chemotherapy patients) or that one or two chemotherapy patients have to be selected from those that match each case (if there are a large number of chemotherapy patients available) while data from the others are discarded. The Mantel-Byar or Cox analysis methods are therefore preferable.

Selection bias

The most difficult problem to deal with is selection bias. Although attempts may be made to ensure that outcome is being compared in similar types of patients, this is often hampered by differing definitions of risk group or stage of disease (Savage *et al.,* 1997) Apparently minor changes in definition can make a substantial difference in outcome.

Even where groups are similar in terms of known risk factors, unmeasured selection factors remain. This has been demonstrated in studies which compare, within cohorts of patients conventionally treated, the group who would have been eligible for intensive treatment and transplant with the rest (Blade *et al.,* 1996; Rahman *et al.,* 1997; Garcia-Carbonero *et al.,* 1997) and, similarly for other intensive procedures (Florell *et al.,*1992; Curran *et al.,* 1993). In all these examples, those eligible for the intensive treatment had a superior outcome, although they received the same treatment as those who would have been ineligible.

Other studies show that a large proportion of patients who are eligible on formal protocol grounds for allogeneic bone marrow transplant may not receive one for a wide variety of reasons (Berman *et al.,* 1992; Graham-Pole, 1989).

Endpoints

The primary endpoint when comparing transplant with other treatment must be survival or event free survival. If event free survival is examined, survival should also be reported, as it may be true that some of the patients with an event can be salvaged. If there is a differential effect according to initial treatment it may be that event free survival is improved without any effect on survival.

When comparing different types of transplant, including HLA matching, graft versus host disease (GVHD) prophylaxis, and T-cell depletion, it may be more appropriate initially to examine effects on other endpoints such as graft failure or GVHD. In this way, it may be possible to identify the best methods of transplant in terms of transplant related mortality, which can then be used in large trials comparing the effect on overall survival of transplant versus non-transplant regimens.

Other endpoints include toxicity and quality of life. These are important, but can only be usefully used in making treatment decisions in conjunction with reliable information on survival benefit.

Conclusions

Most attempts at evaluating the effect of bone marrow transplant are woefully inadequate, either because of poor study design or because of small study size, and often both.

Comparisons of bone marrow transplant with other treatments should be regarded in the same way as other treatment comparisons. This means that the only really reliable way of determining their relative effect is by means of large randomised trials. If two chemotherapy treatments were being compared, a sample size would be calculated prior to initiation of a trial, and the same should be true if one of the treatments is transplant. In the case of related donor transplants use can be made of 'genetic' randomisation by establishing which patients are HLA typed and comparing those with and without a matched sibling donor. However, much larger studies are needed than are currently available.

Appendix

Log rank analysis uses the observed number of deaths in one group (o), the expected number of deaths (e) and the variance of o-e (v) calculated for each time interval. The sum of o-e (O-E) and of v (V) over all time intervals are used to calculate the test statistic $X^2=(O-E)^2/V$ which can be compared with a chi-square distribution with one degree of freedom to obtain a p-value. The ratio of the odds of death in one group to the odds in the other group, together with 95% confidence intervals, can also be calculated from these as $OR = \exp[(O-E)/V \pm 1.96/\mathrm{sqrt}(V)]$.

Allowance for other factors can be made by doing the analyses within strata defined by the factors, obtaining O-E and V for each stratum, and summing these to obtain overall values from which X^2 and OR are calculated.

Acknowledgement

I would like to thank the MRC Childhood Leukaemia Working Party for the use of MRC trial data.

References

Altman, DG. (1992). *Practical Statistics for Medical Research.* Chapman and Hall, London

Anasetti, C., Amos, D, Beatty, PG, Appelbaum, FR, Bensinger, W, *et al.* (1989) Effect of HLA compatibility on engraftment of bone marrow transplants in patients with leukemia or lymphoma. *N Engl J Med* **320**, 197-204

Attal, M, Blaise, D, Marit, G, Payen, C, Michallet, M, *et al.* (1995) Consolidation treatment of adult lymphoblastic leukemia: a prospective, randomized trial comparing allogeneic versus autologous bone marrow transplantation and testing the impact of recombinant interleukin-2 after autologous bone marrow transplantation. *Blood* **86**: 1619-1628

Barrett, AJ, Horowitz, MM, Pollock, BH, Zhang, MJ, Bortin, MM, *et al.* (1994) Bone marrow transplants from HLA-identical siblings as compared with chemotherapy for children with acute lymphoblastic leukemia in a second remission. *N Engl J Med* **331**: 1253-1258

Begg, CB, McGlave, PB, Bennett, JM, Cassileth, PA and Oken, MM. (1984) A critical comparison of allogeneic bone marrow transplantation and conventional chemotherapy as treatment for acute nonlymphocytic leukemia. *J Clin Oncol* **2**: 369-378

Berman, E, Little, C, Gee, T, O'Reilly, R, and Clarkson, B. (1992) Reasons that patients with acute myelogenous leukemia do not undergo allogeneic bone marrow transplanation. *N Engl J Med* **326**: 156-160

Bernasconi, C, Lazzarino, M, Morra, E, Alessandrino, EP, Pagnucco, G, *et al.* (1992) Early intensification followed by allo-BMT or auto_BMT or a secod intensification in adult ALL: a randomized multicenter study. *Leukemia* **6**:(suppl 2): 204-208

Blade, J, San Miguel, JF, Fontanillas, M, Alcala, A, Maldonado, J, *et al* (1996) Survival of multiple myeloma patients who are potential candidates for early high-dose therapy intensification/autotransplantation and who were conventionally treated. *J Clin Oncol* **14**: 2167-2173

Borgmann, A, Schmid, H, Hartman, R, Baumgarten, E, Hermann, K, *et al.* (1995) Autologous bone-marrow transplants compared with chemotherapy for children with acute lymphoblastic leukaemia in a second remission: a matched-pair analysis. *Lancet* **346**: 873-876

Burnett, AK, Goldstone, AH, Stevens, R, Hann, IM, Gray, R, *et al.* (1996) Allo and auto BMT reduce relapse risk in AML in CR1 but do not significantly improve overall survival: results of the MRC AML 10 trial. *Brit J Haem* **93** (suppl 2): a1 184

Burnett, AK, Goldstone, AH, Stevens, RMF, Hann, IM, Rees, JKH, *et al.* (1998) Randomised comparison of addition of autologous bone-marrow transplantation to intensive chemotherapy for acute myeloid leukaemia in first remission: results of MRC AML 10 trial. *Lancet* **351**: 700-708

Chessells, JM, Rogers, DW, Leiper, AD, Blacklock, H, Plowman, PN, *et al.* (1986) Bone-marrow transplantation has a limited role in prolonging second marrow remission in childhood lymphoblastic leukaemia. *Lancet* **May 31**: 1239-1241

Chessells, JM, Bailey, C, Wheeler, K, and Richards, SM. (1992) Bone marrow transplantation for high-risk childhood lymphoblastic leukaemia in first remission: experience in MRC UKALLX. *Lancet* **340**: 565-568

Cox, DR. (1972) Regression model and life tables (with discussion). *J Royal Stat Soc* **B 34**: 187-220

Curran, WJ, Scott, CB, Weinstein, AS, Martin, LA, Nelson, JS, *et al.* (1993) Survival comparison of radiosurgery-eligible and -ineligible malignant glioma patients treated with hyperfractionated radiation therapy and carmustine: a report of radiation therapy oncology group 83-02. *J Clin Oncol* **11**: 857-862

Early Breast Cancer Trialists' Collaborative Group (1992) Systemic treatment of early breast cancer by hormonal, cytotoxic, or immune therapy. 133 randomised trials involving 31,000 recurrences and 24,000 deaths among 75,000 women. *Lancet* **339**: 1-15

Fiere, D, Lepage, E, Sebban C, Boucheix, C, Gisselbrecht, C, *et al.* (1993) Adult acute lymphoblastic leukemia: a multicentric randomized trial testing bone marrow transplantation as postremission therapy. *J Clin Oncol* **11**: 1990-2001

Flemming, DR, Henslee-Downey, PJ, Romond, EH, Harder, EJ, Marciniak, E, *et al.* (1996) Allogeneic bone marrow transplantation with T-cell depleted partially matched related donors for advanced acute lymphoblastic leukemia in children and adults: a comparative matched cohort study. *Bone Marrow Transpl* **17**: 917-922

Florell, RC, Macdonald, DR, Irish, WD, Bernstein, M, Leibel, SA, *et al.* (1992) Selection bias, survival, and brachytherapy for glioma. *J Neurosurg* **76**: 179-183

Garcia-Carbonero, R, Hidalgo, M, Paz-Ares, L, Calzas, J, Gomez, H, *et al.* (1997) Patient selection in high-dose chemotherapy trials: relevance to high-risk breast cancer. *J Clin Oncol* **15**: 3178-3184

Gordon-Smith, EC. for the Consensus Panel (1997) Royal College of Physicians consensus conference on unrelated donor BMT: its use in leukaemias and allied disorders. *Brit J Haem* **96**: 424-425

Graham-Pole, J for the Pediatric Oncology Group (1989) Treating acute lymphoblastic leukaemia after relapse: bone marrow transplantation or not? *Lancet* **Dec23/30**: 1517-1518

Gray, R, and Wheatley, K. (1991) How to avoid bias when comparing bone marrow transplantation with chemotherapy. *Bone Marrow Transpl* **7** (Suppl 3): 9-12

Haioun, C, Lepage, E, Gisselbrecht, C, Bastion, Y, Coiffier, B, *et al.* (1997) Benefit of autologous bone marrow transplantation over sequential chemotherapy in poor-risk aggressive non-hodgkin's lymphoma: updated results of the prospective study LNH87-2. *J Clin Oncol* **15:** 1131-1137

Harousseau, J-L. and Attal, M. (1997) The role of Hematopoietic stem cell transplantation in multiple myeloma. *Seminars Hematol* **34** (Suppl 1): 61-66

Hoogerbrugge, PM, Gerritsen, EJA, Does-van den Berg, A, Berg, H, Zwinderman, A.H, *et al.* (1995) Case-control analysis of allogeneic bone marrow transplantation versus maintenance chemotherapy for relapsed ALL in children. *Bone Marrow Transpl* **15**: 255-259

Horowitz, MM, Messerer, D, Hoelzer, D, Gale, RP, Neiss, A, *et al.*(1991). Chemotherapy compared with bone marrow transplantation for adults with acute lymphoblastic leukaemia in first remission. *Ann Int Med* **115**: 13-18

Mantel, N and Byar, DP. (1974) Evaluation of response-time data involving transient states: an illustration using heart transplant data. *J Amer Stat Assoc* **69**: 81-86

Peto, R, Pike, MC, Armitage, P, Breslow, NE, Cox, DR, *et al.* (1977) Design and analysis of randomized clinical trials requiring prolonged observation of each patient. II. Analysis and examples. *Brit J Cancer* **35**: 1-39

Ravindranath, Y, Yeager, AM, Chang, MN, Steuber, CP, Krischer, J, *et al.* (1996) Autologous bone marrow transplantation versus intensive consolidation chemotherapy for acute myeloid leukemia in childhood. *N Engl J Med* **334**: 1428-1434

Rahman, ZU, Frye, DK, Buzdar, AU, Smith, TL, Asmar, L, *et al.* (1997) Impact of selection process on response rate and long-term survival of potential high-dose chemotherapy candidates treated with standard-dose doxorubicin-containing chemotherapy in patients with metastatic breast cancer. *J Clin Oncol* **15**: 3171-3177

Savage, DG, Szydlo, RM, Chase, A, Apperley, JF and Goldman, JM. (1997) Bone marrow transplantation for chronic myeloid leukaemia: the effects of differing criteria for defining chronic phase on probabilites of survival and relapse. *Brit J Haem* **99**: 30-35

Sebban, C, Lepage, E, Vernant, J-P, Gluckman, E, Attal, M, *et al.* (1994) Allogeneic bone marrow transplantation in adult acute lymphoblastic leukemia in first complete remission: a comparative study. *J Clin Oncol* **12**: 2580-2587

Uderzo, C, Valsecchi, MG, Bacigalupo, A, Meloni, G, Messina, C, *et al.* (1995) Treatment of childhood acute lymphoblastic leukemia in second remission with allogeneic bone marrow transplantation and chemotherapy: ten-year experience of the Italian bone marrow transplantation group and the Italian pediatric hematology oncology association. *J Clin Oncol* **13:** 352-358

Wheeler, K, Richards, S, Bailey, C, Chessells, J. (1998) Comparison of bone marrow transplant and chemotherapy for relapsed childhood acute lymphoblastic leukaemia: the MRC UKALLX experience. *Brit J Haem* **101**: 94-103

Zhang, M-J, Hoelzer, D, Horowitz, MM, Gale, RP, Messerer, D, *et al.* (1995) Long-term follow-up of adults with acute lymphoblastic leukemia in first remission treated with chemotherapy or bone marrow transplantation. *Ann Int Med* **123**: 428-430

Zittoun, RA, Mandelli, F, Willemze, R, De Witte, T, Labar, B, *et al.* (1995) Autologous or allogeneic bone marrow transplantation compared with intensive chemotherapy in acute myelogenous leukemia. *N Engl J Med* **332**: 217-223

CHAPTER 18

HLA AND DISEASE ASSOCIATION: STATISTICAL CONSIDERATIONS

J. H. Barrett, W. Thomson and W. Ollier
ARC Epidemiology Unit
University of Manchester School of Epidemiology and Health Sciences
Stopford Building, Oxford Road
Manchester M13 9PT, England

Introduction

A close relationship between genes in the HLA region and disease susceptibility has gradually emerged since the initial report some thirty years ago, of an association of class I polymorphisms with Hodgkin's lymphoma (Amiel, 1967). It is now clear that the role of HLA genes in the regulation of the immune response is largely responsible for their involvement in the aetiology of autoimmune, malignant and infectious conditions. Many conditions are now known to be associated with particular HLA alleles (Tiwari and Terasaki, 1985). The majority of these have been identified through case-control association studies. Here we suggest how such studies can be designed and discuss approaches which can be used to statistically test whether any association found is real. Although these suggestions have been written with HLA genes in mind, it is important to stress that they apply equally to any genetic association studies, e.g. cytokine gene polymorphisms and disease.

Basic definitions

The terms **association** and **linkage** are often confused and inappropriately used. Classical linkage aims to demonstrate that a locus or a chromosomal region co-segregates with a disease or particular phenotype. The pattern of inheritance of polymorphic genetic markers can be tracked through families that include multiple cases of the disease. Examples of linkage include Huntington's chorea and cystic fibrosis, where a single gene plays a major role. Several approaches have been developed for the investigation of genetic linkage. These will not be discussed here.

In contrast, genetic association relates to the demonstration of a statistical relationship between an allele of a gene and a particular phenotype. The basis for such studies is that if a particular allele (or set of alleles) increases the risk of developing disease, then that allele will be found more frequently in the cases than in the controls. Similarly if a polymorphic marker is located close to and in linkage disequilibrium with a disease locus, then the distribution of that marker's alleles will differ between cases and controls. Association studies are population-based and have provided a useful approach to studying complex diseases, such as diabetes and rheumatoid arthritis (RA), where several genes and environmental factors play a major role.

Necessary preliminaries

Before undertaking any association study it is worthwhile considering a number of important preliminary steps. Firstly it is always advisable to seek professional statistical help regarding study design, control selection, the required sample size and the types of analyses to be used. Statisticians always prefer to be involved at the outset rather than inherit data from a flawed study design.

A second consideration is appreciating the nature of the clinical condition being investigated. Even though a single diagnostic label may be used, many diseases exhibit considerable clinical heterogeneity. This will often be the result of genetic heterogeneity within the condition. Such heterogeneity will dilute the effects of individual genes and make it difficult to demonstrate statistically significant associations. Juvenile chronic arthritis (JCA) is a good example of how clinical heterogeneity can influence the genetic associations observed. If all JCA cases are considered together, it is difficult to detect significant HLA associations. However if specific clinical subsets are considered, such as those children with only limited joint involvement and a very young age at disease onset (less than 6 years), strong associations with HLA-DRB1*11, DRB1*08 and DPB1*0201 are found (Donn and Ollier 1996). Thus it is important that every attempt is made to ensure that cases are as homogeneous as possible. This will influence the criteria used for case selection.

Study design

Overall study design should be carefully considered beforehand. Several issues are of great importance, including the following:

Choice of controls

The appropriate selection of controls is crucial to the design of association studies. As in classical case-control studies, controls should be selected from the same population as cases. Problems can arise if cases and controls are drawn from a stratified population, where different sub-populations have evolved fairly separately. In this case an association study may detect differences in the distribution of alleles which have nothing to do with disease. There are, for example, regional differences within the UK in the frequency of some HLA alleles (Swingler and Compston 1986). One type of design used in epidemiology is the matched case-control study, where each case is matched to one or more controls on potential confounding factors such as age and sex. (A confounding factor is one that is related to both the exposure of interest and the disease). A case-control study in genetic epidemiology may be matched on factors such as ethnic group and place of birth, in order to remove the potential confounding effect of population stratification. An increasingly popular design in genetic case-control studies is to use relatives of the cases as controls. This ensures a similar genetic background and also is often a very practical design, since relatives of cases may be particularly willing to take part in research. This is discussed in more detail below.

Power and sample size

Another important design consideration is the power of the study. The power is the probability that the study will detect an effect of a particular size. Thus for example if a study has 80% power to detect a relative risk of disease of 1.5 to carriers of a particular allele, compared to non-carriers, this means that 80% of studies of that size would be expected to detect a significant association. It is usually assumed that a significance level of 5% is used in the analysis, but this can be altered. A more stringent significance level will require a larger sample size to achieve the same power. Similarly a larger sample size will be needed to maintain the same power to detect a smaller effect.

The power of a genetic association study with a standard case-control design (or the sample size needed to achieve a particular power) can be estimated using the same methods as for conventional case-control studies. Table 18.1 gives the sample size needed to detect various different sizes of effect with 80% power, using a 5% significance level. The effect size is given in terms of the odds ratio, which is the ratio of the odds of disease given the genetic risk factor to the odds of disease without the risk factor. For rare diseases this gives a good estimate of the relative risk of disease to those with the risk factor compared to those without. More details of odds ratios are given in the statistical methods section below.

A worked example explaining how to calculate sample size requirements is given in the Appendix. A simple approach has been used, since sample size calculations are essentially always approximate, depending on many unknowns which have to be estimated. Some refinements can be made, for example taking account of matching in the design, but these rarely make an important difference. Further details on sample size and many other aspects of the design and analysis of case-control studies in a general context can be found elsewhere (Breslow and Day 1980, 1987). Software is also available to carry out sample size calculations for case-control studies, for example Epi Info (Dean *et al.,* 1994), which is freely available and easy to use.

It can be seen from Table 18.1 that sample size requirements are quite sensitive to the specification of parameters which are either only known imprecisely (the population frequency of the genetic risk factor) or are specified somewhat arbitrarily (such as the relative risk of interest). It is therefore important to interpret the results of sample size calculations with a degree of common sense. For example it can be seen that a rare genotype with a modest effect would only be likely to be detected in an extremely large study. However if this is infeasible it

Odds ratio	Population phenotype frequency (%)					
	1	5	10	20	50	70
1.5	7954	1687	910	534	387	499
1.8	3487	746	407	244	187	250
2	2394	515	282	171	136	185
2.5	1245	271	151	94	80	114
3	803	177	99	64	58	85
4	448	100	58	38	38	59
10	112	27	17	14	18	32
50	20	7	6	6	12	23

Table 18.1. Sample size requirements. Figures indicate the number of cases needed to achieve 80% power in a case-control study with equal number of controls, using a two-sided 5% significance level.

may still be worth investigating rare risk factors, since even a modestly sized study would have sufficient power to demonstrate a greatly increased risk.

HLA-DRB1*0401 and *0404 alleles are both implicated in RA susceptibility (MacGregor *et al.,* 1995). In the UK population the frequency of the DRB1*0404 phenotype (i.e. carrying one or more copy of this allele) is about 5%. Hence to have 80% power to demonstrate a modest increase in risk (OR=2.0) associated with this phenotype over 500 cases and 500 controls would be needed. On the other hand a greatly elevated risk (OR=10.0) could be detected with less than 30 cases. The *0401 phenotype is much more frequent at about 25%. In this case even an OR of 2.0 could be detected with about 150 cases.

Statistical methods

Many different approaches are possible to the analysis of data from genetic association studies. The most appropriate method depends on the risk factor(s) under investigation and on the design of the study. If the aim of the study is to examine the effect of a particular allele or genotype, the best approach is to estimate this effect using the odds ratio (Section 1 below), whereas a different approach will be needed to study the overall association between a polymorphic gene and disease (Section 2). The use of family members as controls requires more specialized methods (Section 3).

1. *Two by two tables*

The simplest type of case-control study investigates a *binary* exposure, where each individual is either exposed or not exposed to the risk factor. In genetic studies such an exposure might be a particular phenotype (e.g. carrying at least one copy of a particular allele, such as DRB1*0404), or it might be a particular genotype (e.g. being homozygous for DRB1*0404). In such a situation the results of the

	Case	Control
Exposed	*a*	*b*
Not exposed	*c*	*d*
Total	*n*	*m*

Table 18.2. Case-control data with binary exposure. *a, b, c* and *d* are the number of subjects in each category among *n* cases and *m* controls.

case-control study can be summarized in a two-by-two table, cross-classifying exposure and disease status, as illustrated in Table 18.2.

We are interested in estimating the relative risk R to those who are exposed compared with those who are not exposed.

$$R = \frac{\text{Probability of having disease in those who are exposed}}{\text{Probability of having disease in those who are not exposed}}$$

These probabilities cannot be estimated from case-control data, since subjects have been selected on the basis of their disease status, ensuring that a much larger proportion of our sample are cases than in the wider population.

However from case-control data it is possible to calculate the odds ratio, OR. The *odds* of an outcome means the probability of that outcome occurring divided by the probability of it not occurring. In the above example the odds of exposure in cases in thus a/c. The odds ratio is calculated as follow:

$$OR = \frac{\text{Odds of being exposed in cases}}{\text{Odds of being exposed in controls}} = \frac{a/c}{b/d} = \frac{ad}{bc}$$

This is equivalent to the ratio of the odds of being a case in those who are exposed to the odds of being a case in those who are not exposed. The importance of this is that for rare diseases the odds ratio is a very good approximation to the relative risk. Hence relative risk can be estimated from a case-control study by the odds ratio ad/bc. An odds ratio of 5.0, for example, indicates that a person exposed to the risk factor is 5 times more likely to develop the disease.

Any such point estimate should be accompanied wherever possible by its confidence interval, to give an indication of the range of values of the true odds ratio which are consistent with the data. This is easily calculated, and details are given in the Appendix.

The hypothesis of an association between the exposure and disease (equivalent to an odds ratio not equal to one) can be tested directly using Fisher's exact test or, if the sample size is reasonably large, a chi-squared test with one degree of freedom.

Example:

In a case-control study of RA, subjects are classified according to whether or not they carry a DRB1*0401 allele. Out of 139 controls, 36 carried the allele compared with 99 out of 201 cases. The odds ratio is thus calculated as (99x103)/(36x102) = 2.78, with a 95% confidence interval of (1.74, 4.44).

2. *Several exposure categories*

Case-control studies are often carried out where interest is in examining the effect of more than two categories of exposure. This is particularly common in genetic studies, where the effect of a particular gene or genetic marker may be under investigation, but no particular allele can be selected a priori as a risk factor. In this situation several analytic strategies are possible.

2.1 *Comparison of allele frequencies*

The overall distribution of alleles in cases and in controls can be compared. Data are summarised in a two by k table, where k is the number of distinct alleles. The unit of observation is each copy of the gene, so that each individual contributes two observations to the table. An example is given in Table 18.3.

Differences in the distributions are tested using one overall test. If the sample size is large and no alleles are rare, this can be done using a simple chi-squared test with k-1 degrees of freedom. (A rule of thumb is that no expected frequencies should be less than 5 under the null hypothesis of no difference between the cases and controls). Otherwise, if k is small, use of Fisher's exact test is recommended. However, if the number of alleles is large, this will be infeasible, and Monte Carlo methods should be used to estimate the exact p-value, since the chi-squared approximation may yield incorrect results. These methods are now available in general-purpose statistical packages (e.g. SPSS) as well as specialist software (e.g. StatXact).

If a difference is found between cases and controls, the next step will be to investigate where the difference lies. One systematic approach to this is to compare the observed and expected frequencies of each allele in turn by examining the adjusted residuals from the chi-squared analysis of the table. The formula for these is given elsewhere (Agresti 1996) and many statistical programs will produce them. Using this procedure the alleles contributing most to the overall difference can be identified.

Allele	Case	Control
01	68	38
02	0	6
03	70	50
04	24	44
07	14	34
08	40	2
09	2	2
10	0	4
11	36	8
12	0	2
13	22	6
14	0	2
15	54	36
16	0	2
Total	**330**	**236**

Table 18.3. Comparison of HLA-DRB1 broad allele frequencies in 165 cases of juvenile chronic arthritis and 118 controls.

If many alleles are present, it should be born in mind that this approach, based on a test with many degrees of freedom, will have relatively low power to detect an effect, particularly of a rare allele. This disadvantage must be weighed against the advantage of avoiding the problems inherent in multiple testing. It is particularly appropriate when many genes are to be tested, where the generation of false positive results through multiple testing is potentially a major problem.

2.2. *Comparison of phenotypes one by one*

For each allele, a separate analysis can be carried out, calculating the relative risk to carriers of that allele versus non-carriers, as outlined in the above section on two-by-two tables.

This approach leads to k tests, where k is the number of alleles, so caution must be applied in interpreting the confidence intervals, which are not adjusted for multiple testing. Clearly if one hundred tests are being performed, and a five percent level of significance is applied, you would expect five comparisons to be different by chance alone. These will be false positive associations and are known as type I errors. A number of methods can be used to correct significance levels for the effects of multiple testing. The best known is probably Bonferroni's correction (Bland, 1995) where the levels of significance are multiplied by the number of tests performed. This is an extremely rigorous correction and the value of performing this procedure is discussed later.

2.3. *Comparison of genotypes*

In some cases it may be feasible to classify individuals according to their genotype and to compare genotype frequencies in cases and controls. This will only be feasible where the number of alleles is small, since with k alleles there are potentially k(k+1)/2 distinct genotypes. This gives rise to a table similar in structure to Table 18.3 (although now each individual will only contribute once to the overall sample size) and can be analysed similarly.

3. *Family-based case control studies*

As explained above, there are some advantages to using relatives as controls in association studies. Several methods of analysis have been suggested for studies involving single affected cases and both their parents. In the following discussion it is assumed that the gene or marker is biallelic, or that a hypothesis concerning a particular allele or genotype is to be tested.

3.1 *Ignoring matching*

Falk and Rubinstein (1987) proposed a method of analysis known as the haplotype relative risk (HRR). The idea of this method is to compare the genotypes of cases with artificially constructed control genotypes, consisting of the two parental alleles *not* transmitted to the affected offspring. For example if the case has genotype AB and the parents are AA and AB, then the control genotype contributed by this family group is AA. The proportion of cases carrying at least one A allele is compared with the proportion of control genotypes including an A allele, using the methods applicable to two-by-two tables outlined above.

A variation on this method (Terwilliger and Ott, 1992) is based on the comparison of allele frequencies between cases and parental controls: the haplotype-based haplotype relative risk (HHRR). Unlike the HRR method, this approach does not ignore the distinction between AA and AB genotypes. The unit of observation is the allele, with each case and each control (formed as before from the untransmitted parental alleles) contributing two observations. Frequencies of the two alleles in cases and controls are compared, again using Fisher's exact test or a chi-squared test with one degree of freedom.

Since these methods ignore the matching between cases and their parents, their validity depends upon the assumption of independence between the transmitted and non-transmitted alleles (under the null hypothesis of no association). However in the presence of population stratification, this assumption may not be true. Hence, although under some circumstances the methods outlined here can be more powerful than those using matched sets, a more correct approach is to take account of the matching as described below.

3.2. *Taking into account matching*

In this type of study, each parent contributes one case allele (i.e. the allele transmitted to the affected offspring) and one control allele (not transmitted). In a matched analysis, data are arranged as shown in Table 18.4. Note that a, b, c and d will add up to 2n, where n is the number of cases (and 2n is the number of parents).

		Case allele (transmitted)	
		A	B
Control allele	A	*a*	*b*
(not transmitted)	B	*c*	*d*

Table 18.4. Data from a study of cases and their parents arranged for a matched analysis.

The appropriate method of analysis for matched case-control data is to use McNemar's test (Bland 1995). For large samples, this compares the statistic $(b-c)^2/(b+c)$ with a chi-squared distribution with one degree of freedom. (For small samples it is advisable to use an exact test, comparing b with the binomial distribution with probability ½ and (b+c) trials).

An important feature of this method is that only discordant pairs are used. This means that only heterozygous parents contribute information to the analysis.

This method of analysis is known as the transmission/disequilibrium test (TDT) (Spielmans *et al.,* 1993). A positive test result provides evidence for both linkage disequilibrium and linkage.

3.3. *Multiple alleles*

A range of methods have been proposed for the analysis of case-control data using parental controls where the exposure of interest is a gene or marker with more than two alleles (Sham and Curtis 1995; Bickeböller and Clerget-Darpoux, 1995; Schaid, 1996).

3.4. *Missing parental data*

The methods of analysis discussed in this section were designed for sampling families consisting of independent cases and both their parents. Inevitably it is sometimes possible to obtain data on a case and one parent only. In such one-parent families, it will not always be known which allele has been transmitted to the affected offspring. Including only those cases where this can be determined (e.g. where the parent is homozygous) can introduce bias into the sample and should be avoided. However, in the case of multiallelic markers, it is possible to incorporate one-parent data into the analysis without introducing bias, provided both parent and child are heterozygous and of different genotype (Curtis and Sham, 1995).

3.5. *Interpretation of results*

As mentioned earlier when many tests for association are being performed it is possible that false positive or type I errors are generated by the process of multiple testing. False positive associations can also arise from population stratification leading to subtle differences between cases and controls. Just as important, is the possibility that false negative results can be obtained and studies can be underpowered to detect true associations. These problems leave the researcher with the dilemma of how to interpret their results and how to proceed further.

Some adopt the strategy of basing everything on levels of significance, rigorously correcting these for the amount of multiple testing performed. Whilst this is a legitimate approach it may not represent the best strategy in that true positive associations may be missed if too stringent criteria are applied. Central to this dilemma is the issue of whether one is "hypothesis generating" or "hypothesis testing". Ideally sufficient cases and controls are studied so that a two-stage strategy can be adopted: one data set is used for hypothesis generating and a second data set for hypothesis testing. If an association is detected in the former it can be tested and possibly confirmed in the latter without having to correct for multiple comparisons.

Of relevance to these issues is what importance we place on determining levels of significance, which are open to misinterpretation. For example an extremely low p value is often wrongly interpreted as indicating a strong association rather than a highly significant association. A small difference between cases and controls can be highly significant if very large sample sizes are compared; however the strength of association will be small. The strength of an association is best estimated by calculating odds ratios and the belief that can be placed in them determined from the 95% or 99% confidence intervals. The use of odds ratios and confidence intervals is now the favoured approach by most researchers conducting association studies.

Appendix

Sample size calculations for case-control studies

Assuming the same number of cases and controls are included in the study, the formulae below give the approximate number of cases (n) needed to achieve 80% power of detecting an odds ratio R to those with the genetic risk factor compared to those without. A two-sided test with 5% significance level is assumed. Sample size depends on p_1, the proportion of controls with the risk factor, estimated beforehand by the population frequency, and on p_2, the proportion of cases with the risk factor.

$$p_2 = \frac{R\,p_1}{\left(1 - p_1 + Rp_1\right)} \qquad (1)$$

$$n = \frac{\left(1.96\sqrt{2\bar{p}\bar{q}} + 0.84\sqrt{p_1 q_1 + p_2 q_2}\right)^2}{\left(p_2 - p_1\right)^2} \qquad (2)$$

Where

$$\bar{p} = \left(p_1 + p_2\right)/2, \quad \bar{q} = 1 - \bar{p}, \quad q_i = 1 - p_i \quad \left(i = 1, 2\right)$$

The values 1.96 and 0.84 are obtained from the standard Normal distribution and depend on the significance level and power of the study respectively. To use a significance level α, 1.96 can be replaced by $Z_{\alpha/2}$, the $100(1 - \alpha/2)^{th}$ percentile of the standard Normal distribution. For example the 97.5^{th} percentile has been used above for a two-sided significance level of 0.05. To achieve a 1% significance level, the 99.5^{th} percentile, i.e. 2.58, should be used. Percentiles of the Normal distribution can be found in published tables (e.g. Neave, 1978).

Similarly to achieve a power β, the value 0.84 can be replaced by $Z_{1-\beta}$, the $100(\beta)^{th}$ percentile of the distribution. For example 90% power is achieved by replacing 0.84 with 1.28, the 90th percentile.

Example:

A study is to be carried out to investigate whether a particular candidate gene is involved in the development of RA. Interest is in whether carriers of a particular allele (either one or two copies) are at increased risk of developing RA, and previous studies have estimated that 10% of the population carry this allele. How many cases and controls need to be studied to be 90% sure of detecting a two-fold risk to carriers compared with non-carriers?

$R = 2$, $p_1 = 0.1$

From equation (1),

$$p_2 = \frac{2 \times 0.1}{\left(1 - 0.1 + 2 \times 0.1\right)} = 0.2/1.1 = 0.18$$

$$\bar{p} = (0.1 + 0.18)/2 = 0.14$$

$$\bar{q} = 1 - 0.14 = 0.86$$

$$q_1 = 1 - 0.1 = 0.9$$

$$q_2 = 1 - 0.18 = 0.82$$

Since 90% power is required, replace 0.84 by 1.28 in equation (2).

Then

$$n = \frac{\left(1.96\sqrt{2 \times 0.14 \times 0.86} + 1.28\sqrt{0.1 \times 0.9 + 0.18 \times 0.82}\right)^2}{(0.18 - 0.1)^2}$$

$$= \frac{\left(1.96\sqrt{0.24} + 1.28\sqrt{0.24}\right)^2}{(0.08)^2} = 378$$

Hence in the order of 400 cases and 400 controls are needed for the study.

Confidence intervals for odds ratios

Referring back to Table 18.2 in the text, the relative risk of disease to those exposed compared to those not exposed is estimated by the odds ratio: *ad/bc*. The point estimate should be accompanied by its confidence interval.

The simplest method of calculating a confidence interval for the estimated odds ratio is to use the Woolf approximation (Woolf, 1955).

The variance of the natural logarithm of the odds ratio, ln(*OR*), can be estimated by:

$$1/a + 1/b + 1/c + 1/d$$

Using the normal distribution approximation, a 95% confidence interval for ln(*OR*) is therefore given by

$$\ln(OR) \pm 1.96\sqrt{(1/a + 1/b + 1/c + 1/d)}$$

Taking the anti-logs of these values gives a 95% confidence interval for the odds ratio.

Confidence intervals produced using this approach are only approximate, and may be quite inaccurate for small sample sizes. Alternative more exact methods are available but are less simple to calculate (Breslow and Day, 1980, p128-136).

References

Agresti, A. (1996) *An Introduction to Categorical Data Analysis*. pp.31.Wiley, New York

Amiel, JL. (1967) Study of the leucocyte phenotypes in Hodgkin's disease. In: *Histocompatibility Testing 1967* (Ed. Curtoni, Mattiuz and Tosi), pp.77-81. Munksgaard, Copenhagen

Bickeböller, H and Clerget-Darpoux, F. (1995) Statistical properties of the allelic & genotypic transmission / disequilibrium test for multiallelic markers. *Genet Epidemiol* **12**: 865-70

Bland, M. (1995) *An Introduction to Medical Statistics,* 2nd Edition. Oxford University Press, Oxford

Breslow, NE and Day, NE (1980). *Statistical Methods in Cancer Research, Vol I. The Analysis of Case-control Studies.* International Agency for Research on Cancer, Lyon, France

Breslow, NE and Day, NE. (1987). *Statistical Methods in Cancer Research, Vol II. The Design and Analysis of Cohort Studies.* International Agency for Research on Cancer, Lyon, France

Curtis, D and Sham, PC. (1995) A note on the application of the transmission / disequilibrium test when a parent is missing. *Am J Hum Genet* **56**: 811-812

Dean, AG, Dean, JA, Coulombier, D, Brendel, KA, *et al*. (1994) Epi info, version 6: a word processing, database, and statistics program for epidemiology on microcomputers. Centres for Disease Control and Prevention, Atlanta, Georgia, USA

Donn, RP and Ollier, WER (1996) Juvenile chronic arthritis - a time for change? *Eur J Immunogenet* **23**: 245-260

Falk, CT and Rubinstein, P (1987). Haplotype relative risks: an easy reliable way to construct a proper control sample for risk calculations. *Ann Hum Genet* **51**: 227-33

MacGregor, A, Ollier, W, Thomson, W, Jawaheer, D and Silman, A. (1995) HLA-DRB1*0401/0404 genotype and rheumatoid arthritis: increased association in men young age at onset and disease severity. *J Rheumatol* **22**: 1032-1036

Neave, HR. (1978) *Statistical Tables.* George Allen & Unwin, London

Schaid, DJ. (1996) General score tests for associations of genetic markers with disease using cases and their parents. *Genet Epidemiol* **13**: 423-449

Sham, PC and Curtis, D. (1995) An extended transmission / disequilibrium test (TDT) for multi-allele marker loci. *Ann Hum Genet* **59:** 323-336

Spielman, RS, McGinnis, RE and Ewens WJ. (1993) Transmission test for linkage disequilibrium: The insulin gene region and insulin-dependent diabetes mellitus (IDDM). *Am J Hum Genet* **52:** 506-516

Swingler, RJ and Compston, DA. (1986) The distribution of multiple sclerosis in the UK. *J Neurol Neurosurg Psychiatry* **49:** 1115-1124

Terwilliger, J and Ott, J (1992) A haplotype-based 'haplotype relative risk' approach to detecting allelic association. *Human Hered* **42:** 337-346.

Tiwari, JL and Terasaki, PI. (1985) *HLA and Disease Associations.* Springer Verlag, Berlin

Woolf, B. (1955) On estimating the relationship between blood group and disease. *Ann Hum Genet* **19:** 251-253.

PART 6

MINOR HISTOCOMPATIBILITY ANTIGENS

CHAPTER 19

MINOR HISTOCOMPATIBILITY ANTIGENS

E. Simpson
Transplantation Biology Group
MRC Clinical Sciences Centre
Imperial College School of Medicine
Hammersmith Hospital
Du Cane Road, London W12 ONN

Introduction

Evidence for there being transplantation alloantigens in addition to those encoded within the major histocompatibility complex (MHC: H-2 in mice, HLA in humans) came originally from the work of Snell in mice. He defined transplantation (histocompatibility, H) antigens as those which elicited rejection of skin or tumour grafts from genetically non-identical donors, and devised methods for analysing the genetic loci which encoded them (Snell, 1948). Following the identification of H-2 as the strongest of these H antigens (hence the term "major") the others were termed "minor", since individually they elicit slow graft rejection in comparison with the rapid rejection of H-2 disparate grafts. The chromosomal regions encoding each of the H antigens were genetically isolated by backcrossing to make a series of congenic mouse strains, each differing from the parental strain by expression of the defined minor H alloantigen (Snell and Stimpfling, 1966; Bailey, 1975).

The human counterparts of mouse histocompatibility alloantigens were evident from the rejection of tissues and organs transplanted between genetically dissimilar individuals. That the human MHC, HLA, is the homologue of the mouse H-2 was initially established at the functional level by showing that skin grafts exchanged between HLA-matched siblings (HLA-identical by descent) survived significantly longer than those between HLA-mismatched siblings (Ceppellini *et al.*, 1969). However, these experiments also demonstrated the existence of human counterparts of minor H antigens, since even grafts exchanged between HLA-identical siblings were rejected, albeit at a slower tempo than those between siblings mismatched for one or both HLA haplotypes. In the clinical setting, it is also apparent that minor H antigens are implicated in chronic rejection of HLA-matched organ grafts (Candinas *et al.*, 1995). A more florid and devastating manifestation of immune responses to minor H antigens is seen in graft-versus-host (GVH) disease following bone marrow transplantation (BMT) between HLA-identical donor/recipient sibling pairs (Goulmy *et al.*, 1996).

It was clear from work in both mice and humans that minor H antigens must be the result of genetic polymorphisms. However, their biochemical characterisation lagged behind that of HLA molecules, whose polymorphisms were recognised by both antibodies and T lymphocytes, because minor H antigens elicited only T cell responses (Simpson and Roopenian, 1997), and even with our current abilities to isolate and grow T cell clones specific for these antigens, their use *in vitro* is much less tractable than that of antibodies. It was the MHC-restricted nature of T cell responses to minor H antigens however which gave the first clue about their molecular nature. A minor H antigen consists of a self-MHC (HLA, H2) class I or II molecule plus a component derived from a polymorphic gene (Gordon *et al.*, 1975; Bevan, 1975; Goulmy *et al.*, 1977). T cell responses to minor H antigens are therefore MHC-restricted in the same way as those to viruses (Zinkernagel and Doherty, 1974). Once it was discovered that the virally-encoded component was a short (8-10 amino acid) peptide derived from an intracellularly expressed protein (Townsend *et al.*, 1986), it seemed likely that minor H epitopes presented by self-MHC molecules would also be peptides. This assumption was strengthened by the solution of the crystal structure of the HLA-A2 molecule, showing a peptide binding groove created by folds of the outer two domains (Bjorkman *et al.*, 1987a; Bjorkman *et al.*, 1987b), and was confirmed in principle by the peptide elution studies of Rammensee and his colleagues (Rötzschke *et al.*, 1990; Wallny and Rammensee, 1990). However, it took a little longer to harness two complementary approaches, that of peptide elution and that of expression cloning using T cells, pioneered by Thierry Boon's laboratory for identification of tumour antigens (De Plaen *et al.*, 1988; van der Bruggen *et al.*, 1991; Scott *et al.*, 1992) before it was possible to identify not only the peptide sequences of minor H epitopes but the genes from which they are derived. The list of those currently known is shown in Table 19.1, but it is growing fast. The number of clinically important minor H antigens is still not known but it is the immunodominant (i.e. stronger) ones that tend to be identified first. Since the self-MHC presenting allele (HLA, H2, class I or II) is a crucial component of the minor H antigen, different peptide epitopes will be relevant for each one but the pattern of these combinations will emerge as the list grows. What is currently missing is the identification of any MHC class II restricted peptides

The molecular nature of any minor H epitope is that of a complex between an MHC class I or II molecule and a peptide derived by breakdown from a polymorphic protein in one of the cellular compartments - nuclear, mitochrondrial, cytoplasmic, or one of the cytoplasmic vesicles. In principle one would expect MHC class I molecules to be loaded with endogenous peptide in the endoplasmic reticulum (ER) during biosynthesis, and MHC class II molecules with exogenously derived peptide in an endosomal compartment. However, since traffic between cellular compartments is "leaky", and very small numbers of cell surface MHC molecules loaded with a particular peptide suffice to trigger T cell recognition, it is likely that for some endogenous proteins that comprise components of minor H antigens, the distinction between MHC class I and II peptide loading pathways may be blurred, i.e., not all class I presented minor H peptides may be endogenously derived, and not all those presented by class II may be exogenous to that cell and brought into it by endocytosis. Both pathways could be involved in loading minor H peptides into each type of MHC molecule. From genetic studies of Roopenian (Roopenian, 1992), we know that both CD4 T cells responding to an MHC class II presented epitope and CD8 T cells responding to an epitope presented by MHC class I are necessary *in vivo* components of an effective transplantation rejection response.

Phenotyping

The growth *in vitro* of T cells specific for minor H antigens and the isolation from them of T cell clones which could be expanded and propagated in the presence of appropriate growth factors (e.g. IL2) was the first step to enable individuals, mice or humans, to be phenotyped for the presence of minor H antigens. Previously, the early genetic work had relied on cumbersome *in vivo* methods of skin or tumour cell grafting (Snell, 1948; Snell and Stimpfling, 1966; Bailey, 1975). However, phenotyping with T cells allowed the positional mapping of genes encoding the male-specific antigens, HY, on the mouse and human Y chromosomes (McLaren *et al.,* 1984; Simpson *et al.,* 1987; McLaren *et al.,* 1988; Cantrell *et al.,* 1992; King *et al.,* 1994), as well as the genetic dissection of the region on mouse chromosome 2 in which H3 and H13 lie (Mendoza *et al.,* 1997) which led to identification of the minor H peptides and the genes encoding them (Scott *et al.,* 1995; Greenfield *et al.,* 1996; Mendoza *et al.,* 1997).

Phenotyping has also been used to explore the role of human minor H antigens defined by $CD8^+$ T cell clones in acute and chronic GVH disease (Goulmy *et al.,* 1996). However, this is the pioneering work of a research laboratory with strong clinical links, and it is probably not realistic to envisage typing of patients for minor H antigens using phenotyping with T cells. The isolation of further GVH-associated T cells will however remain key in the immediate future for the identification of further immunodominant epitopes in laboratories with this type of research expertise and interactions with clinical colleagues.

It is the identification and characterisation of polymorphic genes encoding minor H peptide epitopes which opens the door to the possibility of routine minor H typing in patients, by genotyping.

Identification of minor H encoding genes and peptide epitopes

Two different, complementary approaches have been taken to identify genes and peptides of minor H antigens. Both depend on the use of minor H specific T cell clones to determine whether a target or antigen presenting cell expresses the minor H epitope. One approach, pioneered for the identification of the genes encoding tumour antigens (De Plaen *et al.,* 1988; Boon *et al.,* 1989; van der Bruggen *et al.,* 1991; Scott *et al.,* 1992), is expression cloning, in which DNA or cDNA is transfected into recipient cells expressing the relevant MHC restriction element, and transfectants expressing the epitope are identified by peptide-specific T cells. The minimum DNA fragment conferring expression is sequenced and from that information candidate peptides are synthesised and tested by addition over a wide dose range to target cells of the appropriate MHC. The peptide sensitizing the target cells for recognition in the nanomolar or picomolar range is the likely

Chromosome	Common Name	Species	MHC restriction	Gene	Peptide(s)**	Reference
Mitochondria	MTFα, MTFβ	Mouse	H2-M3	*mt-ND1*	f-MFFINILTL, f-MFFINALT	Loveland et al. 1990
Mitochondria	-	Mouse	H2-M3	*mt-CO1*	f-MFVNRW	Morse et al. 1996
Mitochondria	-	Rat	RT1.A[a]	*mt-APTase6*	ILFPSSERLISNR	Bhuyan et al. 1997
Y	HY/K[k]	Mouse	H2-K[k]	*Smcy*	TENSGKDI	Scott et al. 1995
Y	-	Human	HLA-B7	*SMCY*	SPSVDKARAEL	Wang et al. 1995
Y	-	Rat and mouse	HLA-B7 transgene	*Smcy*	SPSVNKARAEL	Simmons et al. 1998
Y	-	Human	HLA-A2	*SMCY*	FIDSYICQV	Meadows et al. 1997
Y	HY/D[b]	Mouse	H2-D[b]	*Uty*	WMHHNMDLI	Greenfield et al. 1996
Y	HY/D[b]	Mouse	H2-D[b]	*Smcy*	KCSRNRQYL	Markiewicz et al. 1998
Y	HY/B27	Rat and mouse	HLA-B27 transgene	Unknown	KQYQKSTER, AVLNKSNREVR	Simmons et al. 1998
16	MX-1	Mouse	H2-K[k]	*Mx1*	Unknown	Speiser et al. 1990
9	B6[dom]/H7	Mouse	H2-D[b]	Unknown	AAPDNRETF	Perreault et al. 1996
2	β_2m	Mouse	H2-K[b] or K[d]	*B2m*	Unknown	Peramau et al. 1990, Rammensee et al. 1986
2	H13	Mouse	H2-D[b]	Novel cDNA 47c1	SSVVGVWYL	Mendoza et al. 1997
2	H3	Mouse	H2-D[b]	Novel cDNA Zfp106	ASPCNSTVL	Zuberi et al. 1998
10	H60	Mouse	H2-K[b]	Novel cDNA 22.26	LTFNYRNL	Malarkannan et al. 1998
Unknown autosome	HA-1	Human	HLA-A*0201	Partial cDNA KIAA0223	VLHDDLLEA	den Haan et al. 1998
Unknown autosome	HA-2	Human	HLA-A*0201	Myosin-related gene	YIGEVLVSV	den Haan et al. 1995

Table 19.1. Current status of minor histocompatibility antigens. **, Antigenicity caused by known change at underlined amino acids

cognate peptide for the T cell recognised epitope. Initial selection of appropriate DNA or cDNA for transfection can assist in this approach, and was used to identify two mouse Y chromosome genes which encode H-Y peptides. One was in a cosmid which mapped to a region on the Y known to be deleted in a mutation which extinguished expression of H-Y (McLaren *et al.,* 1984), the other was a cDNA which was mapped within that deletion interval (King *et al.,* 1994). The cosmid contained the ubiquitously expressed gene *Smcy* and was found to encode the first H-Y peptide to be identified, $H\text{-}Y/K^k$, of which the peptide TENSGKDI is presented by the $H\text{-}2K^k$ allele (Scott *et al.,* 1995). The X homologue, Smcx, has a 3 bp deletion within this stretch of the sequence, resulting in a Y-specific peptide differing at 6 amino acid residues from that of the X. The cDNA was part of the ubiquitously expressed *Uty* gene, which encodes another H-Y peptide, $H\text{-}Y/D^b$, in which the peptide WMHHNMDLI is presented by the $H\text{-}2D^b$ allele. The X homologue, Utx, differs at three amino acid residues from Uty in this part of the sequence (Greenfield *et al.,* 1996). An expression cloning approach has also recently identified a novel gene on chromosome 2 encoding the H-13 minor H peptide antigen in mice, thus clarifying the molecular bases of this autosomally encoded minor H antigen (Mendoza *et al.,* 1997). A conservative single amino acid difference in this peptide accounts for each of the alleles. Remarkably, the peptides do not display the conventional motif even though they both bind the $H\text{-}2D^b$ molecule. An additional male-specific peptide, also presented by $H2\text{-}D^b$, KCSRNRQYL, encoded by Smcy, has also recently been described (Markiewicz *et al.,* 1998).

The second approach to identifying peptide components of minor H antigens was that pioneered by Rammensee and his colleagues. It is based on the elution of peptide from MHC molecules expressing the relevant MHC allele and the minor H epitope in question, and testing of separated peptide peaks for their ability to sensitise targets for recognition by minor H specific T cells. The positive peptide peaks are then sequenced and testing of synthetic peptides of the deduced sequence is the final step in identification of the cognate peptide. Examination of the amino acid sequence can provide clues about the likely DNA sequence from which it is derived, although redundancy of the genetic code makes this step in gene identification dependent on genes already identified and in the DNA database. This method was originally used to establish direct evidence for the peptidic nature of the associated $H\text{-}2D^b$ components of the mouse minor H antigens H-4 and H-Y (Rötzschke *et al.,* 1990). A modification of the method, using mass spectrometric analysis for peptide identification, was used to determine the first human minor H peptide, HA-2, as YIGEVLVSV, which appears to be the product of a myosin-related gene on an unknown autosome, recognised in association with HLA-A*0201 (den Haan *et al.,* 1995). The method was subsequently used to identify two human H-Y peptides, components of H-Y/B7(Wang *et al.,* 1995) and H-Y/A2 (Meadows *et al.,* 1997) as SPSVDKARAEL and FIDSYICQV respectively, both products of different regions of the human *SMCY* gene, which had been mapped to a position on the long arm of the Y chromosome known to contain gene(s) controlling H-Y expression in humans (Simpson *et al.,* 1987; Cantrell *et al.,* 1992; O'Reilly *et al.,* 1992).

From these data it appears that for some peptide components of H-Y at least, a homologous gene, *Smcy/SMCY* in mice and humans, is the source of the endogenous protein from which they are derived. However, the peptide components themselves cannot be the same, since the peptide sequence which allows it to be loaded into the different alleles of the human and mouse MHC molecules is different. It is also clear that *Smcy* is not the only Y chromosome gene to encode H-Y peptide epitopes, since in mice at least, a second gene, *Uty*, encodes at least one (H-Y/D^b) and there are additional linked candidate genes, some of which may encode MHC-restricted class II epitopes which are essential for immunogenicity. However, class II peptide epitopes may also be discovered within genes already identified: *Smcy/SMCY* for example is a large gene (with a 6.5kb cDNA), and has already been found to encode two H-Y peptide epitopes in mice and a further two in humans (Scott *et al.,* 1995; Wang *et al.,* 1995; Meadows *et al.,* 1997; and Scott *et al.*, unpublished). From sequence analysis, both *Smcy* and *Uty* appear to encode regulatory proteins which would be expected to be expressed in the nucleus: *Smcy* shares considerable sequence homology with the retinoblastoma binding protein, RBP2 and that of *Uty* is homologous to a family of tetratricopeptide repeat (TRP) proteins. These gene products may therefore interact with DNA or other proteins and hence play a role in transcription regulation, although their function is quite unknown, and it is unclear whether the Y-specific sequence, differing so little from that of the X homologue, has a male-specific role, for example by involvement in spermatogenesis. It is also of interest that the one crucial male-specific gene on the Y, *Sry/SRY*, which controls testis differentiation during embryonic development (Gubbay *et al.,* 1990), lies outside the region where all the H-Y genes are located in mice. That it is not a minor H peptide encoding gene may however be due to the fact that it is not ubiquitously expressed in mice.

A mitochondrial peptide was the first minor H peptide to be identified (Loveland *et al.,* 1990), some time before those of H-Y described above and also taking a genomic approach. The tracking of a minor transplantation antigen to the small mitochrondrial genome came from studies of a maternally transmitted transplantation antigen, which could also be detected by cytotoxic T cells *in vitro* (Fischer Lindahl, 1985) and these were then used to test candidate peptides derived from examination of sequence differences between alleles of the enzyme gene, mt-ND1. A single amino acid difference in the peptide f-MFFINILTL was found to account for immunogenicity. Subsequently additional mitochondrial genes in mouse and rat have been found to encode minor H peptides, and several are presented to T cells by non-classical, MHC class Ib restriction molecules (Morse *et al.,* 1996; Bhuyan *et al.,* 1997).

Why are endogenous peptides immunogenic?

There are a number of different answers to this, depending on the epitope in question. The first requirement for immunogenicity is that the peptide should be generated in, or transported to, an appropriate cellular compartment for incorporation in the biosynthesis of MHC molecules. The second is that the peptide sequence should be capable of being bound in the MHC peptide binding groove of that allele with an appropriate affinity, and the complex be displayed on the surface of an appropriate antigen presenting cell in sufficient quantity for T cell recognition. Finally, there needs to be in the T cell repertoire sufficient cells able to recognise the complex and be activated by it in a milieu with the right cytokines for clonal expansion and differentiation to effector function.

Negative selection in the thymus will remove from the repertoire those T cells which generate antigen-specific receptors able to interact with high affinity to endogenous peptides expressed by cells in the thymic environment. This will remove most T cells with receptors of high affinity for peptides from ubiquitously expressed genes. This process however may leave T cells with lower affinity receptors for such peptides, that could be triggered by expression of high levels of the peptide/MHC complex in the periphery or in the presence of certain cytokines. This may be the basis of some autoimmune reactions, and may account for some tumour antigens (Boon *et al.,* 1989).

Genes expressed in a tissue-specific manner can generate immunogenic peptides: this accounts for some tumour-specific peptides exemplified by those of the MAGE genes (van der Bruggen *et al.,* 1991; De Plaen *et al.,* 1994) and may contribute to the generation of some autoantigens, although in both instances immunogenicity depends on the cell type expressing the gene also expressing accessory molecules characteristic of effective antigen-presenting cells. There are also reports of tissue-specific transplantation antigens (Steinmuller and Tyler, 1980), although none of these is yet identified at the level of a cloned gene or a peptide.

Differences in peptide sequence due to mutations or allelic differences can result in strong immunogenicity, even when the difference is limited to a single amino acid residue, providing the variant sequence can be loaded into an MHC restriction molecule. This determines some tumour antigens (Boon and van der Bruggen, 1996) and several of the minor H peptide antigens (Loveland *et al.,* 1990; Scott *et al.,* 1995; Wang *et al.,* 1995; Greenfield *et al.,* 1996; Meadows *et al.,* 1997). However, the two alleles of the H13 peptide (Mendoza *et al.,* 1997) are an interesting variation of this, since whilst the T cell clones used to detect them are activated by picomolar quantities of the cognate peptide, that of the other allele will activate at a concentration two logs higher, suggesting the potential importance of quantitative changes in expression, although whether such high levels would be reached by natural processing is unclear. Positive thymic selection on related peptides may however contribute to the presence in the periphery of T cells with receptors of higher affinity for the specific peptide.

There have been a number of estimates made of the number of minor H antigens. From the number of congenic strains created (Snell and Stimpfling, 1966; Bailey, 1975), a minimum estimate of several dozen would follow. From mathematical modelling of genetic grafting data several hundreds have been predicted (Bailey and Mobraaten, 1969), and from existing knowledge of allelic variation of endogenous proteins that might be an underestimate. However, consideration of allelic variation of all proteins does not take into account how many of these variant peptides would be loaded into MHC molecules and presented at the cell surface in a manner that could elicit the attention of T cells, nor how other

MHC/peptide complexes select the T cell repertoire. In practice, in the presence of multiple minor H differences between donor and recipient, as is the case between H-2 matched mouse strains, and HLA-identical siblings, a very small number of them seem to elicit a T cell response (Wettstein, 1986; Yin *et al.,* 1993; Wolpert *et al.,* 1995). These few are dubbed "immunodominant", although the basis of immunodominance is very poorly understood, and under experimental conditions the hierarchy of "dominant" and "dominated" minor H antigens varies according to the combination under test. This could be a reflection of ability of the dominant peptide binding the MHC restriction molecule more avidly, thus augmenting the TCR/peptide/MHC interaction (Pion *et al.,* 1997). With the identification of more of the relevant peptides, this can now be tested.

Genotyping for minor H antigens

The identification of MHC class I and class II peptide-presenting alleles (HLA-A, -B, -C, -DR, -DQ and possibly others) is an integral part of typing for minor H antigens, since the potential peptide epitopes will be determined in relation to the MHC alleles present. Currently, HLA typing uses a combination of serological, cellular and DNA-based methods (see parts 1-3 of this volume) although DNA-based methods are now more widely used. Whilst it is in theory possible to type for minor H antigens using cellular methods (T cell clones), it would not be practical to maintain 'in working order' a bank of indicator clones for this in each of the laboratories typing donor/recipient pairs for bone marrow transplantation. Once the relevant minor H genes have been identified and the basis of the polymorphism defined, it is a simple matter to design PCR primers which will detect it, especially as to date minor H antigens appear to be bi-allelic rather than polymorphic. Clinically, it will not be necessary to determine the presence of Y chromosome HY genes since such 'allelism' is phenotypically apparent. There are already clinical reports of the influence of male-specific transplantation antigens in GVH and host- versus-graft (HVG) responses. The significance of minor H antigens encoded by the mitochondrial genome in humans is unknown. The autosomally encoded minor H antigens are the real challenge. So far only one gene, a cDNA including the sequence encoding HA1, has been identified (Markiewicz *et al.,* 1998, and see Table 19.1). As this appears to be an immunodominant epitope in HLA.A2 individuals, there is every reason to PCR-type relevant donor/recipient pairs for this. Others will undoubtedly follow.

Potential clinical use of minor H peptides: tolerance induction and tetramer monitoring of minor H specific T cell responses

One practical justification of gaining knowledge of the nature and identity of minor H antigens is the potential to manipulate immune responses to such epitopes in clinical situations. These include not only down-modulation in HVG, GVH, autoimmune disease and any novel antigens introduced by somatic gene therapy but also upregulation of immune responses to antigens expressed selectively on tumour cells.

Tolerance induction to transplantation antigens has a long history, from the pioneering experiments of Medawar (Billingham *et al.,* 1953) on induction of neonatal tolerance in mice to the more recent studies of Waldmann and his colleagues on tolerance induction in adult mice under a non-depleting CD4 "umbrella" (Chen *et al.,* 1996; Davies *et al.,* 1996). In each case it has proved easier to induce tolerance to minor H mismatches than those involving MHC differences and, in the former, the tolerance induced is long-lasting. The mechanism is unclear although tolerance can persist in the face of alloreactive cells which appear to have been 'silenced'. However, their presence makes the tolerant state a precarious one. In the multiple minor H mismatches studied by Waldmann and his colleagues (loc.cit.), the peptide identity of the immunodominant minor H epitope(s) has not been determined. In principle, it is now possible to select experimental genetic combinations where this is known, for example female mice given syngeneic male skin, since a number of different HY peptide epitopes have been identified (see Table 19.1). Under these circumstances, manoeuvres to induce tolerance with HY peptide agonists, antagonists, or altered peptide ligands, is an attractive possibility currently under investigation. This approach is also possible experimentally using the autosomally encoded H3, H13 or H7 peptides.

In each of the cases in which the peptide epitope has been identified, it is now possible to monitor the T cell immune response to a transplant expressing that epitope by *ex vivo* enumeration of MHC-restricted peptide-specific T cells using tetramers. Fluorescent tetramers created by folding together recombinantly produced MHC class I heavy chains and β_2m, with cognate peptide, have been used to enumerate viral peptide epitope-specific T cells, which bind the tetramers, in patients with virus infections such as HIV and LCMV (Altman *et al*., 1996; Gallimore *et al*., 1998). Tetramers incorporating selected minor H peptide epitopes are currently under test, to monitor responses to HY in mice, and HY, HA-1 and HA-2 in humans. Such tests would be readily transposable to routine clinical testing for patients at risk for HVG and GVH.

Summary

The molecular identification of minor H antigens and the genes encoding them has confirmed the assumption that they are peptides derived from intracellularly expressed genes, incorporated into the peptide binding groove of MHC molecules during biosynthesis. The number of minor H antigen genes and peptides so identified is currently small but growing. Information gained about the genes will allow genotyping of donors and recipients and could be important in selecting MHC-matched donors for BMT, and in predicting the presence of immunodominant antigens to aid clinical management. Identification of the peptide epitopes may facilitate tolerance induction with peptide and allow *in vivo* monitoring of minor H specific T cell responses by fluorescent tetramers.

Acknowledgements

I would like to thank Dr. Derry Roopenian for interesting discussions on the nature of minor H antigens and the immune responses to them. Mrs. Vivien Tikerpäe has provided invaluable assistance in the preparation of the manuscript, for which I am most grateful.

References

Altman, JD, Moss, PAH, Goulder, PJR, Barouch, DH, McHeyzer-Williams, MG, *et al.* (1996) Phenotypic analysis of antigen-specific T lymphocytes. *Science* **274**: 94-96

Bailey, DW. (1975) Genetics of histocompatibility in mice I. New loci and congenic lines. *Immunogenet* **2:** 249-256

Bailey, DW and Mobraaten, LE. (1969) Estimates of the number of loci contributing to the histoincompatibility between C57BL/6 and BALB/c strains of mice. *Transplantation* **7:** 394-400

Bevan, MJ. (1975) The major histocompatibility complex determines susceptibility to cytotoxic T cells directed against minor histocompatibility antigens. *J Exp Med* **142:** 1349-1364

Bhuyan, PK, Young, LL, Lindahl, KF and Butcher, GW. (1997) Identification of the rat maternally transmitted minor histocompatibility antigen. *J Immunol* **158:** 3753-3760

Billingham, RE, Brent, L and Medawar, PB. (1953) Actively acquired tolerance of foreign cells. *Nature* **172:** 603-606

Bjorkman, PJ, Saper, MA, Samraoui, B, Bennett, WS, Strominger, JL, *et al.* (1987a) Structure of the human class I histocompatibility antigen, HLA-A2. *Nature* **329:** 506-512

Bjorkman, PJ, Saper, MA, Samraoui, B, Bennett, WS, Strominger, JL, *et al.* (1987b) The foreign antigen binding site and T cell recognition regions of class I histocompatibility antigens. *Nature* **329:** 512-518

Boon, T, Van Pel, A, De Plaen, E, Chomez, P, Lurquin, C, *et al.* (1989) Genes coding for T-cell-defined tum$^-$ transplantation antigens: point mutations, antigenic peptides, and subgenic expression. *Cold Spring Harb Symp Quant Biol* **54:** 587-596

Boon, T and van der Bruggen, P (1996) Human tumor antigens recognized by T lymphocytes. *J Exp Med* **183:** 725-729

Candinas, D, Gunson, BK, Nightingale, P, Hubscher, S, McMaster, P, *et al.* (1995) Sex mismatch as a risk factor for chronic rejection of liver allografts. *Lancet* **346:** 1117-1121

Cantrell, MA, Bogan, JS, Simpson, E, Bicknell, JN, Goulmy, E, *et al.* (1992) Deletion mapping of H-Y antigen to the long arm of the human Y chromosome. *Genomics* **13:** 1255-1260

Ceppellini, R, Mattiuz, PL, Scudeller, G and Visetti, M (1969) Experimental allotransplantation in man I. The role of the HLA system in different genetic combinations. *Transpl Proc* **1:** 385-389

Chen, ZK, Cobbold, SP, Waldmann, H and Metcalfe, S (1996) Amplification of natural regulatory immune mechanisms for transplantation tolerance. *Transplantation* **62:** 1200-1206

Davies, JD, Leong, LY, Mellor, A, Cobbold, SP and Waldmann, H (1996) T cell suppression in transplantation tolerance through linked recognition. *J Immunol* **156:** 3602-3607

De Plaen, E, Lurquin, C, Van Pel, A, Mariame, B, *et al.* (1988) Immunogenic (tum^-) variants of mouse tumor P815: cloning of the gene of tum- antigen P91A and identification of the tum^- mutation. *Proc Natl Acad Sci USA* **85**: 2274-2278

De Plaen, E, Arden, K, Traversari, C, Gaforio, JJ, Szikora, J-P, *et al.* (1994) Structure, chromosomal localization and expression of 12 genes of the MAGE family. *Immunogenet* **40:** 360-369

Den Haan, JMM, Sherman, NE, Blokland, E, Huczko, E, Koning, F, *et al.* (1995) Identification of a graft versus host disease-associated human minor histocompatibility antigen. *Science* **268**: 1476-1480

Den Haan, JMM, Meadows, LM, Wang, W, Pool, J, Blokland, E, *et al.* (1998) The minor histocompatibility antigen HA-1: a diallelic gene with a single amino acid polymorphism. *Science* **279:** 1054-1057

Fischer Lindahl, K. (1985) Mitochondrial inheritance in mice. *Trends Genet* **1:** 135-139

Gallimore, A, Glithero, A, Godkin, A, Tissot, AC, Plückthun, A, *et al.* (1998) Induction and exhaustion of lymphocytic choriomeningitis virus-specific cytotoxic T lymphocytes visualized using soluble tetrameric major histocompatibility complex class I peptide complexes. *J Exp Med* **187:** 1383-1393

Gordon, RD, Simpson, E and Samelson, LE (1975) In vitro cell-mediated immune responses to the male-specific (H-Y) antigen in mice. *J Exp Med* **142:** 1108-1120

Goulmy, E, Termijtelen, A, Bradley, BA and van Rood, JJ (1977) Y-antigen killing by T cells of women is restricted by HLA. *Nature* **266:** 544-545

Goulmy, E, Schipper, R, Pool, J, Blokland, E, Falekenburg, JHF, *et al.* (1996) Mismatches of minor histocompatibility antigen between HLA-identical donors and recipients and the development of graft-versus-host disease after bone marrow transplantation. *N Engl J Med* **334:** 281-285

Greenfield, A, Scott, D, Pennisi, D, Ehrmann, I, Ellis, P, *et al.* (1996) An H-YD^b epitope is encoded by a novel mouse Y chromosome gene. *Nature Genetics* **14:** 474-478

Gubbay, J, Collignon, J, Koopman, P, Capel, B, Economou, A, *et al.* (1990) A gene mapping to the sex-determining region of the mouse Y chromosome is a member of a novel family of embryonically expressed genes. *Nature* **346:** 245-250.

King, TR, Christianson, GJ, Mitchell, MJ, Bishop, C, Scott, D, *et al.* (1994) Deletion mapping using immunoselection for H-Y further resolves the Sxr region of the mouse Y chromosome and reveals complexity at the Hya locus. *Genomics* **24**: 159-168.

Loveland, BE, Wang, CR, Yonekawa, H, Hermel, E, and Lindahl, KF. (1990) Maternally transmitted histocompatibility antigen of mice: a hydrophobic peptide of a mitochondrially encoded protein. *Cell* **60**: 971-980.

Malarkannan, S, Shih, PP, Eden, PA, Horng, T, Zuberi, AR, *et al.* (1998) The molecular and functional characterization of a dominant minor H antigen, H60. *J Immunol* **161**: 3501-3509.

Markiewicz, MA, Girao, C, Opferman, JT, Sun, J, Hu, Q, *et al.* (1998) Long-term T cell memory requires the surface expression of self-peptide/major histocompatibility complex molecules. *Proc Natl Acad Sci USA* **95**: 3065-3070.

McLaren, A, Simpson, E, Tomonari, K, Chandler, P, and Hogg, H. (1984) Male sexual differentiation in mice lacking H-Y antigen. *Nature* **312:** 552-555

McLaren, A, Simpson, E, Epplen, JT, Studer, R, Koopman, P, *et al.* (1988) Location of the genes controlling H-Y antigen expression and testis determination on the mouse Y chromosome. *Proc Natl Acad Sci USA* **85**: 6442-6445

Meadows, L, Wang, W, den Haan, JMM, Blokland, E, Reinhardus, C, *et al.* (1997) The HLA-A*0201-restricted H-Y antigen contains a posttranslationally modified cysteine that significantly affects T cell recognition. *Immunity* **6:** 273-281

Mendoza, LM, Paz, P, Zuberi, A, Christianson, G, Roopenian, D, *et al.* (1997) Minors held by majors. The H13 minor histocompatibility locus defined as a peptide/MHC class I complex. *Immunity* **7:** 461-472

Morse, M-C, Bleau, G, Dabhi, VM, Hetu, F, Drobetsky, EA, *et al.* (1996) The COI mitochondrial gene encodes a minor histocompatibility antigen presented by H2-M3. *J Immunol* **156:** 3301-3307

O'Reilly, AJ, Affara, NA, Simpson, E, Chandler, P, Goulmy, E, *et al.* (1992) A molecular deletion map of the Y chromosome long arm defining X and autosomal homologous regions and the localisation of the HYA locus to the proximal region of the Yq euchromatin. *Hum Molec Genet* **1:** 379-385

Perarnau, B, Siegrist, CA, Gillet, A, Vincent, C, Kimura, S, *et al.* (1990) β_2-microglobulin restriction of antigen presentation. *Nature* **346:** 751-754

Perreault, C, Jutras, J, Roy, DC, Filep, JG and Brochu, S (1996) Identification of an immunodominant mouse minor histocompatibility antigen (MiHA): T cell response to a single dominant MiHA causes graft-versus-host disease. *J Clin Invest* **98:** 622-628

Pion, S, Fontaine, P, Desaulniers, M, Jutras, J, Filep, JG, and Perreault, C (1997) On the mechanisms of immunodominance in cytotoxic T lymphocyte responses to minor histocompatibility antigens. *Eur J Immunol* **27:** 421-430

Rammensee, HG, Robinson, PJ, Crisanti, A and Bevan, MJ (1986) Restricted recognition of β_2-microglobulin by cytotoxic T lymphocytes. *Nature* **319:** 502-504

Roopenian, DC (1992) What are minor histocompatibility loci? A new look to an old question. *Immunol Today* **13:** 7-10

Rötzschke, O, Falk, K, Wallny, HJ, Faath, S and Rammensee, HG (1990) Characterisation of naturally occurring minor H peptides including H-4 and H-Y. *Science* **249:** 283-287

Scott, D, Dyson, PJ and Simpson, E (1992) A new approach to the cloning of genes encoding T cell epitopes. *Immunogenet* **36:** 86-94

Scott, DM, Ehrmann, IE, Ellis, PS, Bishop, CE, Agulnik, AI, *et al.* (1995) Identification of a mouse male-specific transplantation antigen, H-Y. *Nature* **376:** 695-698

Simmons, WA, Summerfield, SG, Roopenian, DC, Slaughter, CA, Zuberi, AR, *et al.* (1997) Novel H-Y antigens presented by HLA-B27. *J Immunol* **159:** 2750-2759

Speiser, DE, Zurcher, T, Ramseier, H, Hengartner, H, Staeheli, P, *et al.* (1990) Nuclear myxovirus-resistance protein Mx is a minor histocompatibility antigen. *Proc Natl Acad Sci USA* **87:** 2021-2025

Simpson, E, Chandler, P, Goulmy, E, Disteche, CM, Ferguson-Smith, MA, *et al.* (1987) Separation of the genetic loci for the H-Y antigen and testis determination on the human Y chromosome. *Nature* **326:** 876-878

Simpson, E and Roopenian, D (1997) Minor histocompatibility antigens. *Curr Opin Immunol* **9:** 655-661

Snell, GD (1948) Methods for the study of histocompatibility genes. *J Genet* **49:** 87-103

Snell, GD and Stimpfling, JH (1966) The genetics of tissue transplantation. In: *Biology of the Laboratory Mouse*, 2nd edition (Ed. Green, EL), pp.457-491. McGraw Hill, New York

Steinmuller, D and Tyler, JD (1980) Evidence of skin-specific alloantigens in cell-mediated cytotoxicity. *Transpl Proc* **12:** 107-113

Townsend, ARM, Rothbard, J, Gotch, FM, Bahadur, G, Wraith, D, *et al.* (1986) The epitopes of influenza nucleoprotein recognised by cytotoxic T lymphocytes can be defined by short synthetic peptides. *Cell* **44**: 959-968

Van der Bruggen, P, Traversari, C, Chomez, P, Lurquin, C, De Plaen, E, *et al.* (1991) A gene encoding an antigen recognised by cytolytic T lymphocytes on a human melanoma. *Science* **254:** 1643-1647

Wallny, H-J and Rammensee, HG (1990) Identification of classical minor histocompatibility antigen as cell-derived peptide. *Nature* **343**: 275-278

Wang, W, Meadows, LR, den Haan, JMM, Sherman, NE, Chen, Y, *et al.* (1995) Human H-Y: a male-specific histocompatibility antigen derived from the SMCY protein. *Science* **269:** 1588-1590

Wettstein, PJ (1986) Immunodominance in the T cell response to multiple non H-Y histocompatibility antigens. II. Observation of a hierarchy among dominant antigens. *Immunogenet* **24:** 24-31

Wolpert, E, Franksson, L and Kärre, K (1995) Dominant and cryptic antigens in the MHC class I restricted T cell response across a complex minor histocompatibility barrier: analysis and mapping by elution of cellular peptides. *Int Immunol* **7:** 919-928

Yin, L, Poirier, G, Neth, O, Hsuan, JJ, Totty, NF, *et al.* (1993) Few peptides dominate CTL responses to single and multiple minor histocompatibility antigens. *Int Immunol* **5:** 1003-1009

Zinkernagel, RM and Doherty, PC (1974) Restriction of in vitro mediated cytotoxicity in lymphocytic choriomeningitis within a syngeneic or semi-allogeneic system. *Nature* **248**: 701-702

Zuberi, AR, Christianson, GJ, Mendoza, LM, Shastri, N and Roopenian, DC (1998) Positional cloning and molecular characterization of an immunodominant cytotoxic determinant of the mouse H3 minor histocompatibility complex. *Immunity* **9:** 687-698

INDEX

Standard abbreviations: for explanation, refer to text on cited pages

A

B

C

T

U

V

W

X